Hospice and Palliative Care Handbook

Quality, Compliance, and Reimbursement

D1379091

ABOUT THE AUTHOR

Tina M. Marrelli, MSN, MA, RN,C, is the editor and publisher of *Home Care Nurse News* and the president of Marrelli and Associates, Inc., a health care consulting and publishing firm. Ms. Marrelli is also the author of *The Handbook of Home Health Standards and Documentation Guidelines for Reimbursement* (Mosby, 1998), *The Nurse Manager's Survival Guide: Practical Answers to Everyday Problems* (Mosby, 1997), the *Nursing Documentation Handbook* (Mosby, 1996), the *Handbook of Home Health Orientation* (Mosby, 1998), and the forthcoming *Mosby's Home Care and Hospice Drug Handbook* (Mosby, 1999). She is the coauthor of *Home Health Aide: Guidelines for Care* (Marrelli, 1996), *Home Care and Clinical Paths: Effective Care Planning Across the Continuum* (Mosby, 1996), *Home Health Aide: Guidelines for Care Instructor Manual* (Marrelli, 1997), and the *Manual of Home Health Practice: Guidance for Effective Clinical Operations* (Mosby, 1998).

Ms. Marrelli received a Bachelor's degree in Nursing from Duke University School of Nursing in 1976. She has directed various home care programs and has extensive experience in home care, hospice, and hospital settings. In 1984, she received a Master of Arts in Management and Supervision, Health Care Administration. Ms. Marrelli worked at the central office of the Health Care Financing Administration (HCFA) for 4 years in the areas of home care and hospice policy and operations, where she received the Bureau Director's Citation. She is a member of Sigma Theta Tau and is certified by the American Nurses Association (ANA) credentialing center as a home health nurse. Ms. Marrelli is a clinical instructor at The Case Western Reserve University Frances Payne Bolton School of Nursing and serves on the National Hospice Organization's Standards and Accreditation Committee. In 1996, she completed a Master of Science in Nursing.

Marrelli and Associates, Inc. provides consultative services to hospitals, home health agencies, and hospice programs in the areas of management, accreditation, and other quality initiatives, daily operations, and clinical documentation. Correspondence, including feedback, recommendations, or suggestions about this text, may be directed to the author at the following address: Marrelli and Associates, Inc., P.O. Box 629, Boca Grande, FL 33921-0629. Marrelli and Associates, Inc. can also be reached at 1-800-993-6397 or (941) 697-2900.

Hospice and Palliative Care Handbook

Quality, Compliance, and Reimbursement

TINA M. MARRELLI
MSN, MA, RN,C

Editor, *Home Care Nurse News*
Home Care and Hospice Consultant
Boca Grande, Florida

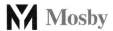 Mosby

St. Louis Baltimore Boston Carlsbad
Chicago Minneapolis New York Philadelphia Portland
London Milan Sydney Tokyo Toronto

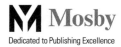

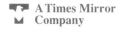

Publisher: Nancy L. Coon
Editor: Loren S. Wilson
Developmental Editor: Brian Dennison
Designer: Renée Duenow
Manufacturing Manager: Linda Ierardi
Cover Design: Elizabeth Young

Printed in the United States of America
Composition/lithography by Clarinda Co.
Printing/binding by R.R. Donnelley & Sons Co., Crawfordsville, IN

Mosby, Inc.
11830 Westline Industrial Drive
St. Louis, Missouri 63146

RA 1000
.M37
1999
0394654436

Library of Congress Cataloging-in-Publication Data

Marrelli, T.M.
   Hospice and palliative care handbook : quality, compliance, and
reimbursement / Tina M. Marrelli.
     p.   cm.
   Includes index.
   ISBN 0-8151-3557-2 (alk. paper)
    1. Hospice care—Standards—Handbooks, manuals, etc.
  2. Palliative care—Standards—Handbooks, manuals, etc.
  3. Medicine—Documentation—Handbooks, manuals, etc. 4. Nursing—
Handbooks, manuals, etc. I. Title.
   [DNLM: 1. Hospice Care—organization & administration handbooks.
2. Documentation handbooks. WB 39M358h 1998]
RA1000.M37 1998
362.1′756—dc21
DNLM/DLC
for Library of Congress   98-35982
                                      CIP

98 99 00 01 02 / 9 8 7 6 5 4 3 2 1

REVIEWERS

Genie Eide, RN, BSN
Certified Nurse Administrator
Scottsdale, Arizona

Carroll Fernstrom, OTR
Occupational Therapist and Consultant
Professional Occupational Therapy
  Services
Richmond, Virginia

Mary M. Friedman, MS, RN, CRNI
Home Care Consultant, Home Health
  Systems, Inc.
Nurse Surveyor, JCAHO
Marietta, Georgia

Laura Friend, RN, BSN
Coordinator of Educational Services
West Virginia Council of Home Health
  Agencies, Inc.
Middleborne, West Virginia

Dorene J. Fankhauser, RN, MS, CRNH
Director, Specialty Systems
  Development
Mount Carmel Health System
Columbus, Ohio

Charlette Gallagher-Allred, PhD, RD
Manager Geriatrics and Long Term
  Care
Ross Products Division
(Volunteer Consulting Nutritionist
Hospice at Riverside)
Columbus, Ohio

Lynda S. Hilliard, MBA, RN, CNAA
Health and Home Care Consultant
Pleasanton, California

Carol Hollingsworth, RN
Performance and Improvement
  Coordinator
St. Joseph Home Health Care
Augusta, Georgia

Linda Krulish, MHS, PT
President, Home Therapy Services
Powell, Ohio

Anne L. Rooney, MPH, MS, RN
Home Care Consultant
Oak Park, Illinois

Mary Deeley-Shoffeitt, BSN, MS
Case Manager, Managed Care
ANA/MNA
Managed Care Nurses Association
Woodbine, Maryland

Anita Thompson, MSW, LISW
Home Health Social Worker
Genesis Health Care System
Chandlersville, Ohio

Carolyn Viall, RN, MSN
Nurse Manager, Pediatrics
Medical University of South Carolina
Charleston, South Carolina

Marilyn Warling, RN, BSN
Director, Benefit Integrity and External
  Relations
Wellmark, Inc.
Des Moines, Iowa

Sandra M. Whittier, RNC, MSN, BSN
Clinical Coordinator, Nursing and
  Rehabilitation
Home Health and Hospice Care
  Network
Whidden Hospital
Swampscott, Massachusetts

Ken Zeri, RN, MS, CRNH
Hospice Consultant
Past President of the Hospice and
  Palliative Nurses Association
  (HPNA)
San Diego, California

PREFACE

Many clinicians and managers who practice in hospice or home care may be familiar with the framework of this book, although the title, the information, and many other features are unfamiliar. During review of the needed revisions for the third edition of "the little red book," the *Handbook of Home Health Standards and Documentation Guidelines for Reimbursement* (Mosby, 1998), it became clear that the changes that needed to be made to meet the changing and growing needs of both home care and hospice clinicians would have made "the little red book" a tome, not a handbook! Therefore it was decided that a new book was needed, one that focuses solely on hospice care and incorporates standards for quality, documentation, and reimbursement while supporting core hospice values.

When the first edition of *Home Health Standards* was written in the mid-1980s, hospice was hardly the common term and specialized service that it is today. As the director of a large hospital-based home health agency and hospice, I wrote that book with a hospice focus directed toward home care services. In fact, at that time, I had trouble explaining what we did in home care, let alone hospice care! A patient's home, where family and friends are available, is often the ideal care setting for hospice and may be more comfortable than traditional health care settings. This trend will only continue to grow as consumers become more active participants and equal partners in their health care management.

This book was written to facilitate the integration of care, standards, and planning for hospice into clinical documentation and forms. The interdisciplinary documentation described in this book will assist health care professionals in providing quality hospice care that meets regulatory standards such as those of Medicare. Although the Medicare program is a medical model, the Medicare framework can lend itself to effectively providing quality hospice care. The interdisciplinary hospice team members have the clinical skills and the information required to identify and address patient and family needs holistically. This book facilitates the integration of hospice nursing with the expertise of other hospice team members, such as physical and occupational therapy, spiritual and psychosocial counseling, nutritional counseling, volunteer support, and speech-language pathology, into a usable format to assist in planning and providing care.

The priority for hospice clinicians and managers is to meet the unique and multifaceted needs of patients and families. The format of this book lends itself to the integration of assessed patient and family needs into a plan consistent with accurate completion of hospice clinical records that support compliance and quality while managing complex care plans. This book assists in the documentation of that process and analysis (e.g., documentation of the care planning process).

This book contains 23 care guidelines that include direction for assessment, documentation, and reimbursement to assist in meeting quality and regulatory standards. These care guidelines give new and experienced hospice clinicians examples of interventions and documentation that may assist in supporting the presence of and continuous need for hospice care. The text is also a way to standardize care and care processes across the organization and among team members. These standards can be reviewed and practiced in orientation, in actual hospice settings, and during clinical case conferences. The generation of appropriate, quality, and reimbursable documentation is a learned process. Like any new skill, learning and improvement occur with practice and positive feedback toward the desired outcome. This book integrates the documentation needed to support covered care and reimbursement while listing the care considerations for patients and their families by clinical problem or diagnosis.

Special features have been included to make this book easy to use. In the clinical care guidelines sections (Parts Four and Five), standard abbreviations are used to simplify the descriptions of hospice care. If any abbreviation is confusing, its meaning can be checked in Part Eight. In addition, the table of contents is alphabetized in the care guidelines sections, and cross-referenced materials are found under the associated or other heading. For example, the care guideline "Breast Cancer and Mastectomy Care" is also listed under "Mastectomy Care," with the page number included for easier identification and retrieval of needed information. This feature should help you find material quickly. Furthermore, each specific care guideline cross-references related care guidelines to assist the reader in accessing additional information. For example, in the guideline for "Depression and Other Psychiatric Care," the reader is also referred to "Alzheimer's Disease and Other Dementias," should that be a related or complicating problem for the patient and his or her family. For a more detailed discussion of how to use this book for planning, delivering, evaluating, and documenting hospice care, see the section "Guidelines for Use." That section details additional features of this new book.

Tina M. Marrelli, MSN, MA, RN,C

ACKNOWLEDGMENTS

A heartfelt thank you to all the clinicians and managers, of all disciplines and professions, who have provided insight and practice examples from their own special hospice experiences. All this information helps keep the focus practical while providing skillful and compassionate hospice care.

Lynda S. Hilliard deserves an award for her ready ear and detail-oriented recommendations for the process and manuscript. Special thanks to Bill and Buddy Glass for humor and support, respectively, and always understanding when deadlines loomed and schedules were out of control.

CONTENTS

GUIDELINES FOR USE

The goal of this book is to assist hospice clinicals and managers meet quality, coverage, and reimbursement standards and requirements through their daily practice, operations, and documentation activities. The Hospice Care Guidelines, or topics, are organized alphabetically for easy retrieval and review of information.

There may be more than one case scenario that is appropriate for your hospice patient. For example, for care of a patient with cancer and an open wound, the following two Care Guidelines could be referred to: "Cancer Care" and "Wound/Pressure Ulcer Care." Depending on the type of cancer, "Brain Cancer," "Breast Cancer," "Head and Neck Cancer," or "Prostate Cancer" could also be appropriate. The information can be individualized for your patients/families, used throughout the clinical record, and serve as a basis for a common glossary in interdisciplinary team or group (IDG) discussions. It is formatted for easy review for care and care planning.

The following information refers to the specifically numbered entries in each of the 23 Hospice Care Guidelines.

1. **General considerations.** This entry contains general information on the designated topic in relation to hospice care. The diagnostic information would be used generally for supporting the medical necessity of hospice care and the reason that the patient was admitted to hospice.

2. **Needs for visit.** This information lists what is generally needed prior to making a hospice visit and supports planning and the securing of physician orders and clinical information needed for the assessment prior to the provision of hospice care.

3. **Safety considerations.** This section lists the general kinds of safety concerns that may impact hospice care, based on the diagnoses or care guidelines problems listed. The information in safety considerations is to be used upon assessment and throughout the care and care planning among the team.

4. **Potential diagnoses and codes.** Depending on the model of hospice provided, the ICD-9 codes may be used on the plan of care, on Health Care Financing Administration (HCFA) form 485, or for billing purposes. If the HCFA form 485 is used or adapted for a Medicare hospice patient, the codes generally will be utilized in item numbers 11, 12, and 13 on the form 485. They are alphabetized to assist in identification and location.

   The source for all codes was the current edition of the IDC-9-CM published by the Commission on Professional and Hospital Activities. The ICD-9-CM system sometimes requires secondary codes for a complete description of the diagnostic entity. For example, pneumonia in the presence of AIDS is coded as both 486 (pneumonia) and 042 (AIDS). It is important, in such instances, to use all the codes given and in the order presented, with or without decimals as listed in the text. If your hospice is a Medicare-certified hospice (or home health agency), your Regional Home Health Intermediary (RHHI) may have preferred or recommended codes, and those codes should be used when appropriate for your patient. These RHHI code updates are usually communicated to your manager through the RHHI's newsletters.

   Codes for associated operations or postoperative care are listed, as appropriate, and surgical codes are marked (surgical) in the text after the ICD-9 number listed. Operation codes may be recognized by their two-digit structure. Diagnosis codes always have three digits before the decimal point and in some cases have no decimal point at all. Operation codes have only two digits before the decimal and are always followed by one or two digits, following the decimal:

Diagnosis: Osteomyelitis, lower leg, 715.96

Surgical procedure: S/P BKA, 84.15

Certain essential assumptions have been made regarding hospice services. These assumptions are that if the patient is a beneficiary of a medical insurance program, such as Medicare, the patient meets recognized hospice and insurer standards and is therefore appropriate for hospice admission and care and justified for reimbursement. Remember that modifiers to diagnosis terms may be important. Modifiers such as acute/chronic, unilateral/bilateral, upper/lower, and adult/juvenile frequently require differentiation in the ICD-9 codes. Similarly, slight variations in terminology may be significant. Please note that the ICD-9 system contains more than 10,000 diagnosis code categories and more than 40,000 cross-referenced diagnosis terms. We have attempted to clearly illustrate such distinctions in the text. Your intermediary may have other or additional specific ICD-9 codes they prefer for you to use. In those cases, use the intermediary's recommended codes. For further information, consult the ICD-9 codes books or a qualified coder.

5. **Associated nursing diagnoses.** This section includes the approved nursing diagnoses that are related to the listed problems in the Hospice Care Guidelines. All the nursing diagnoses listed are approved by the North American Nursing Diagnoses Association (NANDA). The entire list of the NANDA diagnoses appears in Part Ten of this text. These diagnoses are the identified problem and/or focus for care and intervention as identified by the hospice nurse or other team members. The nurse needs to assess the patient and identify those diagnoses that best address the patient's and family's unique problems and situation. These diagnoses may be used in the care planning record, the plan of care, on the problem list, the hospice visit record, or other documentation and communication formats. All or some of these diagnoses may be appropriate for a specific patient and family.

6. **Skills and services identified.** This section lists and identifies the hospice team members and some of their specialized functions or interventions, based on the patient's/family's diagnoses or problems and unique circumstances. The skills and services identified in this section include those of the nurse; aide; social worker; volunteer(s); spiritual counselor; dietitian/nutritional counselor; occupational therapist; speech-language pathologist; bereavement counselor; pharmacist (for some diagnoses); and music, massage, art and other therapists.

Hospice nursing has been listed as the first service. Because of the multifaceted interventions and complex coordination activities that must occur with skillful hospice nursing care, the nursing section is subcategorized into eight areas. These are: (a) Comfort and Symptom Control, (b) Safety and Mobility Considerations, (c) Emotional and Spiritual Considerations, (d) Skin Care, (e) Elimination Considerations, (f) Hydration/Nutrition, (g) Therapeutic/Medication Regimens, and (h) Other Considerations. This specificity should assist in the identification and prioritization of patient/family care interventions.

Interventions for nursing and other services often use verbs in the description of care and to support holistic, skillful interventions. These services may also be used, where appropriate, as the orders for the plan of care. It is important to note that the patient/family care plan must be individualized and based on the assessed needs. This information is provided as a list to assist in the identification of needed hospice care and assists all hospice team members by providing a baseline for services based on the specialized team member's education and professional scope of practice.

7. **Outcomes for care.** Outcomes are quantifiable or measurable goals for care across a time span. The outcomes listed are not lengthy or complex but should be able to be identified generally as met or not met. The outcomes are based on the hospice patient's/family's assessed findings and unique situation. These outcomes are utilized in the interdisciplinary care planning process, planning records, and clinical documentation.

8. **Patient, family, and caregiver educational needs.** This section addresses the unique educational needs of patients, their families, and caregivers. The most common types of information that patients need to safely remain at home are listed in this section. Please keep in mind that this is a handbook, and the listing is by no means intended to be all-inclusive. Your patient and family may have needs that are as varied as their history, with unique learning styles and barriers.

9. **Specific tips for quality and reimbursement.** These tips are often based on diagnoses that contribute to concise, specific documentation assisting in supporting quality, coverage, and reimbursement. This information may be used in the assessment form, visit notes, IDG minutes, care coordination, and planning of activities. Remember that all services need to be based on your patient's/family's unique medical condition and history as determined on the assessment visit(s) and throughout the patient's/family's length of care. Regardless of payor, the documentation must demonstrate the hospice care provided and the patient's/family's response to that care. A more in-depth discussion about the level and specificity of documentation needed in hospice care and the many requirements that effective documentation meets are addressed in Part Two.

10. **Resources for hospice care and practice.** Informational resources are listed to assist the clinician and patients/families with educational and other needs, based on the unique care diagnosis. For example, under this section in the "Renal Care (End Stage)" guideline, there are resources listed from the National Kidney Foundation brochure entitled *When Stopping Dialysis Treatment Is Your Choice* and other patient education materials available through their 800 number. Similarly, in the "Care of the Child with Cancer" guideline, resources listed include *Radiotherapy Days,* a colorful book that explains radiation to young patients and specialized pain resources, as well as supportive organizations such as the Make-A-Wish Foundation and the Candlelighters Childhood Cancer Foundation. These resources have been specially chosen to support patient and clinician education needs. Readers are encouraged to write to the author should they have additional resources they believe should be included in a subsequent edition. Send the resource or the information about the resource to the following address: P.O. Box 629, Boca Grande, FL 33921-0629 or FAX to (941) 697-2901.

PART ONE

HOSPICE
A Unique Practice Specialty

When I was first introduced to hospice, I remember thinking this is how we should care for all patients—truly individualized care; comfort and symptom relief; a collaborative, caring team effort; special volunteers; and spiritual support.

TINA M. MARRELLI

Hospice is a special kind of care and support that is primarily provided in the privacy and comfort of the patient's home. According to the National Hospice Organization (NHO), 77% of hospice patients died in their own personal residences.[1] For this reason and others, hospice is a special type of home care. Simply put, hospice is an organized method of providing care, directed toward comfort and support, to patients with a limited life expectancy. Hospice focuses on making every remaining day the best it can be.

Approximately 28% of *all* Medicare costs goes toward care of people in their last year of life; almost 50% of those costs are expended in the last 2 months of life.[1] Significant savings are seen when terminally ill cancer patients are cared for at home. Carney and Burns[2] calculated savings of 39% to 51% for patients in home hospice care.

The hospice focus, very different from the curative-focused rescue medicine mentality of the U.S. health care system, is causing a groundswell of support for palliative care and hospice services. As a result, hospice is projected to have significant growth in the coming years.

Part 1 provides an overview of hospice care and seeks to explain the special aspects of hospice care that contribute to the high-quality care given to patients and their families. Part 1 also defines the hospice specialty for those wishing to move into this unique and satisfying professional career.

WHAT IS HOSPICE?

Hospice has strong roots in history. *Hospice* is derived from a term used historically to designate a resting place for weary travelers. Today, hospice is a multidimensional and interdisciplinary package that provides a rest for weary patients and their families. Hospice patients have usually been through different treatments for curative purposes, including any combination of chemotherapeutic protocols, radiation therapy, and surgeries, and may have been on multiple regimens. Some patients have been battling cancer, AIDS, cardiac disease, pulmonary disease, or other diseases for years, and have come to hospice when the medical model could no longer in good conscience continue curative treatment.

Hospice then moves in to help patients focus their limited time on themselves, their partners, and their loved ones while optimizing quality of life in the manner that they and their families choose. The NHO sets out standards, including the following[3]:

Hospice provides support and care for persons in the last phases of incurable diseases so that they may live as fully and comfortably as possible. Hospice recognizes dying as part of the normal process of living and focuses on maintaining the quality of remaining life. Hospice affirms life and neither hastens nor postpones death. Hospice exists in the hope and belief that through appropriate care and the promotion of a caring community sensitive to their needs, patients and families may be free to attain a degree of mental and spiritual preparation for death that is satisfactory to them.

These standards provide the framework for hospices as they seek to provide the best possible care for patients and their families.

HOSPICE CARE

Hospice is a special approach to caring for terminally ill individuals that stresses palliative care (relief of pain and uncomfortable symptoms) as opposed to curative care. In addition to meeting the patient's medical needs, hospice care addresses the physical, psychosocial, and spiritual needs of the patient's family/caregiver. The emphasis of the hospice program is on keeping the patient at home with family and friends. It is important to note that although some hospices are located in hospitals, skilled nursing facilities (SNFs), and home health agencies (HHAs), Medicare requires that hospices must meet specific Medicare Conditions of Participation (COPs) and be separately certified and approved for Medicare participation. With this definition and structure come requirements that may be a part of the organization's orientation program, and the roles and nuances of coverage provided throughout the care guidelines that follow.

THE GROWTH OF HOSPICE

Many changes have occurred in the external health environment that continue to make home care and hospice two of the fastest-growing segments of the health care industry for professional clinicians and managers (see Figure 1-1 for an illustration of the growth of hospice). Some of the most appealing aspects are the interdisciplinary focus, the clinician and family/caregiver interactions, the range and diversity of skills and knowledge employed, and the sense of satisfaction that accompanies caring for patients and their families as equal partners in care and care planning.

The following list contains some of the factors contributing to the rapid growth of hospice:

- The changing health care delivery system
- The shift from inpatient care to outpatient and community-based care, such as home care
- The search for alternative methods of care and treatment
- The growth of managed care and lower cost-setting implications
- Technological advances
- Legal and risk-management issues
- Ethical dilemmas relating to end-of-life issues
- The patient's emergence as an educated consumer seeking value and service
- General dissatisfaction with end-of-life care
- The changing belief systems of patients and their families relating to death and illness
- The renewal of spirituality as an important part of life and illness
- The grassroots efforts contributing to hospice's being seen as a valuable and caring alternative for many patients and families

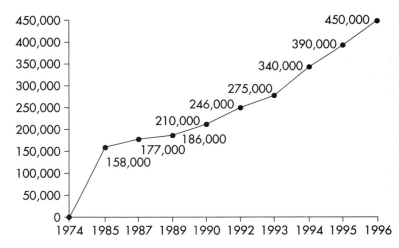

Figure 1-1 Hospice patients—United States. (From *NHO Newsline,* 7[20], 1997. Copyright © National Hospice Organization. All rights reserved.)

- The desire of patients and families to make their limited time valued and affirming
- Demographic changes, including:
  The growing number of the frail and elderly
  The growing number of AIDS patients seeking hospice
- Cost savings
- The trend toward improving quality of life, an ethic that hospice espouses and actualizes in communities across the country

HOSPICE SETTINGS

Hospice can be provided to patients and their families in any setting and transcends traditional care settings and boundaries. Because most hospice care is provided in the privacy and comfort of the patient's home, the emphasis of this book is on home hospice care, although the care and standards addressed apply to all care settings. The term *hospice* is used in its broadest sense and includes community-based free-standing hospices, home health agency–based hospices, volunteer hospices, facility-based hospices, and other organizational models providing or supporting hospice care services. Regardless of care site, hospice is a special kind of care that emphasizes making each day the best it can be for patients and their loved ones.

PATIENTS SEEN IN HOSPICE

The problems of patients seen in hospice care are in many ways similar to those of the general home care patient population. Admission to hospice is predicated on the poor prognosis of the patient; a poor prognosis is generally stated as "6 months or less if the disease runs its expected course." Infants, children, and adults are cared for by hospice. Some hospices, such as a pediatric hospice, may have a specialized focus, but most hospices generally have admission policies that state their mission and the specific patient populations served. Diseases of patients cared for by hospices include various cancers; AIDS; end-stage renal, cardiac, and lung diseases; dementia; and other diseases that are associated with a limited life expectancy.

THE TYPES OF HOSPICE ORGANIZATIONS

The different types or "auspices" of programs providing hospice care include the following:

- An inpatient hospice unit at a facility such as a hospital, nursing home, or subacute unit
- A community-based hospice, such as a not-for-profit volunteer organization serving a defined rural geographical area
- A freestanding inpatient hospice, such as a hospice that cares for patients through death in a large metropolitan area
- A home care organization that provides hospice care with specially trained home care hospice nurses, volunteers, and other team members
- Corporations that provide hospice care
- Other models, such as health maintenance organizations (HMOs)

As managed care continues to grow, other systems, such as alliances or network hospices, are expected to emerge to provide this special care to patients.

THE INTERDISCIPLINARY HOSPICE TEAM

The interdisciplinary team is a key component of hospice care. This team and its members' roles are explained in depth in this section. The hospice team members include the following:

Patients and families
Nurses
Social workers
Physicians (including hospice medical directors)
Dietitians/dietary counselors
Bereavement counselors
Spiritual counselors/chaplains
Volunteers
Physical therapists
Occupational therapists
Speech-language pathologists
Home health aides
Homemakers
Pharmacists
Other team members, depending on the hospice's unique mission and population served

Depending on the size of the hospice, some team members may have more than one role and not all hospices may have easy access to these specialists and services. The hospice team works in collaboration with the patient and family to define and plan care throughout the hospice patient's length of stay.

Administrative staff may include the following:

Administrators and managers

Secretaries and office support team members

Bereavement coordinators

Volunteer coordinators

Billing personnel

Other team members as the hospice organization's mission requires (e.g., massage, pet, and music therapists)

Hospice care is a team effort. To work effectively, meet patient needs and goals, and ensure smooth operation, hospice care depends on clear, open, and positive communications among team members. Team conferences or interdisciplinary group (IDG) meetings should occur on an ongoing basis and according to the hospice organization's policy. Figure 1-2 presents an example of an IDG form that shows communications and coordination among the team members.

Therapists, nurses, volunteers, the physician, the aide or certified nursing assistant (CNA), and other personnel involved with a particular hospice patient all participate in developing the plan of care (POC). It goes without saying that hospice patients and their families or designated caregivers are the focus around which the other team members revolve. This ensures that hospice care is client centered and directed.

All hospice team members providing care must maintain liaison with each other to ensure that their efforts are coordinated effectively and support the objectives outlined in the IDG and the patient's clinical record or minutes of care conferences. The documentation should establish that effective interchange, reporting, and coordination of patient care occur.

The Roles of Hospice Team Members

The following are the members of the hospice care team:

1. **Nurses**

   Nursing care must be provided by or under the supervision of an RN functioning within a medically approved plan of care. Just as (or even more than) in the hospital, physician orders are needed for all care or changes to the plan of care. Hospice nurses should be experienced in the art and science of pain and symptom management and have well-developed physical assessment skills.

   Nursing care in hospice may be provided by clinicians and/or specialists. Some hospice nurses may be master's prepared or have additional training and education and certification for their chosen areas of specialization. Certification is available through the Hospice and Palliative Nurses Association. (See the Resources in Part 9 for more information.)

   Services provided by the nurse are as varied as the hospice patient population. They may include the following:
   - Comforting an end-stage heart failure patient
   - Observing and assessing a patient through such data sources as weight, pedal edema, patient history and input, shortness of breath, and respirations
   - Administering medication and managing symptoms
   - Monitoring the patient's status and reporting to the physician

IDG/IDT MEETING NOTES

Date _____ / _____ / _____

MEETING TYPE:	☐ INITIAL/NEW PATIENT ☐ REVIEW/FOLLOW-UP START OF CARE DATE _____ / _____ / _____
CARE PLAN:	☐ NEW ☐ NO CHANGE—Continue Current Care Plan
	☐ CARE PLAN CHANGES NOTED—See Individual Discipline Notes

Check if discipline representative is present. For each applicable discipline, document current problem(s) and intervention(s) or resolution of problem(s) and intervention(s) used. Include visit frequency, as applicable. Check if notes include changes to Care Plan.

DISCIPLINE	PROBLEM(S)/RESOLUTION(S)/INTERVENTION(S)
RN/NURSING: ☐ Present ☐ Care Plan Change	
SOCIAL SERVICES: ☐ Present ☐ Care Plan Change	
HOME HEALTH AIDE SERVICES: ☐ Present ☐ Care Plan Change	
VOLUNTEER SERVICES: ☐ Present ☐ Care Plan Change	
CHAPLAIN/ CLERGY: ☐ Present ☐ Care Plan Change	
OTHER (Specify): ☐ Care Plan Change	

INTERDISCIPLINARY TEAM SIGNATURES/TITLES

Signature	Title	Signature	Title	Signature	Title
Signature	Title	Signature	Title	Signature	Title
Signature	Title	Signature	Title	Signature	Title

☐ Discipline Representative Signatures on Separate Sheet   DATE OF NEXT REVIEW _____ / _____ / _____

PATIENT NAME—Last, First, Middle Initial   ID#

Form 3455P © 1995 Briggs Corporation, Des Moines, IA 50306   **IDG/IDT MEETING NOTES**
To order, phone 1-800-247-2343   PRINTED IN U.S.A.

Figure 1-2 IDG/IDT meeting notes form. (Courtesy Briggs Corporation, Des Moines, Ia.)

- Teaching an elderly caregiver how to care for a loved one with end-stage disease

2. **Medical social workers**

   The medical social worker is an important member of the hospice team. Support, active listening, and resource identification are just some of the services that medical social workers provide to hospice patients and their family members. Problems addressed by social work in hospice include financial, housing, and caregiver status concerns. Most social workers in hospice are master's prepared and have clinical experience in addressing the counseling and other needs of terminally ill patients and their families.

3. **Physicians**

The physician is a key member of the team and the interdisciplinary group and plays an important role in the care plan and the review of care. Medicare and other medical health insurance plans cover or pay for "medically necessary" care. They require that the physician (1) certify that the patient needs the services and (2) sign the plan of care supporting the care. Some hospices have their own forms, and others use a facsimile of the Health Care Financing Administration's (HCFA) form 485, also called the Home Health Certification and Plan of Care. Medicare law requires that payment for services can be made only if a physician certifies the need for services and establishes a plan of care. All care, changes in the plan of care, and changes in the patient's condition must be reported to the physician and documented in the patient's clinical record. It goes without saying that all verbal orders or any changes must be obtained, put in writing, and sent to the physician for signature. The organization will have policies relating to the forms and process for receiving and documenting verbal and other physician orders. From legal, quality, and standards of practice perspectives, it is very important that the hospice team members communicate and coordinate care with the patient's physician(s).

Many hospice organizations have a medical director or advisor. For Medicare-certified hospice this is a requirement of the COPs. This is an important role and has numerous responsibilities, including acting as a resource to the organization's management and clinical team members and providing direction related to clinical services. Although specific roles, programs, and practices vary, the following are some of the important responsibilities of the hospice medical director:

- Providing guidance about the development of new or revised policies and procedures
- Serving on the hospice advisory committee or other boards or committees
- Collaborating and consulting with the managers and facilitating problem solving toward meeting the patient's needs
- Participating in team conferences
- Serving as the liaison between the hospice organization and physician members of the medical community
- Supporting the hospice organization through teaching, public relations endeavors, education of physicians about hospice and palliative care in the community (e.g., who is appropriate, needing MD orders, communications)
- Acting as a role model by making home visits if possible and attending scheduled team and other meetings and other activities that support the mission of the hospice organization

The physicians will look to the hospice clinicians for recommendations and solutions to care needs for their patients.

The physicians most involved with hospice are the hospice organization's medical director and the local community physicians who refer patients and families for specialized hospice care. The medical director's role varies among hospices but is always very important to the operations of the hospice and effective hospice and family care. The following are some of the multifaceted responsibilities of the medical director, as based on the unique needs of the hospice:

- Providing direction and acting as a resource to hospice team members on palliative care and practice
- Providing guidance about the development of medical and clinical policies relating to the provision of hospice
- Providing insight and feedback from a physician perspective about clinical and administrative areas
- Serving as a member of the hospice advisory board or performance improvement (PI) committees
- Collaborating with the hospice managers to facilitate problem solving toward meeting patient and family needs
- Participating in team or IDG meetings
- Consulting with other hospice team members
- Serving as the liaison between the hospice program and members of the medical community
- Supporting the tenets of hospice in the community through education and public relations endeavors
- Educating physicians and other health care professionals about hospice and the care of the terminally ill patient in the community
- Contacting new physicians who refer patients to hospice, assisting them through the process, answering their questions, and coordinating care
- Assisting in the resolution of difficulties that may arise between members of the team and physicians in the community
- Acting as a role model by making home visits if possible to hospice patients and their families

Counseling includes dietary counseling with respect to the care of the terminally ill individual and bereavement counseling with respect to the survivors' adjustment to death. Although Medicare hospice puts dietary counseling and bereavement counseling together under the heading "counseling," these important counseling services are very different.

4. **Dietitians/dietary counselors**

   Dietary counselors are very important for the provision of quality hospice care. Many hospice patients have symptoms and side effects that have an impact on their nutritional status. Anorexia, mouth sores and pain, swallowing disorders, diarrhea or constipation, and nausea are common symptoms and challenges in hospice. The nutritional status of the patient and the family/caregiver response to nutritional changes often are a source of conflict and uneasiness with the unit of care and among caregivers. The importance of educating patients and family members about nutritional and dietary changes cannot be overemphasized. Hospice dietary counseling is usually provided by a dietitian. Depending on the state and licensure requirements, the dietitian may be a licensed dietitian (LD) and/or registered dietitian (RD).

   The role of the professional dietitian in hospice home care is expanding as more patients are cared for in the community setting or at home. One important part of the role of the dietitian is to make home visits to patients and families and provide consultative services to promote optimal comfort and nutrition to hospice patients. Another important part of the role of the dietitian is to be an inservice educator for the other hospice team members. The dietitian assists in the development of educational policies, procedures, and tools for use by clinicians and patients and families.

Many home care and hospice programs have dietitians available to make home visits and provide consultative services to promote optimal nutrition. To determine whether nutritional services or intervention is required, nurses in hospice assess patients for being at risk for conditions such as cachexia by monitoring weight loss and checking that the refrigerator is stocked with an adequate supply of food. For accreditation, standards require that the patient's nutritional status be assessed, interdisciplinary nutritional care planning be performed, counseling or nutrition intervention be carried out, and appropriately qualified staff members be designated to coordinate services. Hospice has traditionally relied upon hospice nurses to identify, coordinate, and implement nutrition-related services. Hospice organizations may need the dietitian for diet modification and counseling and use of oral supplements. The dietitian may also make recommendations relating to enteral and parenteral nutrition therapies. Other services include teaching about complex diets, identifying educational materials for use with patient teaching, and acting as an inservice educator and resource on nutrition services. Resources relating to hospice nutritional services are listed in Part 9; Part 6 is a guide to planning and implementing hospice nutritional care.

5. **Bereavement counselors**

   Bereavement counselors are important to comprehensive hospice care. The standards for bereavement counseling and care include that bereavement care be provided for 1 year after the patient's death to bereaved survivors. This counseling is based on an assessment performed when the patient is initially admitted to hospice. High-risk and other problematic areas are identified on admission and updated through the length of hospice care to best address the needs of the bereaved family members.

   Bereavement counseling is a part of the hospice organization's planned intervention program for the survivors and is a key indicator of the quality of hospice services. Components of the bereavement program may include a standardized assessment tool to identify at-risk families or family members, organized support meetings, cards and letters, and counseling services. Services may be provided by specially trained bereavement volunteers under the direction of the hospice and by social workers, psychologists, or others with a background in counseling, grief, and loss. See Figures 1-3 and 1-4 for examples of a bereavement assessment tool and a follow-up tool.

6. **Spiritual counselors/chaplains**

   Spiritual counseling is a core component of quality hospice. A spiritual assessment should be part of the comprehensive assessment that is performed upon evaluation and admission to hospice. The spiritual care services provided should be consistent with the belief systems of the patients and family. Many hospices have a network of community clergy who provide support and spiritual care to patients according to their own beliefs or the religious community. Other hospices have their own chaplain team, which works with the local community spiritual representatives.

   Hospice spiritual services are varied. For purposes of clarity only, the term *chaplain* will be used, though a rabbi, minister, or priest also could fill this important role. The chaplain (or other spiritual counselor) serves a popu-

BEREAVEMENT ASSESSMENT

Date of Contact _____ / _____ / _____

☐ Home Visit ☐ Telephone Consult

GENERAL INFORMATION

Name of Bereaved: _____

Address: _____

City/State/ZIP: _____

Telephone No.: (_____) _____

Age: _____ Sex: ☐ Male ☐ Female

Bereaved's Relationship to Deceased: _____

Length of Relationship: _____

Patient Address: _____

City/State/ZIP: _____

Date of Patient's Death: _____ / _____ / _____

Place of Patient's Death: _____

Circumstances of Death (Describe): _____

SUPPORT SYSTEMS

Person(s) Providing Support:

Spouse: _____

Family Member(s): _____

Friends: _____

Clergy: _____

Professionals: _____

Others: _____

Support Person(s) Available:

☐ Daily ☐ Several Times a Week ☐ Once a Week

☐ Other (Specify): _____

Meaningful Activities (Describe): _____

Important Dates:

Birthdays: Patient _____ Bereaved _____

Other (Specify): _____

EMPLOYMENT

Employment Situation (Describe): _____

PHYSICAL STATUS

Sleep Patterns: ☐ Unchanged ☐ Changed Comments _____

Appetite: ☐ Unchanged ☐ Changed Comments _____

Appearance: ☐ Neat ☐ Unkempt ☐ Not Observed

Recent Illnesses: ☐ None ☐ Present ☐ Describe _____

Weight: ☐ Gain ☐ Loss ☐ Unchanged

Additional Comments: _____

BEHAVIOR OBSERVED/FEELINGS EXPRESSED

Behavior Observed: ☐ Depressed ☐ Guilty ☐ Angry ☐ Withdrawn ☐ Denial ☐ Tearful ☐ Restless ☐ Talkative

Other (Specify): _____

Comments: _____

Suicide Considered: ☐ No ☐ Yes Comments: _____

Alcohol Intake: ☐ None ☐ Occasional ☐ 2 or more times a week ☐ Daily

Comments: _____

Drug Intake: ☐ None ☐ Occasional ☐ 2 or more times a week ☐ Daily

Comments: _____

PATIENT NAME—Last, First, Middle Initial ID#

Form 3451HH ©1995 Briggs Corporation, Des Moines, IA 50306
To order, phone 1-800-247-2343 PRINTED IN U.S.A.

BEREAVEMENT ASSESSMENT
☐ Continued on Reverse

Figure 1-3 Bereavement assessment tool. (Courtesy Briggs Corporation, Des Moines, Ia.) *Continued*

lation that spans the life continuum from infancy through death. The chaplain, like other hospice team members, interfaces with patients and their family members during some of the most difficult times of their lives. This struggle with the meaning of life, a common experience among patients who have significant health concerns, is the work of the chaplain, regardless of any formal religious beliefs the patient may have. The chaplain's role varies depending on the patient and family and their unique belief systems and needs. Responsibilities may include providing bereavement counseling, serving on ethics committees, supporting hospice staff and attending team meetings, performing the sacraments for the sick, and intervening in other

BEREAVEMENT ASSESSMENT

PSYCHOSOCIAL

History of Ability to Cope: ☐ Poor   ☐ Fair   ☐ Good   ☐ Excellent

Comments:_____

Assessment of Coping Ability:_____

OTHER STRESS SOURCES

Additional Recent Losses:_____

Finances: ☐ Unchanged   ☐ Changed   ☐ Sufficient   ☐ Insufficient

Comments_____

Living Situation: ☐ Unchanged   ☐ Changed   ☐ Stable   ☐ Uncertain

Comments_____

Health: ☐ Unchanged   ☐ Changed   ☐ Improved   ☐ Deteriorated

Comments_____

PROBLEMS

Major Problems:_____

BEREAVEMENT FOLLOW-UP

Is Bereaved Interested in Follow-Up?   ☐ Yes   ☐ No

Does Bereaved Feel a Need For Immediate Support?   ☐ Yes   ☐ No

Others Needing/Desiring Follow-Up (Indicate name and relationship):

_____ Phone _____

_____ Phone _____

PLAN/INTERVENTION

Plan/Intervention:_____

COMMENTS

Signature and Title of Assessor _____   Date ___/___/___

BEREAVEMENT ASSESSMENT

Figure 1-3 cont'd, For legend see previous page.

ways. The chaplain facilitates patients' and families' movement toward their own resolution of life's questions. A spiritual assessment form follows (Figure 1-5). It is completed initially by admitting team members and later reviewed and addressed/completed in detail by the chaplain.

7. **Volunteers**

Volunteers and their supportive care and services are a unique and valued part of hospice care. Conceptually the role of the specially trained hospice volunteer varies among hospices. Some hospices have volunteers who are

BEREAVEMENT FOLLOW-UP

Date of Contact _____/_____/_____

☐ Visit ☐ Phone ☐ Letter ☐ Other

Name of Bereaved _____

INSTRUCTIONS: For each area addressed, check the box(es) which most closely describes the changes that have occurred since the original Bereavement Assessment or last Bereavement Follow-up was completed.

PHYSICAL STATUS

Sleep Patterns	☐ Unchanged	☐ Changed	Comments _____
Appetite	☐ Unchanged	☐ Changed	Comments _____
Appearance	☐ Neat	☐ Unkept	☐ Not Observed
Recent Illnesses	☐ None	☐ Present	Describe _____
Weight	☐ Unchanged	☐ Gain	☐ Loss

Additional Comments _____

BEHAVIOR OBSERVED/FEELINGS EXPRESSED

Behavior Observed: ☐ Depressed ☐ Guilty ☐ Angry ☐ Withdrawn ☐ Denial ☐ Tearful ☐ Restless ☐ Talkative

Other _____

Suicide Considered: ☐ Yes ☐ No

Comments _____

Alcohol Intake: ☐ None ☐ Occasional ☐ 2 or more times a week ☐ Daily

Comments _____

Drug Intake: ☐ None ☐ Occasional ☐ 2 or more times a week ☐ Daily

Comments _____

OTHER STRESS SOURCES

Additional Recent Losses _____

Finances: ☐ Unchanged ☐ Changed ☐ Sufficient ☐ Insufficient

Comments _____

Living Situation: ☐ Unchanged ☐ Changed ☐ Stable ☐ Uncertain

Comments _____

Health: ☐ Unchanged ☐ Changed ☐ Improved ☐ Deteriorated

Comments _____

GENERAL AREAS OF CONCERN

Has survivor resumed previous lifestyle? _____

Are all members of family coping? ☐ Yes ☐ No

If no, is intervention desired by bereaved? ☐ Yes ☐ No

Comments _____

PLAN/INTERVENTION

Plan/Intervention: _____

_____

_____

_____

_____

_____

_____

Planned Date of Next Contact _____/_____/_____

Signature and Title of Assessor _____ Date _____/_____/_____

PATIENT NAME—Last, First, Middle Initial _____ ID# _____

Form 3452P © 1995 Briggs Corporation, Des Moines, IA 50306
To reorder call 1-800-247-2343 PRINTED IN U.S.A.

BEREAVEMENT FOLLOW-UP

Figure 1-4 Bereavement follow-up tool. (Courtesy of Briggs Corporation, Des Moines, Ia.)

dietitians, nurses, and social workers providing some of the patient and family care and support. The primary role of these volunteers is to offer respite for the family. Other hospices have volunteers who are specialized in areas such as bereavement, spiritual support, and art or other therapies. Still other hospices "pair" volunteers, having them work together with an assigned hospice patient and family. Most try to match the hospice patient to the volunteer, depending on availability. An example is a hospice volunteer who is an engineer paired with a patient who shares the same profession and/or background. Hospice volunteers make an important difference

SPIRITUAL ASSESSMENT

Information Obtained By: ☐ Phone   ☐ Visit

GENERAL INFORMATION

	Patient	Primary Caregiver	Family
Faith/Denomination			
Church Affiliation			
Name of Pastor/Priest/Rabbi			
Phone No.	( )	( )	( )
Contact Requested	☐ Yes ☐ No	☐ Yes ☐ No	☐ Yes ☐ No
Hospice Chaplain Referral Requested	☐ Yes ☐ No	☐ Yes ☐ No	☐ Yes ☐ No
Importance of Religion in Life: (Great, Moderate, Unimportant, Unknown)			

PATIENT ASSESSMENT

Current Support Systems:

☐ Family   ☐ Friends   ☐ Community Groups   ☐ Religious Groups
☐ Prayer/Meditation   ☐ Worship Services   ☐ Religious Rituals (sacraments, etc.)
☐ Other (Specify) _____

Patient is satisfied with current spiritual support: ☐ Yes   ☐ No (Explain) _____

INDICATORS OF SPIRITUAL STRENGTH (Check all that apply)	INDICATORS OF SPIRITUAL DISTRESS (Check all that apply)
Patient demonstrates/expresses:	Patient demonstrates/expresses:
Acceptance of Reality	Depression
Eternal Life Beliefs	Anxiety
Spiritual Discipline	Guilt
Serenity/Peace	Shame
Life Meaning/Purpose	Anger
Hope	Hopelessness/Despair
Forgiveness	Powerlessness
Reconciliation	Meaninglessness
Acceptance of Limits	Grief
Self Worth	Denial of Reality/Pain
Unknown at This Time	Withdrawal/Isolation
Other (specify)	Self Pity
	Suicidal Thoughts
	Fear of (specify)
	Other (specify)

Overall patient demonstrates: ☐ Spiritual Connection   ☐ Spiritual Distress   ☐ Uncertain
Further spiritual follow-up desired: ☐ Patient   ☐ Primary Caregiver   ☐ Family
Specify type of follow-up desired: _____

Comments/Counseling/Care plan implementation: _____

Signature and Title of Assessor _____ Date __/__/__

PATIENT NAME—Last, First, Middle Initial   ID#

Form 3468P   © 1995 Briggs Corporation, Des Moines, IA 50306
To order, phone 1-800-247-2343   PRINTED IN U.S.A

SPIRITUAL ASSESSMENT

Figure 1-5 Spiritual assessment tool. (Courtesy Briggs Corporation, Des Moines, Ia.)

in the quality of life for hospice patients and families. A frequent sentiment heard from families is, "I could not have done it without my volunteer(s)."

Hospice volunteers are special people who are specially trained in this poignant work. Activities that a volunteer might assist with include listening, reading, transportation, meal preparation, plant care, and numerous other tasks, depending on the patient's needs and the relationship forged.

New hospice team members, such as new nurses, may be a part of the volunteer training program. Some hospices use this mechanism as a way for new team members to get to know the new hospice volunteers.

Figure 1-6 Volunteer care plan. (Courtesy Briggs Corporation, Des Moines, Ia.)

The team concept is at the core of all hospice care and is particularly important for relations between the hospice nurses and volunteers because the volunteers must be comfortable reporting changes and generally updating and reporting on the patient's progress to the nurse. In addition to fulfilling their all-important role in patient care, other volunteers may participate in fund-raising, bereavement counseling, spiritual support, massage, and committee work. Examples of a volunteer care plan and an activity record are presented in Figures 1-6 and 1-7 for review.

Other services, depending on physician orders the hospice, and the patient's and family's unique needs, may include the following:

VOLUNTEER ACTIVITY RECORD

DAY→	SUN	MON	TUE	WED	THU	FRI	SAT	WEEK OF
Date								/ /
Time In								
Time Out								THROUGH
SITE OF SERVICE:								
Home								/ /
Nursing Home								
Hospice Office								
Other (Specify)								

PATIENT-RELATED ACTIVITIES	SUN	MON	TUE	WED	THU	FRI	SAT	COMMENTS (All comments must be dated)
Companionship—Patient								
Respite—Primary Caregiver								
Emotional Support:								
Patient								
Primary Caregiver								
Bereavement:								
Telephone Call								
Support								
Attend Funeral								
Shopping								
Meal Preparation								
Light Housekeeping								
Yard Work								
Laundry								
Other (Specify)								

(Left margin labels: PSYCHOSOCIAL SUPPORT, ACTIVITIES)

ORGANIZATIONAL ACTIVITIES	SUN	MON	TUE	WED	THU	FRI	SAT	
Fund-raising Assistance								
Answer Phone								
Clerical Work								
Other (Specify)								

(Left margin label: HOSPICE)

VOLUNTEERS ASSIGNED			
INITIALS	VOLUNTEER NAME		DATE
			/ /
			/ /

PATIENT NAME—Last, First, Middle Initial   ID#

Form 3469P   © 1995 Briggs Corporation, Des Moines, IA 50306
To order, phone 1-800-247-2343   PRINTED IN U.S.A.   VOLUNTEER ACTIVITY RECORD

Figure 1-7 Volunteer activity record. (Courtesy Briggs Corporation, Des Moines, Ia.)

8. **Physical therapists**

Physical therapists (PTs) are sometimes called *licensed physical therapists* (LPTs). Members of the rehabilitation team have very important roles in hospice. Physical therapy in hospice home care is based on the patient's problems, and its goals are usually directed toward safety and comfort. An example is the patient who has a pathological hip fracture but refuses surgical intervention. The therapist in this case teaches the nurse, aide, and other team members safe positioning, movement, and pain control. One of the primary skills of the PT in hospice is teaching the family or caregivers the home exercise program (HEP) to promote comfort and safe care at home. The PT, like other team members, provides input into the plan and any necessary revisions of the plan, prepares clinical documentation, and participates in inservice programs.

9. **Occupational therapists**

   Occupational therapists (OTs) assist the hospice patient to attain the maximum level of physical and psychosocial independence. Areas of expertise generally include fine motor coordination, perceptual/motor skills, sensory testing, adaptive techniques, assistive devices, activities of daily living (ADLs), and specialized upper extremity/hand therapies. Problems frequently seen in hospice care that may require OT intervention include end-stage lung processes such as chronic obstructive pulmonary disease (COPD). OT can train patients in diaphragmatic breathing and relaxation techniques for comfort and energy conservation training. Safety assessments for hospice patients wishing to remain at home also are appropriate for the OT who specializes in safety measures relating to daily function.

10. **S-LP Speech-language pathologists**

    Speech-language pathology (S-LP) services are an important part of therapy for patients with various speech and swallowing problems. Patients who may need specialized S-LP services in hospice include those with cerebral vascular accidents (CVAs), tracheostomies, laryngectomies, or various neuromuscular diseases such as ALS and MS. Like all the team members, the S-LP creates clinical documentation, provides input into the plan of care, and attends case conferences about the patient's status and progress on a regular basis for care coordination.

11. **Home health aides**

    Home health aides (HHAs), or certified nursing assistants (CNAs), as they are called in some states, provide what is probably the most important service for many patients. HHAs are truly the "eyes and ears" of the hospice organization. They are often the team members who visit the patient the most because they provide personal care and assistance in the activities of daily living to support the patient in maintaining comfort at home. The HHA's role and functions are pivotal in the determination of whether hospice patients can remain at home safely. Because the HHA usually spends more time with the patient and family than any other team member, the HHA's contribution is invaluable to both the team process and patient and family satisfaction. The Medicare standards for home health aides require that they be specially trained. Home health aides are selected on the basis of such factors as a sympathetic attitude toward the care of the sick; the ability to read, write, and carry out directions; and the maturity and ability to deal effectively with the demands of the job. From a Medicare perspective home health aides must be proficient or competent in 12 subject areas:

    1. Communication skills
    2. Observation, reporting, and documentation of patient status and the care or service furnished
    3. Reading and recording of temperature, pulse, and respiration
    4. Basic infection control procedures

5. Basic elements of body functioning and changes in body function that must be reported to the aide's supervisor
6. Maintenance of a clean, safe, and healthy environment
7. Recognition of emergencies and knowledge of emergency procedures
8. Physical, emotional, and developmental needs of hospice patients and families and ways to work with the populations served by the hospice, including respect for the patient and the patient's privacy and property
9. Appropriate and safe techniques in personal hygiene and grooming, including:
   Bed bath
   Sponge, tub, or shower bath
   Shampoo, sink, tub, or bed
   Nail and skin care
   Oral hygiene
   Toileting and elimination
10. Safe transfer techniques and ambulation
11. Normal range of motion and positioning
12. Adequate nutrition and fluid intake

HHAs should also be proficient in any other task that the organization may choose to have aides perform. Home health aides are closely supervised by the RN or other team members to ensure their competence and comfort in providing the best hospice care to patients.

12. **Homemakers**

Homemakers maintain the patient care area in a manner acceptable to provide safe and effective hospice care. Some hospices define homemaker services as those services required to keep patient care areas maintained. Homemaker services may include housekeeping duties such as cleaning, vacuuming, and grocery shopping.

13. **Pharmacists**

The important role of the pharmacist is growing as the complexities of drug–drug, drug–disease, and drug–food adverse reactions increase. In home hospice care, nurses are acutely aware that many patients are inappropriately medicated or overmedicated. Traditionally most hospice patients are elderly and have multiple risk factors for therapeutic misadventures secondary to drug therapy. They may have multiple pathologies, have different prescribers, and exhibit polypharmacy (both prescription and nonprescription medications), and they are at greater risk for adverse effects from medications because of altered physiology secondary to aging and disabilities (e.g., poor eyesight, impaired hearing, arthritic fingers).

The nurse in the community sees the whole picture, including the shoeboxes full of medications given to patients by multiple physicians. It is in this instance that the hospice nurse addresses safety concerns related to medications, acts as the patient's advocate to clarify medications and orders, and consults with the pharmacist, who can effectively evaluate the multiple medication regimens.

Traditionally the pharmacist has been considered simply the provider of a product; that is, drugs. While this is certainly one of the pharmacist's roles, the pharmacist, as a drug expert, can offer many other services to the hospice care team, including the following:

- Providing the hospice care team with inservice education and information about drugs
- Reviewing medication regimens and screening for interactions and incorrect doses or dosage forms
- Suggesting simplifying medication regimens by altering drug delivery systems or medication administration scheduling
- Monitoring and assessing the therapeutic or toxic effect of drugs
- Participating in case conferences, hospice rounds, and IDG meetings
- Perhaps most importantly, acting as a resource for pain and other symptom control for hospice patients, their families, and the hospice team

14. **Other services**
   Other services may be available, such as music or art therapy or massage, depending on the hospice organization's mission and specialty programs.

   Although the entire team is very much involved with the patient's care, hospice nurses make most visits in the community. Safety is an important issue in hospice home care, as it is in all our communities. Information for the entire team about home care safety follows.

DEFINING HOSPICE NURSING

Whatever the organizational structure of the hospice, the hospice nurse plays a key role on the team. Hospice nursing practice is the provision of palliative nursing care for the terminally ill and their families, with the emphasis on their physical, psychosocial, emotional, and spiritual needs.[5] Hospice nursing is a synthesis of special skills that are used to create the environment for the best outcomes for the hospice patient and their families.

The hospice nurse's role is often that of case or care manager as the nurse coordinates the implementation of the plan of care. Whatever the role defined by the organization, the following are key aspects of the hospice home care specialty that must be learned, nurtured, and improved through continued education and experience. Experienced nurses new to hospice may be paired with an experienced hospice nurse as a preceptor through the new nurse's orientation. It goes without saying that, as with any specialty, home care nurses without additional orientation, education, and experience cannot successfully make the transition to hospice. Hospice is very different from home care nursing practice, even though some of the care interventions appear similar.

HALLMARKS OF EFFECTIVE HOSPICE NURSING CARE

The following are some of the areas in which hospice nurses must be proficient when caring for hospice patients and their families.

1. **Pain and symptom management skills**
   This is a specialty area in hospice. Because of the teamwork in hospice, this is often an interdisciplinary effort with input from the hospice nurse, the physi-

cian, the pharmacist, and other team members, such as a social worker and a spiritual counselor. Because the focus of care is palliative and supportive, it is imperative that hospice nurses be competent in pain assessment, intervention, and evaluation. Pain is emerging as the fifth vital sign that should be assessed during every patient encounter. Modalities for pain relief and optimal comfort range from pharmaceutical agents to acupuncture, imagery, massage, and other care interventions. Most patients receive a complement of pain solutions (e.g., massage and analgesics). Readers are referred to the Agency for Health Care Policy and Research's *Clinical Practice Guidelines Number 9: Management of Cancer Pain,* which is free and can be obtained by calling 1-800-358-9295. This fact-filled text of over 200 pages has numerous recommendations and pain assessment models, resources, and tools to improve pain control and patient comfort. Examples of pain assessment tools are included in Part 7. Please refer to the "Pain" care guideline for an in-depth discussion on pain.

2. **Knowledge of concepts related to death and dying**
   Hospice integrates the dying process as a part of life. The nurse's philosophy and belief system should be congruent with the basic tenets of hospice care. Dr. Elisabeth Kübler-Ross's research on the stages of dying and other studies may be incorporated into patient care and care planning. The theoretical framework in Kübler-Ross's work provides the rationale for intervention and identification of resolutions to challenges that patients and families face.

3. **Stress management skills**
   Hospice nurses and colleagues have varied mechanisms for providing support to themselves and each other. Hospice care may be stressful for nurses and other hospice workers. Hospices provide staff support mechanisms to assist in the resolution of problems and for review of care and feelings raised through hospice care. Staff support may be structured, such as scheduled meetings with a trained facilitator, or may be volunteer-initiated, with varying models. It is important that all hospice team members take care of themselves and find activities and events that promote emotional well-being, nurture, and support. Whatever model staff support takes, it is a means for sharing, caring, team building, validating, and processing the important work of hospice.

4. **Sensitive communication skills**
   Communication skills are essential for effective hospice team members. There is untold intimacy and poignancy in hospice. A nurse walks into the homes of patients who may have been battling cancer for years and are now ready to change the focus from fighting the disease to enjoying their last days in their chosen way. The patient's sole priority while beginning growth work through hospice may seem to be the care of their pets or the maintenance of a garden. These values also become the hospice team's priority to support care and respect the patient's wishes. The psychosocial and spiritual components of hospice are very important to quality of life and patient and family satisfaction. Hospice staff can facilitate closure or the mending of difficult relationships. Figure 1-8 presents an example of an initial psychosocial assessment tool.
   Communication skills include active listening, realizing the work of "getting things in order," presence as an intervention, and being sensitively

INITIAL PSYCHOSOCIAL ASSESSMENT

PRIMARY CAREGIVER INFORMATION

Name _____

Address _____

City/State/ZIP _____

Phone No. (_____) _____

Age _____ ☐ Male ☐ Female

Relationship to Patient _____

Health Status _____

_____

_____

_____

SOCIAL HISTORY ASSESSMENT

Family System Background (General History) _____

_____

Family Stability _____

_____

Caregivers and Supporters (in Addition to Primary Caregiver) _____

_____

_____

Members of Immediate Family/Significant Others Living with Patient

_____   _____

_____   _____

_____   _____

Members of Immediate Family/Significant Others NOT Living with Patient

_____   _____

_____   _____

_____   _____

Patient's Most Significant Relationship _____

　Length of Relationship _____

Patient's Educational History (Indicate Number of Years Completed)

　　Elementary _____ Jr. High/Middle School _____ High School _____ College _____ Vocational _____

Patient's Occupational History _____

_____

Ethnic and Cultural Considerations _____

_____

Significant Losses/Crises Experienced with Family or Other Significant Others _____

_____

_____

_____

_____

PATIENT NAME—Last, First, Middle Initial | ID#

Form 3457HH　© 1995 Briggs Corporation, Des Moines, IA 50306
To order, phone 1-800-247-2343　PRINTED IN U.S.A.

INITIAL PSYCHOSOCIAL ASSESSMENT

Page 1 of 4

Figure 1-8 Initial psychosocial assessment tool. (Courtesy Briggs Corporation, Des Moines, Ia.) *Continued*

cued to what the patient and family are saying (and sometimes asking for). An example is Sarah, a 39-year-old woman with an aggressive, recurrent breast cancer. At a nursing visit, Sarah said to the hospice nurse, "Anne, I want to renew my vows with my husband before I die." Anne said that she would talk to her later about that because she was doing her dressing change. However, this discussion did not occur, and Sarah later expressed the same wish to the home health aide, who reported it at the patient care conference. Because of this team effort, Sarah did renew her vows before her death. Especially in hospice, because of the limited time factor, patient and family needs must be

SUPPORT SYSTEM ASSESSMENT
Discuss the questions listed below with the patient and family. Summarize their responses in the space provided.

What has this experience been like for you? Do(es) family/patient talk about illness with you? How is that for you?

Patient:_____

_____

_____

Family: _____

_____

_____

Have there been changes in the roles of members of your family? Changes in family plans/routines?

Patient:_____

_____

_____

Family: _____

_____

_____

What are the reactions to increased dependency?

Patient:_____

_____

Family: _____

_____

Who/what in your community can you count on in hard times?

_____

_____

RISK ASSESSMENT						
Check the appropriate response for each question below. A "yes" response indicates a risk potential.						
	PATIENT			**PRIMARY CAREGIVER**		
	YES	NO	Uncertain	YES	NO	Uncertain
Are there children/adolescents in immediate family?						
Are there dependent family members (handicapped, elderly, sick)?						
Is a parent still alive?						
Will death result in loss of financial provision?						
Will death mean loss of constant companion/emotional support?						
Will death mean loss of home (feared or actual)?						
Does the family have difficulty making decisions?						
Is family unable to share feelings?						
Is there reluctance to face facts of illness?						
Is there marital or family discord?						
Are there communication difficulties in the family?						
Is there a concurrent life crisis?						
Has there been difficulty in dealing with previous losses?						
Is the family inflexible?						
Has the patient or family members had excessive or prolonged emotional problems/mental illness?						
Is there a lack of community support?						

INITIAL PSYCHOSOCIAL ASSESSMENT

Page 2 of 4

Figure 1-8 cont'd, For legend see previous page.

addressed in a timely manner and followed up on. In addition, this example shows an important component of hospice, spiritual care.

Patient and family needs, both those clearly articulated and those that are more veiled, should be identified to ensure that the hospice team is meeting them. These spiritual and other psychosocial needs are a key component in the provision and evaluation of high-quality hospice nursing.

Another challenge is family members asking, "When is he/she going to die?" Box 1-1 (p 25) provides a useful list of some of the signs that family members may expect to see with the approach of death.

PHYSICAL RESOURCE ASSESSMENT

Environmental Factors _____

Source and Adequacy of Income _____

Other Financial Factors _____

SERVICE NEEDS

Does the patient need assistance in any of the areas listed below?

	YES	NO	TYPE OF ASSISTANCE/REFERRAL NEEDED
Budget Counseling			
Other Financial Need			
Social Services			
Funeral Arrangements			
Legal Will Preparation			

EMOTIONAL ASSESSMENT

Is the patient exhibiting or experiencing the following?

	YES	NO		YES	NO		YES	NO
Memory Problems			Withdrawal			Feelings of: Loneliness		
Changes in Sleep Patterns			Hostility			Isolation		
Anxiety			Anger			Guilt		
Alertness			Irritability			Moodiness		
Lethargy			Depression			Hallucinations		

Does the patient have impaired comprehension, judgment, or reasoning?   ☐ Yes (If yes, explain)   ☐ No

_____

COMMENTS ON PATIENT/FAMILY RISK POTENTIAL AND EMOTIONAL STATUS (Discuss risk potential of patient/family and the primary problems observed. Include family dynamics, present and anticipated coping, support systems, etc. Also include grief potential within the family and any factors that would influence the intensity or level of grief.)

_____

Page 3 of 4   **INITIAL PSYCHOSOCIAL ASSESSMENT**

Figure 1-8 cont'd, For legend see p. 21.

5. A sense of humor

It is only in the past few years that the healing power of laughter has finally come to be recognized. A kind sense of humor helps the entire team and patients and their families on particularly rough days or in meeting unique challenges.

6. Flexibility

Patients and families in hospice control their care and care planning. Because the days shared with the hospice team are the patient's last months or weeks, the patient calls the shots. This includes scheduling, visit times, length of

ASSESSMENT SUMMARY AND PLAN

Signature and Title
of Assessor _____ Date ____ / ____ / ____

INITIAL PSYCHOSOCIAL ASSESSMENT   Page 4 of 4

Figure 1-8 cont'd, For legend see p. 21.

visits, and a myriad of other decisions. Respect for and acceptance of the patient's choices and decisions are part of effective daily operations in hospice and are required by law through patient self-determination acts.

7. **Hospice knowledge**

It is very important that the hospice nurse have a strong base of knowledge grounded in hospice care and practice. A body of literature is emerging related to hospice, and all team members must keep current.

BOX 1-1

APPROACHING DEATH
Signs and Symptoms

The following are some of the signs and symptoms as death approaches. It is important to note that not all of these symptoms may ever appear, nor will they appear at the same time. Some of the most common symptoms are as follows:

1. *Cooling of the extremities* means that the patient's hands, arms, or feet are cool to the touch, and mottling or a purplish coloring may appear. Sometimes the skin also darkens with the decrease in circulation as death approaches. Interventions are related to keeping the patient warm, but electric blankets should not be used for safety reasons.

2. Breathing slows and becomes irregular. Cheyne-Stokes breathing may occur as the cerebrum, the control center for respirations, begins to fail. This breathing is usually characterized by irregularity and apnea, sometimes with long periods between breaths.

3. The patient sleeps almost all the time. This occurs as the slow but progressive failure of body systems occurs and metabolic needs decrease proportionately toward death.

4. Fluids begin to build up in some patients. This may appear as increased secretions in the throat or create a sound like a "rattle." The body can no longer absorb the secretions, and the fluid is heard as a result. The rattle, which can be distressing to family members, can sometimes be controlled with medication. The patient may also be suctioned or repositioned for comfort in some instances.

5. The patient may appear confused or restless. Confusion states are a common part of the death process and may be very upsetting to family members. Caregiver and family members may want to reassure the patient or provide presence to the patient. It is important that the restlessness be assessed as being caused by the lack of oxygenation and not from pain or other discomfort.

6. No matter what the symptoms or signs of approaching death, it is important that family members support the patient through this changing period with their presence and support. Patients can still hear even if their eyes appear glassy and unresponsive.

IDENTIFIED DIFFERENCES BETWEEN HOME CARE AND HOSPICE NURSING

Because of the growth of hospice and the bulk of care being provided in the patient's home, it is important to note that many patients may be in home care or a home care oncology program and have been receiving home visits. Patients and nurses seeking to make the transition to hospice commonly want clarification of the major differences. The following information seeks to address some of the many differences. It is important to note that the dimensions of scope, depth, and breadth of quality hospice care extend well beyond those of the standard medically directed and focused home care program.

1. *In home care:* The patient is the unit or focus of care. Patient care is usually directed toward health and ultimately self-care. Care is the traditional medical model, as Medicare, a medical insurance program, pays for medically necessary care. Care in home care is usually related to illness and therapeutic, curative, interventions.

   In hospice: The patient, partner, family, and/or identified caregivers are a single unit and are the recipients of care. Hospice is what all nurses learned in nursing school; here the patient and family are an inseparable unit of care, and the patient is an equal partner in determining that care and making choices related to care and care planning.

2. *In home care:* Much of the care is medically focused on curative interventions and outcomes. Care and programs are structured for reimbursement and regulatory reasons.

   In hospice: The care and outcomes are focused on comfort and relief of suffering, pain management, and other palliative or symptom-control interventions. Because of this, hospice nurses and their hospice teammates are often experts in symptom management and care planning. Because hospices have historically grown out of grassroots initiatives to provide special supportive care in a local community, they have a flexibility and creativity unknown to most traditional health care models. This means that there are unique programs to support patients, their families, and surviving loved ones. Creative programs offered by hospices include specialized bereavement camps for children, music therapy programs, art therapy interventions, and others. In fact, some hospices continue to be community- and volunteer-based, are not Medicare certified, and do not provide "insurance-covered" care, with its attendant rules and structures.

3. *In home care:* In the best organizations, home care is a team effort.

   In hospice: In hospice, care and care planning are truly a team effort. A standard in all hospice programs is that the patient and family care is planned and provided by an interdisciplinary team.

4. *In home care:* Medicare has traditionally been a cost-based reimbursement system that sometimes reinforced unneeded or medically unnecessary visits. As home care becomes a prospective payment system, the need for efficiencies becomes paramount.

   In hospice: The Medicare hospice benefit is a managed care system of reimbursement. An in-depth discussion about Medicare hospice can be found on page 27. The Medicare/Medicaid certified hospice program is reimbursed on a daily capitated rate (amount per day) to provide palliative care related to the terminal illness.

5. *In home care:* In home care, it can be frustrating when a patient chooses not to have hospice when the nurse has determined that the patient and family (and the care team) would have additional support and that needed care cannot be provided under the auspices of regular home care. For this reason, some programs have a "bridge," or "pre-hospice," program.

   In hospice: Volunteer support, staff support mechanisms, and the true team concept all assist and support the nurse and other team members through the patient's death and beyond. Continuity and closure are also offered through bereavement services for the patient's survivors with trained bereavement counselors for a year after death. The supportive and nurturing nature of the team encourages members to support each other, avoiding the "I'm out there alone" feeling.

6. *In home care:* Productivity and other parameters of effectiveness are designated by time frames (e.g., 6-7 visits per day on average, or 25-30 visits per week on average).

   In hospice: Time frames may be more difficult to project in hospice because of lengthy or extended visits. The initial visit to hospice may take more than 1 visit and may be over 2 hours. Hospice nurses may make only three to four visits a day, depending on the patient/family needs and status. Although there may be productivity standards, the hospice nurse stays and visits as long as reasonably needed to meet patient/family needs.

Not only is there much information to provide on admission; it must be provided in a sensitive manner with the patient and family usually setting the pace. Some hospices have both a nurse and a social worker admit the patient for the first or initial admitting visit. If the hospice is Medicare certified and the patient is admitted under the hospice benefit, the rules must be explained, multiple forms, such as a hospice consent, must be signed, and clinical and physical assessment data must be gathered. All this is labor intensive. It is only with experience that admission and subsequent visits become more efficient and effective.

MEDICARE HOSPICE 101

Many insurers now cover or reimburse hospice programs for hospice services. How hospice services are defined may vary, as may the specific coverage and documentation requirements. Medicare has a Medicare hospice benefit (MHB), which many state Medicaid programs mirror. The hospice nurse is often the expert on communicating coverage and other information to patients and families in the advocacy role. It is for this reason that hospice nurses should know the fundamentals of the Medicare hospice program.

Congress enacted the benefit in 1983 and made it a permanent program in 1986. The following five requirements must be met for a patient to be eligible for the hospice Medicare benefit.

1. The patient is eligible for Medicare Hospital Insurance (Part A)
2. The patient is certified by an attending physician and the hospice medical director to have a limited life expectancy with a poor prognosis (usually 6 months or less if the disease runs its expected course)
3. The patient resides in a geographic area where there is a Medicare-certified hospice program
4. A written plan of care is established and regularly reviewed
5. The patient elects the hospice Medicare benefit.

Simply put, the patient who elects the hospice benefit "gives up," or "waives," regular Medicare benefits for the admitting disease or diagnosis. This is usually not a problem unless the patient wants more care than can be delivered through hospice. Patients who elect the benefit receive palliative and noncurative care and support for certain benefit periods. These periods are for two initial 90-day benefit periods, followed by an unlimited number of subsequent 60-day periods. The benefit periods may be used consecutively or at intervals. Regardless of whether patients use the benefit periods consecutively or at different times, they must be certified each time

Figure 1-9 Hospice benefit certification form. (Courtesy Briggs Corporation, Des Moines, Ia.)

(by the physician) as terminally ill. Patients can "revoke" the benefit should they wish to withdraw from the hospice program and revert to standard Medicare coverage. A hospice benefit certification form and revocation form are presented in Figures 1-9 and 1-10. Note that if a patient revokes in the middle of a benefit period, the remaining days in that benefit period are lost. In addition, some of the requirements of regular Medicare home care are waived for these patients. For example, the patient does not have to be homebound or meet skilled care requirements as skilled care is defined in the Medicare home health benefit.

HOSPICE MEDICARE
BENEFIT REVOCATION

STATEMENT OF REVOCATION

Effective ___/___/___, I, _____, choose to revoke
　　　　　Date of Revocation　　　　　　　Patient's Name

election for Medicare coverage under the Hospice Medicare Benefit.

1. I understand that I am revoking Hospice Medicare Benefit for the remainder of the current benefit period.

2. I understand that if I am in the first, second or subsequent benefit periods, as listed below, I can at any time in the future elect Hospice Medicare coverage for the remaining benefit period(s). I am, however, forfeiting Hospice Medicare coverage for the days remaining in the current benefit period.

The benefit periods are as follows:

First Benefit Period — 90 Days
Second Benefit Period — 90 Days
Subsequent Benefit Periods — Unlimited 60 Day Periods

3. I understand that the Medicare health care benefits I waived to receive Hospice Medicare coverage will be resumed after the effective date of this revocation.

Signature of Patient
or Legal Representative _____ Date ___/___/___

Signature of Witness _____ Date ___/___/___

Signature of Witness _____ Date ___/___/___

PART I — Clinical Record	PART 2 — Physician	PART 3 — Patient/Representative
PATIENT NAME—Last, First, Middle Initial		ID#

Form 3456/3P   © 1995 Briggs Corporation, Des Moines, IA 50306   HOSPICE MEDICARE BENEFIT REVOCATION
R196   To order, phone 1-800-247-2343   PRINTED IN U.S.A.

Figure 1-10 Hospice Medicare benefit revocation form. (Courtesy Briggs Corporation, Des Moines, Ia.)

The strength of the Medicare hospice program is that it is a comprehensive managed care program where all services and care are coordinated through one entity—the hospice organization. Coverage for services related to the terminal illness generally includes physician services, nursing care, medical supplies and equipment, short-term inpatient care (including respite care), home health aide services, physical therapy, speech-language pathology services, and medical social services and counseling, including dietary counseling. Patients have limited cost-sharing for drugs and inpatient respite care. The hospice program is the expert on the rules related to the Medicare hospice program. Although the Medicare hospice program is a needed and viable program for some Medicare beneficiaries seeking hospice, it may not be appropriate for all patients, some of whom may desire curative care or treatment through death.

SKILLS AND KNOWLEDGE NEEDED IN HOSPICE CARE

1. **A knowledge of the core care standards and rules for hospice care**
   These consist of both administrative and clinical information and are important to being an effective hospice nurse. For Medicare-certified hospices or hospices that are also home health agencies (HHAs), knowledge of the following is required:
   • The Medicare Conditions of Participation for hospice (and home care if dually certified)
   • The Hospice Manual provisions about hospice coverage
   • If dually-certified, the section of the home health agency manual that addresses the correct completion of the 485 series and forms
   • The Medicare Hospice Manual.
   Other important core care standards are the National Hospice Organization's (NHO) *Standards of a Hospice Program of Care* and relevant accreditation standards related to hospice, such as those issued by the Joint Commission on Accreditation of Healthcare Organizations (JCAHO).
   Because Medicare sets many standards, it is important to be familiar and up to date with these rules. Some other insurers also use Medicare's criteria for qualifying and/or coverage. In addition, many insurers, such as state Medicaid programs or private insurers, use facsimiles of the HCFA form 485 as the plan of care (POC) and provide hospice services that mirror the Medicare coverage. In hospice the HCFA form 485 is not mandated, but a plan of care is.

2. **A repertoire of service-driven and patient-oriented interpersonal skills**
   Community liaison and public relations activities are a part of the hospice home care clinician's busy day.

3. **The ability to pay incredible attention to detail**
   This is true both in addressing complex patient and family care needs and in documentation. Both are equally important, and they go hand in hand in the provision of high-quality hospice care.

4. **The possession of multifaceted skills accompanied by flexibility**
   It is the hospice clinician who must "bend" or renegotiate to meet patient and family needs and achieve patient-centered outcomes. This flexibility usually includes visiting times and scheduling but can also include aspects that center on accommodating patient and family/caregiver needs.

5. **The possession of a reliable car and safe, effective driving skills**
   The hospice nurse in the community must like, or at least not mind, driving (even in inclement weather), have a good sense of direction (or a map!), and be willing to take risks.

6. **The ability to assume responsibility for the patient and family's care and the patient's POC**

   Holistic care is a reality in quality hospice care. From the initial hospice assessment through the identification of patient and family needs and challenges, the hospice nurse assumes the planning and follow-through for care. Sometimes only a limited number of core hospice team members are involved in the care, depending on the patient and family needs. Because of these factors, the hospice nurse in the community setting can directly affect the care and see the results of that planned and continually evaluated care. Close communication is required between the hospice nurse and the other team members and any case managers involved with the care. This patient-management function, with its associated prioritizing and sometimes complex decision making, makes hospice practice unique. It is from this aspect that hospice team members often receive personal satisfaction and positive feedback from patients and their families, friends, and caregivers.

7. **Strong clinical skills and the ability to function as both a specialist and a generalist nurse**

   Hospice patients may be of all age groups, from infants to the elderly. In addition, the diagnoses and care needs of patients may vary from day to day. Within the hospice organization, a wide range of clinical problems and nursing diagnoses may exist. Developing an area of expertise and acting as a resource for nurses new to hospice care are important assets for the individual clinician or manager's own professional growth.

8. **Self-direction and the ability to function autonomously in a nonstructured atmosphere**

   Self direction means having well-developed and effective time-management skills to address the many aspects of care, including visits scheduled, documentation, and detail-oriented administrative duties (e.g., completing and updating plans of care, returning phone calls).

9. **The desire to continue learning and being open to new information and clinical skills**

   This is particularly important given the many new kinds of technologies being used in the home setting. Dobutamine management, new pain- and symptom-management methods, and ethical dilemmas are just some of the care problems competent clinicians and managers address daily. For this reason, "resources for care and practice" are listed in each care guideline, and journal articles, books, and other resources that may assist in lifelong education are listed in Part 6.

10. **A sincere appreciation of people**

    This includes interacting positively with and being empathetic to all patients, families, and caregivers, who are often in the midst of crises. Because many family caregivers continue to work outside the home, hospice team members use their observation, assessment, teaching, and training skills to maintain patients safely in the home. This teaching or consulting role brings job satisfaction as well as comfort and security to the families.

11. **The ability to be open and sincerely accepting of people's unique and chosen lifestyles and of the effects that these lifestyles have on their health**
    Being accepting is easier said than done! We have all cared for patients with end-stage COPD who continue to smoke two to three packs a day and do not adhere to the safety instructions they have been taught regarding oxygen. These ethical dilemmas of safety versus self-determination are a part of professional hospice home care practice.

12. **The awareness and acceptance that a constant balance must be maintained between clinical and administrative demands**
    In addition, the clinician must know that both demands are equally important, but in different ways and for different reasons.

13. **The knowledge that change can be difficult**
    The hospice home care culture is very different from the "down the hall" camaraderie, supervision, and peer consultation available in the inpatient hospice setting.

14. **The possession of a kind sense of humor that can help patients, families, and peers get through the rough times**
    This sense of humor is finally being recognized for its healing power when used appropriately.

15. **Knowledge of the economics of health care and the larger environment that is affecting home care and hospice specifically**
    A basic knowledge of reimbursement, including differences among payer sources, utilization, and payment mechanisms and what this means to hospice patients and their families, is very useful in the nurse's role as admission and insurance specialist on the initial visits.

16. **Time-management skills to be able to prioritize and manage diverse and sometimes equally important tasks and responsibilities**
    The best nurses and other clinicians in hospice home care are very well organized and use their organizational skills in their daily routines. They create and keep detailed schedules, document at the patient's home (unless there are safety concerns), and generally seek to do things right the first time. Day scheduling calendars, cellular phones, voice mail, and other technological tools also assist in these important endeavors.

17. **The practical wisdom hospice care and practice**
    Practical wisdom is information that comes with reading and practice. It may be called "the best way to do things." Much of this knowledge base comes from watching and learning from experienced hospice nurses. It includes such practical tips as always having two supplies with you (the Noah's Ark approach) because the time you don't will be the time you'll need that second catheter or other item. Other areas where experience helps include organizing paperwork, setting up your schedule, and tracking physician orders. Try also to remember what it felt like to be a new nurse, and try to impart to others the information you needed then and have now.

THE HOSPICE ORIENTATION

All new hospice team members need an appropriate orientation period. A high-quality orientation is important to being successful and feeling comfortable in the hospice team member role. No matter how understaffed the program may be, prospective team members should, when possible, try to define or address their orientation (including time span and content) before accepting the position. The following list addresses some of the information that an orientation should include. Obviously, if the clinician or manager has been in hospice home care for some time, it may not be appropriate or necessary to review all this information; however, it is important that all team members have an understanding of these hallmarks of hospice.

- The organization's orientation manual
- The Medicare Conditions of Participation (COPs) for Hospice (and/or Home Care if the organization is a dually Medicare-certified program)
- The schedule of hospice team and staff support meetings
- The Medicare hospice and/or HHA manual (the coverage of services sections) if the organization provides hospice services as a Medicare-certified hospice and/or HHA
- The hospice clinical and administrative policy and procedure manual(s)
- An overview of the organization's clinical records, documentation system, and required forms, including where the paperwork goes and when it must be completed and submitted
- Guidelines for hospice home visits and what they entail including verbal orders, the referral process, and scheduling
- The opportunity to "buddy" with an experienced hospice clinician from the organization
- The hospice's required forms
- Hospice coverage and documentation requirements, including confidentiality and the timeliness of physician orders
- Administrative details and processes (e.g., payroll, on-call scheduling, mileage reports)
- Equipment and supply acquisition (e.g., venipuncture supplies, personal protective equipment [PPE], lab forms, and drop-off locations)
- The specific automated clinical documentation system, where applicable
- Performance improvement (PI) activities and processes and the clinician's role in identifying and reporting information (e.g., patient infection, falls, missed visits, adverse drug reactions)
- Benefits, employee handbook, mileage, on-call process and pay, lab pickup schedules, and other miscellaneous information unique to the program
- Occupational Safety and Health Administration (OSHA) requirements, including (1) hepatitis B virus vaccination, (2) the HHA-related policies and supplies for bloodborne pathogens and tuberculosis, (3) standard precautions supplies with appropriate barriers and related disposal of supplies, and (4) record-keeping activities
- Completion of a skills checklist or proficiency testing and ongoing educational plan
- Information related to compliance with laws and regulations (e.g., home health aide supervisory visit frequency, timeliness for obtaining physician orders)
- Pain- and symptom-management skills

- On-call strategies and skills
- The roles of the other team members of the hospice IDG

A more in-depth narrative discussion about hospice orientation follows.

HOSPICE ORIENTATION CONSIDERATIONS

Hospice orientation varies in scope, depth, and time span, depending on the organization. Remember that you are not alone in making the transition to a new area of care or practice and that orientation and education continue long after the formal orientation period. In fact, the best hospice clinicians and managers truly make learning a lifelong endeavor. There is always more to know!

Everyone knows how exciting and difficult it can be to leave what is known and familiar and move on to learn new skills in a foreign environment. The challenge is well worth the work. *It goes without saying that no nurse new to home care or hospice should care for patients without an effective orientation.* The *Webster's Collegiate Dictionary* definition of *orient* is "to acquaint with the existing situation or environment." The American Nurses Association (ANA) defines *orientation* as "the means by which new staff members are introduced to the philosophy, goals, policies, procedures, role expectation, physical facilities and special services in a specific work setting." The information in this section provides a framework for review and reference during this transition.

Orientation is perhaps the most important period in the role transformation to hospice nurse, and the initial information presented may set the stage for future growth and professional development. The orientation period is the time designated for honing clinical skills, taking the time to find answers, and developing new relationships with peers and managers. It has been said that excellence "is in the details," and this is very true in hospice care. During orientation, information will be provided about documentation, detailed assessments, thoughtful data analysis, and the importance of clear communications to other hospice team members. These are the kinds of details that contribute to effective and quality hospice care. Perhaps most important, orientation is the time to be detail oriented and acquire the knowledge that constitutes the "practical wisdom" of hospice.

DEFINING THE HOSPICE ORIENTATION

Many important aspects of hospice care must be covered in the limited "official" orientation period. Overall behavioral outcomes or goals for the transitioning clinician include:

- Completing the orientation within the time allocated
- Identifying key staff members and customers (defined by the organization)
- Describing and explaining new patient assignment processes
- Demonstrating clinical competence in the home hospice setting
- Adhering to policies and procedures as observed/monitored
- Knowing where to go for questions or challenges related to practice and operations
- Other goals defined as policies and procedures by the individual hospice organization

COMPETENCY ASSESSMENT AND VALIDATION

Nurses new to hospice can expect their new or existing employer to check their references and request completion of a self-assessment tool or checklist. These checklists identify specific skills or areas of knowledge and education, including areas where the nurse may need to review or be observed. They are also a way to validate competency, which is a hallmark of quality in hospice practice. The process of identifying educational and orientation needs is a way for the organization to ensure competency by hiring qualified team members.

It is important to note that some organizations identify their own list of high-risk, low-volume skills and may have all nurses demonstrate competency in these skills. Examples include tracheostomy care and specialty assessments. A preceptor may accompany the new nurse in the field to observe certain skills and thereby ensure safe and effective patient care and standardization of care and care processes among team members and across the organization.

ORGANIZATIONAL ORIENTATION TOPICS

The topics that may be addressed by the organization's orientation program cover a broad range of content. The information under these topics is prioritized in this section to emphasize the regulatory aspects interfacing with clinical patient care that must be understood to function safely in hospice. This section then lists topics and areas that should be addressed for quality, safety, practice, and accreditation reasons.

Although this looks like a voluminous amount of information, it all will make sense over the months to come (see Box 1-2 for orientation tips). In fact, colleagues who have successfully made the transition are likely to say that "about 6 months into this, it all came together and made sense." This information is presented in a functional format to make sense to nurses making this important transition. There are numerous policies in hospice, but those listed below and their associated processes/outcomes provide a practical overview of the hospice nursing specialty. This list is by no means all-inclusive but identifies those areas with the most direct impact on hospice clinicians.

Orientation may include, in addition to nurses, other new hospice team members, such as therapists, social workers, pharmacists, spiritual counselors, volunteers, home health aides or certified nursing assistants, intake coordinators, and clinical managers or educators. This is a great way to meet new colleagues and team members in a new hospice organization. From the beginning, you will see that the best hospice care is truly a team effort and that "everyone works from the same page."

As health care moves to the standardization of care and care processes for quality purposes, much of the same information must be provided to all the team members. Some organizations provide an orientation that is standardized for all new employees at the beginning and then, as the information becomes more specific, such as for nursing, the orientation continues with only the nurses.

1. **Mission, vision, values, philosophy**
   Hospice organizations have their own unique mission. Simply put, the mission is the bottom line of what the organization does and why it exists. The

---

BOX 1-2

ABSORBING IT ALL
Five Tips for Orientees

1. Complete assessment (or weekly evaluation forms, etc.) questions completely and accurately. This assists you and your manager/instructor/preceptor in goal revision.
2. Take notes. Orientation presents voluminous and important information, and it is sometimes difficult at the beginning to see the bigger picture. These notes can refresh your memory.
3. Ask questions. Others may have the same questions and not ask them. As well as addressing any confusing issues, your questions may inspire additional explanations that will help you remember certain information.
4. Listen actively. The depth and breadth of information demand this level of participation.
5. Provide feedback at the conclusion or after a defined time period. When the evaluation process occurs, complete evaluation forms and provide comments to assist the organization in its ongoing efforts to improve the orientation program and related processes.

Reprinted with permission, Marrelli and Associates, Inc. (Modified from *Home Care Nurse News* 3[8], 1996.)

mission statement can be one sentence or a few sentences long if it articulates the vision and values to which the organization ascribes. Examples of mission statements include the following: "XYZ Hospice provides the best palliative care with the most competent staff"; "St. Elsewhere Home Care follows the mission of St. Elsewhere Hospital into the community, where we provide comprehensive and high-quality health care services, including hospice, in the community."

Process/outcome: The orientee may receive a copy of the mission statement in the orientation packet with the history of the hospice organization. Sometimes the mission statement is written on the back or front of the identification/name badge, on business cards and letterhead of the organization, or on the agency's brochures. All team members in hospice must work together, and the mission can help in this quest. The new orientee should be able to restate the hospice mission statement and goals on completion of the orientation.

2. **Hospice brochure**
   The organization's brochure contains important information about the services provided. This is the information shared with patients, discharge planners, and other customers who may be interested in hospice services. This brochure indicates whether the organization is state licensed or Medicare-certified and/or accredited; how patients reach the organization; the on-call system and how to access care after regular business hours; the specific services their organization provides through its program; and any specialty programs or other information. Usually the brochure is provided during or before the application process. However, it may be given during the formal orientation as part of the packet

of materials for new team members. The geographical areas covered by the hospice also may be listed in the brochure or provided as a policy.

Process/outcome: This information is also provided initially and is explained by the nurse during the admitting visit and reinforced on subsequent visits. The new orientee should be able to list and describe the services and other information in the brochure about the hospice organization.

3. **Organizational chart**

The new employee's position in relation to the hospice organization is very important for reporting, operational, and communication reasons. The organizational chart or table of organization clearly shows the lines of communications and the manager to whom the new hospice team member will report. Keep in mind that in some larger hospice organizations, new nurses may spend more time with the preceptor or instructor than with their immediate supervisor, particularly during orientation, depending on the size and organizational structure of the hospice.

Process/outcome: The hospice nurse or other new team member in orientation should be able to identify managers, peer interdisciplinary patient care providers, and organizational operations.

4. **Office information**

Office information includes the business hours of hospice operations (i.e., when the office is open), time card and payroll processes, beeper or pager acquisition, car phone and/or allowance, equipment and supply closet/acquisition process, mileage reimbursement, nurse bag signout or purchase procedure, schedule of staff meetings, and other processes and details.

Process/outcome: The new team member should be able to obtain needed supplies or equipment for hospice patients and families using the standard process provided in the orientation and should know whom to call with a question or for assistance related to these important processes.

5. **Personnel or human resource (HR) information**

The personnel staff can be very important to making a successful transition. Physical exams, any required lab tests, TB testing, hepatitis B vaccine acceptance or declination statement, benefit information, CPR certification, license verification, professional liability policy, dress code, safety training, standards of conduct, the organizational grievance process, and other areas may all be under the purview of human resources (HR). HR may also request background checks, car insurance, and a valid driver's license. Many of these requirements are based on compliance requirements under individual state laws, organizational policies, and others (e.g., CDC, OSHA).

6. **Position description**

Orientees usually receive and may sign a copy of their position description and contract, if applicable.

Process/outcome: An evaluation tool may be included with or as a part of the position description for the hospice team members at the organization. The new team member should identify the values of the organization and work toward achieving high scores on the behaviors and skills listed on the performance appraisal tool.

7. **Important policies and procedures**
   The orientee will review and may be asked to sign numerous but important policies and procedures. In addition, the new hospice clinician may be given an orientation manual that contains the specific applicable clinical and administrative policies. It is very important that the new orientee thoroughly review this information and demonstrate an ability to describe and adhere to these policies from accreditation, state survey, and risk management perspectives. Some of these policies follow.

• *Patient Rights and Responsibilities*
   The Patient Rights and Responsibilities policy is listed first because it is an important requirement of the Medicare Conditions of Participation (COPs). This information is usually explained to the patient and family or other responsible person and read aloud if the patient needs assistance or has visual problems. This policy provides the patient and family with written notice of the patient's rights.
   An example of a patient rights and responsibility form is found in Figure 1-11. The five components of the bill of rights that may be the most important are as follows: (1) the patient and family are given a signed copy of their notice of rights; (2) the rights explain the respect that the organization will have for patients, their belongings, and their property; (3) patients should be notified of their right to confidentiality of medical record information, a policy that is upheld by hospice team members; (4) patients must be kept apprised of financial arrangements related to care and coverage, and changes must be communicated to patients per the rights and responsibility document; and (5) if the hospice is home health agency based, patients and caregivers must be made aware of the home health hotline, a 1-800 phone number in each state that patients can use for complaints related to home care and/or advance directives and for questions about local home health agencies.
   Process/outcome: The intent of this process is to ensure that at all times patients understand their rights and team members respect patient choices and decisions. Attitude is essential. Nurses must know that they enter the home as guests, with services to offer that patients are free to accept or reject. The nurse should be able to describe the intent and the process at the hospice organization for explaining patient rights and responsibilities.

• *Patient consent for hospice care*
   A written consent must be obtained for patients admitted to hospice. It is very important that the patient and family understand hospice, including the intent of the services, the hours of care available (as opposed to regular organizational office hours), and the roles of the hospice in the care of the patient and family. An example of a patient consent for care form is given in Figure 1-12.
   Process/outcome: The information on the consent form should be reviewed with the patient or family before the provision of hospice care, the form should be signed by the hospice patient, and the patient or the patient's representative should be given a copy.

• *Infection Control*
   There are very specific infection control processes unique to caring for patients in the home environment. The Occupational Safety and Health Admin-

**HOME CARE PATIENT/CLIENT
RIGHTS AND RESPONSIBILITIES**

As a home care patient/client, you have the right to be informed of your rights and responsibilities before the initiation of care/service. If/When a patient/client has been judged incompetent, the patient's/client's family or guardian may exercise these rights as described below. As they relate to:

PATIENT/CLIENT RIGHTS, you have the right:

1. To receive services appropriate to your needs and expect the home care organization to provide safe, professional care at the level of intensity needed, without unlawful restriction by reason of age, sex, race, creed, color, national origin, religion or disability.
2. To have access to necessary professional services 24 hours a day, 7 days a week.
3. To be informed of services available.
4. To be informed of the ownership and control of the organization.
5. To be told on request if the organization's liability insurance will cover injuries to employees when they are in your home, and if it will cover theft or property damage that occurs while you are being treated.

PATIENT/CLIENT CARE, you have the right:

1. To be involved in your care planning, including education of the same, from admission to discharge, and to be informed in a reasonable time of anticipated termination and/or transfer of service.
2. To receive reasonable continuity of care.
3. To be informed of your rights and responsibilities in advance concerning care and treatment you will receive, including any changes, the frequency of care/service and by whom (disciplines) services will be provided.
4. To be informed of the nature and purpose of any technical procedure that will be performed, including information about the potential benefits and burdens as well as who will perform the procedure.
5. To receive care/service from staff who are qualified through education and/or experience to carry out the duties for which they are assigned.
6. To be referred to other agencies and/or organizations when appropriate and be informed of any financial benefit to the referring agency.

RESPECT AND CONFIDENTIALITY, you have the right:

1. To be treated with consideration, respect, and dignity, including the provision of privacy during care.
2. To have your property treated with respect.
3. To have staff communicate in a language or form you can reasonably be expected to understand and when possible, the organization assists with or may provide special devices, interpreters, or other aids to facilitate communication.
4. To maintain confidentiality of your clinical records in accordance with legal requirements and to anticipate the organization will release information only with your authorization or as required by law.
5. To be informed of the organization's policies and procedures for disclosure of your clinical record.

FINANCIAL ASPECTS OF CARE, you have the right:

1. To be informed of the extent to which payment for the home care services may be expected from Medicare, Medicaid or any other payer.
2. To be informed of charges not covered by Medicare and/or responsibility for any payment(s) that you may have to make.
3. To receive this information orally and in writing before care is initiated and within 30 calendar days of the date the organization becomes aware of any changes.

Form 3531 © 1994 Briggs Corporation, Des Moines, IA 50306
To order, phone 1-800-247-2343 PRINTED IN U.S.A.

RIGHTS AND RESPONSIBILITIES
Continued on Reverse

Figure 1-11 Example of a patient rights and responsibilities form. (Courtesy Briggs Corporation, Des Moines, Ia.) *Continued*

istration (OSHA) is the government department responsible for defining occupational safety for workers. Universal/standard precautions are the method used for infection control, and these protection and prevention guidelines related to bloodborne pathogens are also outlined by OSHA. Various policies addressing the identification, handling, and disposal of biohazardous wastes in the home setting will be provided to new clinicians. Other policies and activities are education related to infections, sharps disposal, prevention, reporting, identification and tracking of infections in hospice patients, a tuberculosis exposure control plan, disinfection of supplies, and other aspects of infection control.

SELF-DETERMINATION, you have the right:

1. To refuse all or part of your care/treatment to the extent permitted by law and to be informed of the expected consequences of said action.
2. To be informed in writing of rights under state law to formulate advance directives.
3. To have the organization comply with advance directives as permitted by state law and state requirements.
4. To be informed of the organization's policies and procedures for implementing advance directives.
5. To receive care whether or not you have an advance directive(s) in place, as well as not to be discriminated against whether or not you have executed an advance directive(s).
6. To be informed regarding the organization's policies for withholding of resuscitative services and the withdrawal of life-sustaining treatment, as appropriate.
7. To not participate in research or not receive experimental treatment unless you give documented, voluntary informed consent.
8. To be informed of what to do in an emergency.
9. To participate in consideration of ethical issues that may arise in your care.

COMPLAINTS, you have the right:

1. To voice complaints/grievances about treatment or care that is (or fails to be) furnished, or regarding lack of respect for property without reprisal or discrimination for same and be informed of the procedure to voice complaints/grievances with the home care organization. Complaints or questions

   may be registered with _____
   Define individual(s)
   by phone, in person or in writing. The address and phone are _____

   _____.

   The organization investigates the complaint and resolution of same.

2. To be informed of the State Hotline. The _____ also has a State Hotline for complaints
   Define entity

   or questions about local home care agencies as well as to voice concerns regarding advance directives.

   The State Hotline number is **1-800-**_____

   and the days/hours of operation are _____

   _____

PATIENT/CLIENT RESPONSIBILITIES

As a home care patient/client, you have the responsibility:

1. To provide complete and accurate information about illness, hospitalizations, medications, and other matters pertinent to your health; any changes in address, phone or insurance/payment information; and changes made to advance directives.
2. To inform the organization when you will not be able to keep your home care appointment.
3. To treat the staff with respect.
4. To participate in and follow your plan of care.
5. To provide a safe environment for care to be given.
6. To cooperate with staff and ask questions if you do not understand instruction or information given to you.
7. To assist the organization with billing and/or payment issues to help with processing third party payment.
8. To inform the organization of any problems or dissatisfaction with services.

RIGHTS AND RESPONSIBILITIES

Figure 1-11 cont'd, For legend see previous page.

Process/outcome: The organization should have proper personal protective equipment (PPE) available to hospice team members. This equipment includes disposable latex gloves, masks, aprons, goggles, and other coverings; mouthpieces for CPR; and other equipment as necessary. CPR masks should be kept on the nurse's person (e.g., not in the car parked in front of the patient's home). Infection control related to the home visit bag and equipment must be maintained. The contents and equipment must be protected from contamination, particularly because they can be sources of cross-contamination. The organizational policies related to the cleaning of

PATIENT CONSENT FOR CARE

I, _____, hereby consent to admission to and care by
                     Patient's Name
_____ Hospice. I understand that:

1. Hospice's goal is not to cure my terminal illness. The goal of hospice is to maintain quality of life through the management of pain and other symptoms when no further curative measures are planned. Hospice staff will also provide emotional and spiritual support (when requested) to me and my family and/or primary caregiver.

2. _____ will be considered my
                                    Name
"primary care person." This means he/she will be the person mainly responsible for overseeing my care at home.

3. Hospice services are provided by a team of staff specially trained in hospice care. Services may include medical, nursing, social work, homemaker/health aide, dietary, pastoral/ spiritual and volunteer. The role of each hospice team member has been explained to me.

4. Care will be provided by scheduled appointment, but assistance is available 24 hours a day, 7 days a week. I can reach Hospice by calling (_____)_____.

5. While I am enrolled in this hospice program, a hospice team of caregivers will manage my care whether I'm being cared for in my home or in a hospital or nursing home.

6. The hospice medical record will contain information about me, my family and/or my primary care person. Every effort will be made to keep this information confidential. However, I authorize the organization to disclose and release information contained in my clinical record to the health care providers involved in my care, third party payers, utilization review and professional standard review organizations, regulatory review entities and any other organizations, companies, community resources, etc. that may/will assist me to meet my hospice care and/or health needs. Information about me will be exchanged with my family.

7. This consent may be withdrawn at any time.

8. Hospice does not take the place of the caregiver, but rather, supports the caregiver.

In summary, I have been advised of my rights and responsibilities. All services have been explained to me and I have had ample opportunity to ask questions.

Signature of Patient
or Legal Representative _____ Date ____/____/____

Signature of Witness _____ Date ____/____/____

PART 1 — Clinical Record   PART 2 — Patient/Family

PATIENT NAME–Last, First, Middle Initial   ID#

Form 3460/2P © 1995 Briggs Corporation, Des Moines, IA 50306
To order, phone 1-800-247-2343   PRINTED IN U.S.A.   PATIENT CONSENT FOR CARE

Figure 1-12 Patient consent for care form. (Courtesy Briggs Corporation, Des Moines, Ia.)

supplies and the frequency of these cleanings should be reviewed. Some organizations have designated "bag check" days when an inventory of the contents is made and the process for retrieval and storage of equipment is reviewed.

Effective and regular handwashing is critical to the provision of high-quality care. Organizations provide paper towels and soap or alcohol-based soap ("waterless wash"). Team members should use the paper towels instead of the patient's cloth towels (unless they are known to be clean) and liquid soap instead of the bar of soap in the patient's home. Infection control and adherence to related policies are standards heavily weighted by accreditation surveyors as well as important indicators of quality. On completion of the orientation the orientee should be able to describe infection control practices as specified by the hospice (Box 1-3) and verbalize and correctly demonstrate bag technique.

- *Self-Determination/Advance Directives*
  The Federal Patient Self-Determination Act of 1990 was designed to enable patients to decide in advance what health care decisions are to be made should the patient lose the capacity to do so. A goal of hospice is that the patient's self-determined choices be upheld and implemented in the framework of quality care. All Medicare-participating entities, such as hospices and home care agencies (HHAs), must comply with the advance directive provisions of the OBRA law. This policy is usually distributed to new team members during orientation.

  Most hospices have the admitting nurse or other hospice team member provide this information to the patient. The law requires that the hospice or HHA inform patients in writing of its policies regarding the implementation of advance directives and educate staff and the community on issues concerning advance directives.

  Process/outcome: Many times, patients who have come out of the hospital are well aware of advance directives and may have thought about and/or discussed them with their family members or physician. The admitting nurse's role is usually to provide an informational flyer identifying resources should the patient wish more information. Upon completion of orientation the nurse orientee should be able to describe the intent of the self-determination law and the hospice team member's role in implementing and complying with this requirement.

- *Community resources*
  A listing of available community resources may be given during orientation. This list should provide linkage to services in the community and may include such educational and/or financial support resources as the local cancer or other societies, community loan closets, and area offices on aging.

  Process/outcome: The hospice nurse in the case manager role coordinates care for the patient across health care settings and notifies patients of services available. Linkage and rapport with available community resources assist in ensuring effective communications and assisting patients and families in accessing needed services. Upon completion the nurse orientee should be able to reference and identify possible resources based on examples or patient cases discussed during orientation.

- *Emergency preparedness*
  The hospice organization should have a process prepared in case an emergency occurs where the normal operations of the organization or office are shut down. Examples include fire, floods, hurricanes, ice storms and blizzards, power outages that affect local phone service, and earthquakes. The process has a plan that is practiced should such a case occur.

BOX 1-3

NINE TIPS FOR INFECTION CONTROL

When the hospice patient is cared for at home, one hallmark of quality care is infection control and related practices. The following nine tips may contribute to improved practice and patient care while supporting accreditation and other standards.

1. Although it is well known that handwashing is the most effective way to prevent the spread of infection, numerous studies show that it is not always performed or is not performed enough.

   Tip: Wash hands, apply clean gloves, provide care, discard gloves, and wash hands. Always wash hands (and change gloves) between patient contact, even between tasks or procedures on the same patient to prevent cross-contamination. If there is no running water or paper towels, use foam or waterless soap/cleansing agents and paper towels from your bag. Do not use bar soap. Do not use the patient's towel unless you know it is clean (e.g., right out of the washer and dryer).

2. Urinary tract, wound, infusion site, or strep infections may appear to be isolated cases until looked at from a trending perspective.

   Tip: Report patient or staff infections to your manager for data collection, analysis, and trending within the organization.

3. The new term from the Centers for Disease Control (CDC) to replace *Universal Precautions* is *Standard Precautions*. This means that every patient cared for is automatically provided with Standard Precautions.

   Tip: Use Standard/Universal Precautions at all times and always carry your personal protective equipment (PPE) in your bag.

4. Equipment may be a source of cross-contamination in households and among patients.

   Tip: Clean thermometers and scissors after each use. When possible, have the patient keep his or her own thermometer and scissors for use in home care. Follow your organization's policies on the cleaning of blood pressure cuffs, stethoscopes, and the nursing bag.

5. Hazardous waste management is an important part of infection control and risk management. The most common and problematic area is needles and other sharps.

   Tip: Never recap needles. Use the biohazardous sharps container provided by the hospice. These containers are usually hard plastic and should be leak resistant and puncture proof for safety. It goes without saying that overfilling these containers is to be avoided.

6. The clinician's bag is an important part of the nurse's equipment and is usually divided into clean and dirty sides for infection control purposes. It may be a challenge to know where to place the bag once inside the home.

   Tip: Try to identify a clean surface in the home for the bag and needed supplies. A barrier should be placed under the bag, such as a chux, a piece of plastic, or a newspaper. If there is no clean spot or there are many roaches or other obvious infestations, the bag may be hung on a doorknob or only what is needed may be brought into the home in a clean plastic bag.

Continued

BOX 1-3

NINE TIPS FOR INFECTION CONTROL—cont'd

7. There is much discussion in conference rooms and in medical literature about aseptic versus sterile techniques in wound care at home. For this reason specific orders are needed from the physician for the patient's care.

    Tip: Obtain specific orders from the physician about dressing changes, including whether to use sterile or aseptic techniques. Consider speaking with your manager about working with an enterostomal therapist about problematic wounds in hospice patients and possible inservice education about the many options for wound care supplies and products now available.

8. In caring for patients with various cancers and other illnesses necessitating immunosuppression, it is important to be aware of terms such as *pathogens* (i.e., disease-producing microorganisms), *contamination* (i.e., introducing harmful or infectious material), and *cross-contamination* or *cross-infection* (i.e., moving or transferring pathogens from one site or source to another).

    Tip: There is clearly a higher risk of cross-contamination when the infection is especially virulent. There recently has been much information disseminated about infections resistant to certain antibiotics. With this in mind, try to schedule immunosuppressed patient care before visiting and caring for patients with infected or difficult wounds or other sources of known infection.

9. Caring for challenging hospice patients and their families can be difficult on certain days. Infection control is an important component for both patients and clinicians.

    Tip: Take care of yourself by eating properly, exercising regularly, getting plenty of sleep, practicing effective infection control on and off the job, and taking time for yourself to rejuvenate.

Modified from *Home Care Nurse News* 4[5] May 1997.

Process/outcome: Patient care will continue as far as possible, patients will be prioritized based on their needs, and hospice team members will know their roles and activities in the process. Cellular phones, telephone trees for communications, a listing of the patients with an assigned priority number in the on-call book, and mock fire drills or other drills should all be part of an emergency preparedness and safety plan that works should an unforeseen event occur.

Many other policies may be provided to the new hospice nurse for review. Some organizations may also have a scavenger hunt to test team members' ability to locate and identify these policies, procedures, supplies, or equipment.

SAFETY IN HOSPICE

Personal safety is an appropriate concern in community-based practice when making home visits to hospice patients and families. It is particularly important to nurses and other team members entering unfamiliar geographical areas at unusual hours.

BOX 1-4

PERSONAL SAFETY TIPS

When going anywhere for the first time, get specific, detailed, and correct directions to the patient's home and have them validated by the patient or caregiver.

If you are unsure of a neighborhood or have heard about problems, talk with your supervisor, who may contact the local police. The police know the communities and the problems best and can be very helpful in identifying problem areas and working with the care team on solutions.

Organizations may have contracts with security staff. Your supervisor will know of such arrangements and the process for their use.

Know the community. As you are driving, always be aware of your surroundings.

You may want to call patients and families before leaving so they can be watching for you. Ask about parking too.

Lock the car doors and keep any valuables, such as purse, supplies, and any patient information, out of sight.

Wear a seatbelt while driving.

When nearing the home, look for the landmarks described and address numbers on houses.

Keep maps out of sight where possible and try to avoid looking as though you are unfamiliar with the area.

Try to park in well-lit areas and in front of the home or as close as possible. Lock the car and identify your route to the front door.

Be cautious when boarding elevators.

When making evening or night visits, let your family know where you are going and when you expect to return.

When walking to your car, have your keys out, ready to unlock the car. Many of the newer car models have "keyless entry," which works with a computer chip and unlocks the door when the mechanism is pointed toward the car and pressed.

Before getting back in the car, check the back seat and floor areas.

If you feel unsafe, you probably are. Trust your feelings and intuition and call your supervisor from a safe spot.

Speak with your supervisor about your organization's unique policies relating to home visiting safety.

The clinician should review any protocols the hospice organization has related to staff safety and home visits. Organizational procedures such as calling in a schedule to coordinators may assist in staff safety, as may beepers, pagers, and car phones. Some organizations have local law enforcement persons who provide training and education about home visiting and safety. The information shared is valuable to team members both as clinicians and as members of a community.

Personal safety starts with awareness of the surroundings (see Box 1-4 for a list of personal safety tips). Use those well-honed skills of observation and assessment wherever you are!

BOX 1-5

CAR SAFETY TIPS

Car safety is also very important. It begins with a knowledge of the strengths and weaknesses of your car. Successful and safe home visiting team members have good driving records and reliable cars that are usually not gas guzzlers. A small car can make it easier to find a spot on snowy streets or downtown in metropolitan areas. Always make sure you have enough gas. Some hospice nurses make it a habit never to let the gas tank get below one half full. Do not make visits running on empty!

Carry one gallon of water, a blanket, and a first aid kit. A candle in a coffee can can help heat your car in cold weather, but be careful! Lock all car doors when entering or leaving the car.

Store sand, rug mats, or kitty litter in your trunk to assist you out of ice and snow.

If your organization gives you a sign that identifies you as a health care worker, use it per program policies. Sometimes these signs help you obtain and keep a parking spot in front of the hospital or lab.

Consider obtaining gas credit cards and joining an automobile club for assistance in emergencies such as towing, running out of gasoline or fuel, and/or dead batteries.

Take good care of your car, winterize it if you live where the weather is cold, and maintain it well.

Have the oil and fluid levels checked regularly.

Make sure that your spare tire is in good condition and inflated and that you have the tools to change a flat tire.

MAP READING:
UPDATE OF AN IMPORTANT SKILL

A skill needed for all team members making home visits is map reading. Many organizations cover a large and diverse geographical catchment area that may cover urban, suburban, and rural areas. With this in mind, you cannot know every side street or bridge in a given area. Experienced clinicians and managers have found the ability to navigate and read maps sorely tested. In communities where there is rapid growth, sometimes the newer roads and access routes may not even be on the map. For that reason the large county book maps that are updated fairly frequently seem to work well. When taking directions from patients or their family members or caregivers, write down landmarks such as schools, playgrounds, trash dumps, marinas, shopping centers, or other identifying information that will confirm that you are on the right track.

Personal safety is enhanced by the ability to get from one patient and family's home to the next easily (see Box 1-5 for car safety tips). Supervisors or experienced colleagues will know the nuances of any community that can plague a planned day. These include when and where streets are cleaned, making parking almost impossible; snow emergency routes where cars seemingly are towed when the first snowflake falls; or streets that change direction during rush hours to accommodate the traffic so that "you can't get there from here." These challenges can tax the most experienced visiting staff. Be prepared!

SUMMARY

The kinds of patients and families cared for through hospice have grown and changed. Historically hospice has provided care primarily to patients with cancer. Patients and families of patients with Alzheimer's, amyotrophic lateral sclerosis (ALS), and end-stage heart disease and other organ failures are now finding support and care through hospice. All kinds of patients of varying ages and problems who are seeking comfort and care with a limited life expectancy are turning to hospice. Hospice care is limited by the prognosis, not the disease.

The special qualities, skills, and characteristics of caring people go into making up the hospice team. The nurse has the unique role of case manager at many hospices. As such, the nurse coordinates and clarifies the desires of patients and their families or partners. Expertise in symptom control, the desire for continued learning about pain and its relief, flexibility, and a sense of humor are all assets for nurses wishing to make the transition to a practice setting where nurses and other hospice workers make an important difference in care and life through the dying process for patients and their families. Whatever the role of the nurse at an individual hospice, the focus is always centered on the patient and caregiver and their unique, individualized choices and journeys.

Orientation is an important period in a new hospice team member's tenure. It is the time when the organization's standards and other information are provided. Orientation varies among organizations, and the orientation may set the precedent for and establish the value of the care and education that the organization espouses. Everyone comes with different skills and competencies, so orientation is the time to identify areas for improvement and provide needed education and information. Welcome to hospice home care!

REVIEW EXERCISES

1. List six of the services offered by hospices.
2. Describe the basic tenets of hospice.
3. Identify the reason that documentation is an important component in hospice care.
4. List three reasons for the growth in hospice.
5. Define hospice and hospice nursing.
6. Describe the different kinds of hospice organizations.
7. Identify four of the differences between home care and hospice nursing.
8. What is the focus of hospice?
9. Who is the unit of care in hospice?
10. What kinds of patients and families are cared for through hospice?

References

1. National Hospice Organization: *Hospice fact sheet,* Arlington, Va, October 10, 1995, The Organization.
2. Carney K, Burns N: Economics of hospice care, *Oncology Nursing Forum* 18:761-786, 1991.
3. National Hospice Organization: *Standards of a hospice program of care,* Arlington, Va, 1998, The Organization.
4. Hospice and Palliative Nurses Association: *Standards of hospice nursing practice and professional performance,* Pittsburgh, 1995, The Association.

PART TWO

AN OVERVIEW OF HOSPICE DOCUMENTATION

Part 2 seeks to assist both new and experienced hospice nurses in meeting various requirements and documenting the specific information required by any payor, illustrating the patient's condition and responses to interventions, and accurately chronicling the patient's care and course.

HOSPICE DOCUMENTATION

Hospice team members and their clinical practice are described every day to surveyors, peers, and managers through the review of clinical records. Visit records, notes, and other information that appear in the record reflect the standard of hospice and nursing care as well as the particular care provided to a specific patient. Hospice clinicians must be able to integrate knowledge of regulatory criteria, care coordination, and practice into effective documentation that supports coverage while demonstrating quality to any reviewer. Today numerous third-party payors make quality and reimbursement decisions based on the care the patient received as evidenced in the medical record.

The clinician's entries in the patient's clinical record are recognized as a significant contribution that documents the standard of care provided to a patient. As the practice of nursing and hospice has become more complex, so too have the factors that influence documentation. These factors include requirements of regulatory agencies and accreditation bodies (e.g., JCAHO, CHAP, state licensure departments, governmental entities), consumers of health care, and legal entities. Hospice clinicians must try to satisfy these various requirements all at once, often with little time in which to accomplish the important task of documentation. Fortunately, many organizations have integrated these requirements, where possible, into the organization's policy and/or procedure manuals and documentation forms. Nurses must remember that the written clinical record is their best defense against malpractice or negligence litigation.

The increased specialization of practice and the complexity of patient problems contribute to the provision of multiple and varied services to patients. The clinical record is the only source of written communication—and sometimes the only source of any communication—for all team members. The team members not only contribute their unique and individual assessment findings, interventions, and outcomes, but also may actually base their subsequent actions on the events documented by another hospice team member.

A hospice chart audit tool is a way to assist in evaluation of the overall clinical record (see Figure 2-1). This review may be useful as a way to identify areas that may need improvement, such as care coordination, pain and medication management, and spiritual and psychosocial support.

Why Is the Clinical Record So Important?

The clinical record is a legal document, and it is the only document that chronicles a patient's stay from start of care through discharge. As such, it should be completed as soon as possible per rules, regulations, standards of practice, and organizational policy. This includes beginning and completing the physician's orders, plan of care, or other required forms and the daily visit record or nursing notes as soon as possible. It is recommended that the documentation be completed at the time the care is provided. Many nurses remember performing rounds with

Date of Review _____
Reviewer _____
Team _____

Patient Name _____   Medical Record # _____
SOC Date _____ D/C Date _____
Primary Dx _____   Secondary Dx _____

Hospice Admission and Benefit Election	Yes	No	N/A	Comments (describe any missing components, opportunities for improvement)
Attending MD and medical director certification of terminal condition (certification obtained within state licensure and federal guideline requirements)				
Informed consent for hospice				
Election statement with date				
Evidence that rights and responsibilities were reviewed				
Documentation of terminal diagnosis and prognosis				
Assessment of advance directive (e.g., DNR, Living Will, etc.)				
If patient has advance directive, copy or written documentation of content				
Team Assessments and Care Planning				
Complete nursing assessment, including comprehensive pain and symptom assessment and assessment of HHA need				
Home environment and safety assessment				
Assessment and appropriate ordering of DME				
Assessments comprehensive and timely (evidence of contact within ___ days from SOC)				
Spiritual assessment				
Assessment for volunteer need				

Figure 2-1 Hospice chart audit tool. (Courtesy Anne L. Rooney, RN, MS, MPH.)
Continued

the physician in the inpatient setting, where it would have been unheard of not to complete the documentation as care and plans for care were developed for the patients.

Important facets of hospice documentation include the patient's condition, the status (e.g., psychosocial, spiritual) of the family or other caregivers, the environment of care, a description of the specific care provided, the patient's pain and symptom presentation and associated interventions and evaluations, communications with the physician or other team members, and the observed or verbal patient/family response(s) to interventions and care.

Other assessments when ordered (e.g., dietary, physical therapy, occupational therapy, speech therapy)				
Interdisciplinary team care plan, including clear and measurable goals, signed by MD				
Evidence of patient/family involvement in care planning				
Signed and dated verbal orders when needed for changes in frequencies, medications, treatments, etc.				
Care plan revised when necessary				
Current HHA or HCA plan of care, if applicable				
Do progress notes for all team services reflect implementation of the plan of care as written? Are interventions appropriate to the assessed needs? *Note:* Address visit frequencies, planned follow-up interventions. Note discrepancies under comment section.				
Care Coordination				
Ongoing care conference notes that reflect updates to plan of care				
Progress notes that reflect ongoing interdisciplinary communication				
Communication with the MD for significant changes or concerns				
Evidence that hospice team assumes professional management responsibility for care, regardless of setting				
Evidence of care coordination with other involved organizations (e.g., SNFs, case managers from other agencies)				
Evidence of communication with receiving organization when patient transfers between settings (e.g., transfer summary)				

Figure 2-1 cont'd, For legend see previous page.

Factors Contributing to More Emphasis on Documentation

The following discussion addresses five specific areas that have increased the importance of clinical documentation.

1. **The current economics of our health care system and the emphasis on utilization management**

   Patients continue to be discharged sooner or stay home while they are considerably ill. In response to spiraling health care costs, third-party payers, such as

Pain and Symptom Management and Medication Monitoring				
Current medication profile that matches MD orders *Note:* Check travel chart for current profile				
Allergies noted				
Progress notes that reflect ongoing assessment of pain and other symptoms (e.g., pain scale, usage of breakthrough pain medication, monitoring of bowel status)				
Progress notes that reflect evidence of education on medications, management of side effects, etc.				
Documentation of all medications administered by hospice staff				
Reassessment and Recertification				
Evidence of ongoing interdisciplinary assessments				
Documentation that reflects assessment of continued appropriateness of hospice care (e.g., according to NHO guidelines, especially for noncancer diagnoses)				
Communication with attending MD and medical director before recertification				
Bereavement Care				
Risk assessment completed for at least PCG and other at-risk survivors (e.g., children)				
Bereavement plan of care appropriate to assessed survivor risk and needs				
Documentation of bereavement care as described in bereavement plan of care				
Appropriate intervention when complicated grief identified (e.g., suicidal ideation)				
General Issues				
HHA supervision documented every 2 weeks				

Figure 2-1 cont'd, For legend see p. 51.

government, commercial, and business self-insurers, have increased their scrutiny and control of limited resources. Initially these programs, called *utilization review* or *utilization management,* were influential in decreasing hospital lengths of stay. This review of care then moved into the outpatient, home care, and hospice arenas.

The phrase often heard to describe this phenomenon is "quicker and sicker." In general, the decreased length of hospital stays has increased the acuity levels of patients at home. This often translates into increased care needs, as is evidenced by the increase in the number of visits or hours patients are seen. In addition, some managed-care programs are decreasing their

Documentation legible, dated, authenticated by signatures				
Errors corrected according to policy (e.g., no correction fluid; item should be crossed through with "error" written above)				
Other technical documentation issues				
Revocation form signed and dated, if applicable. Does documentation reflect reason for revocation?				
In reviewer's opinion, were the patient's/family's needs addressed and coordinated?				
In reviewer's opinion, were the utilization of hospice services and level of care appropriate?				
General comments/suggestions				

Figure 2-1 cont'd, For legend see p. 51.

number of home visits while also limiting the patient's inpatient stay, which places stress on team members as they continue to provide needed care and, many times, "negotiate" for the patient so that the appropriate levels of safe, effective care are provided. Third-party payers often need substantiating evidence and documentation clearly showing that appropriate care was provided.

The information in the clinical record is one of the sources with which third-party payers make payment or denial decisions. It is important to note that Medicare, by law, can pay only for covered care. It is primarily the clinical documentation that is the objective basis for payment determinations. These notes reflect the care (admission, visit notes, discharge, and ordered services) provided to hospice patients at home.

2. The emphasis on performance improvement (PI)

As quality initiatives in all health care settings evolve, patient outcomes are being recognized as valid indicators of care. Hospice care is concerned with patients and families having and retaining self-determined courses of care and death with comfort and dignity at home. Clinical documentation is the written record demonstrating the care or nursing process, based on the hospice interdisciplinary plan of care, and movement toward achieving patient-centered, quantifiable goals of care. The nursing and other documentation must reflect the patient's condition and, in essence, paint a clear picture for any reviewer assessing for coverage and quality reasons. Because the reviewer has not seen the patient, it is important to express objectively the way the patient looks throughout the clinical documentation.

The interdisciplinary focus on quality efforts creates an incentive for the entire hospice team to work together to achieve these outcomes for hospice patients and their loved ones. The clinical documentation in the written record demonstrates care coordination, and this collaboration is in the format of IDG or team meetings, conferences, or other team activities and communications.

Performance improvement (PI) is based on data measurement and assessment. PI addresses what is actually done and how well it is accomplished and focuses on the design (or redesign) of processes or functions within the hospice organization. Examples of PI activities include revamping the patient education tools, the documentation system, and the comprehensive orientation program or redesigning the physician order retrieval process to improve the timely returns of hospice physician orders.

3. **The emphasis on standardization of care, policies and procedures, and processes**

   All patients are entitled to a certain level or standard of nursing and hospice care. Operationally this means that regardless of which nurse is assigned, the patient receives the same level of care and the same interventions in the same order as designated by our organizations and managers. This ensures standardization of care and related processes across the organization. This standardization ensures that the same "brand" of hospice care is provided in a community by all team members. In fact, the use of a text such as this by all clinicians in a given organization contributes to standardization of patient care.

   As patients and their families become more proactive consumers in their purchase of health services, patient satisfaction with the care provided becomes key to any organization's reputation and ultimate survival. More patients are demanding care in their own homes. Because of their healing skills and other areas of professional proficiency, hospice nurses are pivotal in fostering patient satisfaction. Further, the role of the nurse as patient advocate, listener, and teacher has become widely accepted in recent years. In general, it also is known that satisfied patients are less likely to sue. A hospice satisfaction questionnaire is provided in Figure 2-2.

4. **The further recognition and empowerment of the nursing profession**

   Although more nurses are in the work force than ever before, qualified professional hospice nurses continue to be needed.

   The nurse's notes can become the factor by which documented quality becomes demonstrated quality. All health care professions, including nursing, have recognized standards of care. As society becomes more litigious, the hospice nurse must become aware of state practice and other accepted standards of care. Standards of care represent the minimum level that any patient can expect in similar circumstances. Other standards include policies and procedures, state or federal regulations, and the published standards of professional nursing organizations. These standards necessitate keeping current with and informed of the standards of practice through affiliation with specialty groups or other professional groups.

   An example of a hospice organization's standards of care is as follows: Every patient and family shall have an assessment that is comprehensive, on a standardized form that is completed in the same way, addresses specific patient needs, is performed by a registered nurse on admission, and is documented in the clinical record by a set time line. Through complete, effective documentation the hospice clinicians demonstrate that the standard of care has been maintained.

HOSPICE SATISFACTION QUESTIONNAIRE

DATE ___/___/___

Thank you for allowing us to provide hospice services to your family. We are interested in your ideas or opinions about our care/services. Please take a moment to answer the following questions. Additional comments are welcome and can be recorded on the back of this form. If you need assistance in completing this form, please feel free to contact our office.

For questions 1 - 10, please circle the appropriate number that best describes your opinion.
1-Strongly Agree 2-Agree 3-Disagree 4-Strongly Disagree 5-No Opinion or Not Applicable

1. We are satisfied with the care provided by the:	
a. Nurse(s)	1 2 3 4 5
b. Physical Therapist/Occupational Therapist	1 2 3 4 5
c. Medical Social Worker	1 2 3 4 5
d. Home Health Aide(s)	1 2 3 4 5
e. Hospice Volunteer	1 2 3 4 5
f. Chaplain	1 2 3 4 5
g. Physician	1 2 3 4 5
2. We were involved in decision-making regarding the plan of care for our family.	1 2 3 4 5
3. Staff treated our family, our home and belongings with respect.	1 2 3 4 5
4. Staff explained care services, rights and responsibilities, and other procedures related to the care provided.	1 2 3 4 5
5. The staff generally arrived as scheduled.	1 2 3 4 5
6. We were able to reach the hospice staff promptly and phone calls were returned.	1 2 3 4 5
7. When we called the hospice, office staff were courteous and available and directed calls correctly.	1 2 3 4 5
8. We would use this hospice again.	1 2 3 4 5
9. We would recommend this hospice to friends and relatives.	1 2 3 4 5

10. Suggestions for improvements/additional comments:

11. What most impressed us about the agency's care/service was:

Thank you for your valuable feedback. This confidential information will be used only in efforts to improve care/service.

Sincerely,

____
Organization Director or Administrator Signature

We ☐ would/☐ would not like to discuss our responses further.

Please return the completed questionnaire in the enclosed, self-addressed, stamped envelope.

_______________________ ___/___/___
Optional Signature of Person Completing Form Date

Form 3471 HOSPICE SATISFACTION QUESTIONNAIRE

Figure 2-2 Hospice satisfaction questionnaire. (Courtesy Briggs Corporation, Des Moines, Ia.)

5. **The emphasis on effectiveness and efficiency in all settings in health care, particularly community-based care**

   As organizations continue to streamline their operations, administrative tasks historically performed by clinicians are being reconsidered for their effectiveness. Repetition or duplication of documentation has been an area of appropriate concern to both nurses and their managers. Some organizations have moved toward automation to help prevent the duplication of much clinical and administrative information needed for effective daily operations. Quality, not quantity, is now emphasized with regard to documentation. Effective documentation may not need to be lengthy or wordy; it needs only to support appropriate and covered care.

All the previously discussed factors have created an environment in which the hospice nurse and other clinicians have increased responsibilities to complete in a shorter time period.

The Importance of the Hospice Record

The importance of documentation in the clinical record relates to the fact that this record has the following characteristics:

• It is the only written source for reference and communication among members of the hospice care team
• It is the primary source (written or verbal) for reference and communication among the members of the hospice team
• It is the text that supports insurance coverage or denial
• It is the evidence of the basis on which patient care decisions were made
• It is the only legal record
• It is the primary foundation for the evaluation of the care provided
• It is the basis for staff education or other study
• It is the objective source for the organization's licensing (where applicable), certification, accreditation, and state surveyor review

The Health Care Financing Administration (HCFA), which manages the Medicare programs, instructs the fiscal intermediaries on the administration of the Medicare hospice program. These instructions have implications for hospice nurses who provide care to patients covered under the Medicare hospice benefit. Regional Home Health Intermediaries (RHHIs) are specialized fiscal intermediaries that have contracts with HCFA to process and make payment determinations on all hospice (and home care) claims from across the country.

The RHHIs can pay only for hospice care under Medicare provisions that are covered by law. They look to the hospice's clinical documentation in the medical record to decide whether to support covered care.

Because of the high volume of claims, the RHHIs cannot look at each hospice claim individually. The RHHIs direct their medical review efforts toward areas and claims where the greatest risk of inappropriate payment exists. This process is called *focused medical review* (FMR). Hospice claims are subject to FMR based on the RHHIs initiatives and findings identified in claims processing. FMR entails the screening of claims with the greatest risk of overutilization of program payment. This happens through database analysis and referrals. In addition, the government, under Operation Restore Trust (ORT) and other initiatives, is increasing its scrutiny of hospice and other Medicare services and claims. Because of this heightened review, it is more important than ever that hospices effectively document and manage clinical records. All government or Medicare reviewers hold Medicare-participating hospice organizations to the Medicare Conditions of Participation (COPs) for hospice.

Documentation: The Key to Coverage, Compliance, and Quality

Documentation is critical to the positive outcome of the FMR process. Paint a picture with your documentation from the onset of care through continuation of hospice services. Distinguish clearly in your documentation between the chronic and termi-

---

BOX 2-1

DOCUMENTATION TIPS

- Write legibly or print neatly. The record must be readable.
- Use permanent ink.
- For every entry identify the time and date; sign the entry and include your title.
- Describe care or interventions provided or mark appropriate box on flow sheet and the patient's response to care.
- Write objectively when describing findings (e.g., behaviors).
- Document in consecutive and chronological order with no skipped areas.
- Document or data-enter information either at the patient's home (if safe and appropriate) or as soon as possible after care is provided.
- Be factual and specific.
- Use patient, family, or caregiver quotes.
- Use the patient's name (e.g., "Mr. Smith").
- Document patient complaints or needs and their resolutions. (Remember to discuss the complaint with your manager, who may also document it in the complaint log and note the resolution or follow-up actions taken and any trends.)
- Make sure the patient's name is listed correctly on the visit record, daily note, or other form.
- Be accurate, complete, and thorough.
- Write out what you are saying if anything is questionable. (Avoid potentially confusing abbreviations.)
- Chart only the care that you provided.
- Promptly document any change in the patient's condition and the actions taken based on such a change.
- Document the patient's, family's, or caregiver's response to teaching or any other care intervention.
- To correct an error: (1) draw a line through the erroneous entry, (2) briefly describe the error (e.g., wrong date, spilled coffee on visit record), and (3) add your signature, the date, and the time (or as per organizational policy).

Try to Avoid the Following:
- Relying on memory.
- Whiting out or erasing any entries; such changes may appear to be an attempt to cover up incriminating entries.
- Crossing out words beyond recognition.
- Making assumptions, drawing conclusions, and blaming.
- Leaving blank spaces between entries and your signature.
- Waiting too long to record entries.
- Leaving gaps in documentation.
- Using abbreviations except where they are clear and appear on the organization's list of approved, acceptable abbreviations.

nal phases of a disease, especially if it is long and chronic in nature. Specify any patient periods of exacerbation, stabilization, and further deterioration. Document the
way treatments and medication play a palliative role in the POC. Remember that
notes from all caregivers are usually reviewed in FMR and documentation in all
notes should complete the picture of the terminally ill patient. Remember that what
is "normal" and "stable" to a hospice nurse or other team member may still indicate
a clearly terminal patient if the details are provided in the documentation. Avoid gen-
eralizations such as "no change" or "as tolerated"; the payors need to pay for covered care and the nurse's documentation plays an important role.

Because home care and hospice nurses often need to meet these documentation
requirements simultaneously, they are appropriately concerned about their ability to
do so. Clinicians in practice today can meet these needs and produce clear, effective
documentation. The tips in Box 2-1 can assist in this goal.

HOSPICE DOCUMENTATION 101

Medicare, like any medical insurance program, has both covered services and exclusions. For payers, documentation is the only paper trail of the care provided and the
patient's response to that care.

To qualify for the Medicare hospice benefit, a patient must have Medicare and
be terminally ill, the physician must certify that the patient is terminally ill, the
patient must choose to receive hospice care instead of the standard Medicare
benefits for the illness, and the care must be provided by a Medicare-participating
hospice program.

For documentation purposes the patient is considered terminally ill under the
Medicare guidelines if one of the following conditions applies:

- The medical documentation meets the criteria in the National Hospice Organization (NHO) prognosticating guidelines and supports that the patient is terminally ill (i.e., there is no conflicting or inconsistent information in the record
  to suggest that the patient is not terminally ill even though the guidelines are
  met).
- The medical documentation in the record supports that the patient is terminally ill even though criteria in the NHO guidelines are not met or the patient's condition is not covered by the NHO guidelines.
- The patient dies from the illness for which he or she elected the hospice
  benefit.
- Medical documentation is insufficient to make a decision, but the hospice
  medical director or attending physician provides clinical documentation to
  support the certification of terminal illness. The documentation should be clear
  and in the records.

Documentation may include results of tests or narrative descriptions of the clinical
indicators or progression of disease.

The patient must have a prognosis of 6 months or less for most hospice
programs, including those under Medicare. If on admission the family member
states, "Grandma's been like this for 3 years," the nurse must identify the changes
that now make this patient appropriate for hospice. Remember that the recertifi-
cation process confirms the patient's projected length of care or time limits related
to the prognosis.

Always try to review the documentation objectively after completion. Remember that the clinical documentation and the record must support that the patient under care has an illness of a terminal nature and the progress and other notes must describe the condition.

The RHHIs, when reviewing Medicare hospice claims, look to the following items, at a minimum, to support covered hospice services:

- Hospice admission history and physical (including the assessment)
- Election form with designated effective date
- Certification of the terminal illness with clinical indicator(s) supporting justification
- Visit, prognosis, and other notes describing the patient's condition
- Recertification(s)

Some hospice organizations also provide a written summary that shows the hospice benefit is appropriate for the patient's condition. *Remember that by law the RHHIs can pay only for covered care and the documentation is the source that supports the covered hospice care.* When summaries are written, the following may be included:

- Patient diagnoses, including any illness affecting the terminal diagnoses
- Any co-morbidity that affects the prognosis
- History and progression of the illness
- Physical baseline (e.g., weight and weight changes, vital signs, heart rhythms, rales, edema sites and amount)
- Physician's prognosis stating rationale for life expectancy of 6 months or less

Medicare Hospice Documentation: A Checklist Approach

✔ Are the physician's certification, assessments, and recertification(s) of terminal illness complete and included?

✔ Are all discipline visits notes and/or telephone calls signed, dated, legible, and descriptive of the course of care related to the patient, family, and caregivers?

✔ Has the physician provided written material that chronicles the patient's course of illness and care to date?

✔ Are all the laboratory or other test results included?

✔ Is the hospice election form signed and dated by the hospice provider and the patient/family or other responsible party?

✔ Is the effective date for the care clearly marked?

✔ Has the hospital provided a discharge summary, history, and results of a physical?

✔ Is the POC established, updated, and being followed?

✔ Has a copy of the election form been left with the patient, family, or other responsible party?

✔ If and when different levels of care are used, is there documentation of the date, time, and reason for the change in the level of care and services?

✔ Does the documentation support that the patient is terminally ill?

✔ Is the certification obtained on a timely basis?

✔ Do patient assessments paint a clear picture of the patient's status, including the following core aspects of hospice care: functional, spiritual, nutritional, clinical, emotional, psychological, and physical assessments and plans?

Effective Hospice Documentation:
A Checklist Approach

✔ Are handwritten notes or other entries legible to team members or others who may require the information?

✔ Are data elements or areas requiring completion addressed in an understandable manner? For example, is a legend or a list of acceptable abbreviations included in instances where abbreviations occur?

✔ Does the care plan reflect the problems identified during the comprehensive assessment?

✔ Are new team members oriented to forms and provided with accurately completed examples?

✔ Does the clinical record paint a clear picture of the hospice patient and family, interventions, responses, and outcomes (or quantifiable goals of care)?

✔ Do the hospice record and the documentation overall pass the test of effective care planning and coordination? Could another colleague, in your absence, review the record and be able to continue effectively with the hospice plan of care?

✔ Does the clinical documentation support the level of service provided (e.g., continuous care, inpatient care)?

✔ Does documentation show the active and ongoing management and reassessment of pain and symptoms?

✔ Are the prevention and treatment or interventions related to secondary symptoms such as constipation carried out and documented in the clinical notes?

✔ Are the psychosocial and spiritual concerns of the patient and family receiving acknowledgment and follow-up?

✔ Are initial and ongoing assessments of the dying patient clearly identified in the clinical record?

✔ Are interventions based on the patient's/family's needs as documented in the comprehensive assessment and the subsequent entries throughout the patient's care?

✔ Does the documentation emphasize the reasons that the patient/family needs or continues to need hospice services?

✔ Does the documentation support covered care as defined by Medicare, the case manager, or payor?

✔ Are the clinical records reviewed on an ongoing and timely basis for quality, completion, and identification that the patient either (1) has met predetermined goals or (2) needs continued care with possible changes to the plan based on the ongoing assessment findings and response to interventions? This includes dates, communications, and physician order follow-procedures.

✔ If a surveyor, payer, patient, or accreditation entity were to review your record, would the clinical documentation reflect the provision of safe, quality, and effective hospice patient care?

✔ Does the documentation simultaneously do the following:
1. Demonstrate the care provided and the patient's response to that care?
2. Show that the current standards of care are maintained?
3. Meet documentation requirements for Medicare and other payers?

✔ Are the clinical record and entries legible, neat, and organized consistently? How the clinical record looks may be seen as an indicator in assessing care and the organization.

✔ Are telephone calls and other communications with physicians, community agencies, and other team members documented? Do they explain what occurred with the patient, what actions were ordered, modified, and implemented, and what the patient's/family's response was to these interventions?

✔ Is the nursing process demonstrated in the record? Look for the nursing diagnoses or problem identification, the assessment, evidence of care planning, implementation of ordered interventions and actions, movement toward patient-centered goals, assessment of the patient's response, and continued evaluation.

✔ Are goal achievement and/or progress toward goals and outcomes documented? Are the goals realistic, quantifiable, and patient and family centered?

✔ Are family/caregiver teaching and their responses/demonstration of behavior and learning documented?

✔ Is the patient's response to care interventions and nursing documented?

✔ Are the interventions modified based on the patient's response, where appropriate?

✔ Is evidence of interdisciplinary team conferences and discussions documented?

✔ Are continuity of care planning goals and consistent movement toward outcomes/goal achievement by all members of the team shown?

✔ Does the record tell the story of the patient's care, needs, and progress while the patient/family was receiving hospice services?

✔ Is compliance with organizational, regulatory, licensure, and quality standards demonstrated?

Clinical Path Considerations

As hospice and home care organizations seek to become more efficient, new models of care and documentation are emerging. Clinical paths, or care pathways, are a way to ensure that all team members are on the same page as they work together to achieve patient goals. More paths are emerging in hospice and becoming available to all the staff involved in the plan of care and the patient and family. Clarifying the expectations for care, integrating standards of care into the path, and identifying quantifiable patient goals at the onset create an environment for improved communications and care. The National Hospice Organization (NHO) has a path specifically designed for hospice.

Clinical paths are one way of defining a clinical budget or the amount of resources needed to care for a particular patient or group of patients. The reason clinical paths are initiated is to improve quality of care; the main focus must be on the patient.

Defining Clinical Paths

Clinical paths are tools that organize, sequence, and time the major interventions of clinicians for a particular case type, medical condition, diagnostic category, or functional diagnosis. They identify and standardize tools and information, interventions, and processes for achieving predetermined outcomes (quantifiable goals of care). The development and implementation of clinical paths are similar to project management, wherein certain key processes that are mapped out schematically can be used to monitor the effectiveness of the plan and determine progress through a process of quality improvement to positively impact and improve patient care.[1]

Clinical paths demand the standardization of care and care processes. For example, goals are clearly defined, and all care to be provided is specifically explained, laid out in a linear design, and based on the organization's historical data. Your organization may have paths for certain groups of patients or diagnoses as a way to ensure quality care for patients with those particular problems. Not all patient problems will have a path; the course of some medical problems cannot be easily projected.

The Future Is Here: Computerization and Documentation

There is no question that we need to be more effective in health care; automation or computerization is one method to increase efficiency while enabling team members to provide more detailed and accurate documentation. However, computers are not the answers to all care planning and scheduling issues in hospice. Data, whether documented on paper or keyed into a computer, must be correct for the entire process to flow toward billing and discharge.

To be able to compare "apples to apples," everyone must collect the same information in the same format and manner while using the same glossary in communications. Benchmarking with peers, performance improvement activities, and data management and collection will only become more important in the coming years. Dr. Deming[2], the guru of quality, has been credited with saying, "In God we trust; all others must have data." Only through standardized data collection tools, methods, and definitions are valid comparisons for cost and care efficiencies possible. These data will help direct our collective efforts to improve hospice care for patients and their loved ones.

SUMMARY

The hospice nurse plays an important role in supporting coverage of hospice through the generation and maintenance of effective documentation. Hospice documentation should reflect that the patient clearly has a terminal illness with a limited life expectancy of less than 6 months. The hospice documentation should emphasize the patient's prognosis, whatever the diagnosis; this is the reason for hospice.

Hospice team members practicing in the community must be service oriented, flexible, strong clinically, and able to document effectively. Payers and insurers must continue to address spiraling health care costs. The customary way to do this has been to decrease authorized visits and services and add additional review levels. The emphasis on the collection of data quantifying the impact of care will only increase in the coming years.

The professional nurse can validate the need for skillful hospice care and back it up with effective documentation. Nurses and other clinicians must know the coverage criteria for specific insurers, such as Medicare, and the documentation needed to support covered care. The documentation and related coverage criteria go hand in hand, and their importance cannot be overstated. They assist in meeting patients' needs, marketing services, safeguarding team members and the organization against alleged Medicare fraud or abuse claims, and ensuring reimbursement for services. They also provide the baseline for community education related to hospice services and a benchmark for reviewing visit utilization.

Clinical documentation continues to be an important indicator of the quality of care provided. In community-based hospice home care, in which a reviewer or surveyor cannot walk down inpatient halls and see patients receiving care, the clinical record and its format, organization, and timeliness of filing become important as the link to the quality of the care provided. From this perspective, with the spiraling costs of health care, the clinical record reflects the organization and their belief that "excellence is in the details." In hospice care the details of clinical documentation are a driving force toward payment and certification; more important, they help ensure that patients and families receive quality hospice care.

REVIEW EXERCISES

1. Explain the following statement: "Hospice and clinical practice are described every day through review of patient records."
2. List three reasons for the importance of clinical documentation and the record.
3. Who are the Regional Home Health Intermediaries (RHHIs), and what important role do they play in hospice?
4. Explain the following statement: "The RHHIs can pay only for hospice care under Medicare that is covered by law."
5. List the hallmarks of effective hospice documentation.
6. Describe the hospice documentation needed to support covered care.
7. What is the test of effective care planning and care coordination?
8. Define a clinical path and the role it plays in effectively managing a patient's care across the care continuum.
9. Explain the rationale that supports the standardization of care and care processes.
10. Describe the clinician's role in compliance related to Medicare and documentation requirements.

References

1. Marrelli T, Hilliard L: *Home care and clinical paths. Effective care planning across the continuum,* St Louis, 1996, Mosby.
2. Deming WE: *Out of the crisis,* Cambridge, Mass, 1986, Massachusetts Institute of Technology Center for Advanced Engineering Studies.

PART THREE

PLANNING AND MANAGING CARE
IN HOSPICE

PLANNING AND MANAGING CARE IN HOSPICE

Frequency of visits and length of service are usually based on the hospice team's assessment and ongoing evaluation of the patient and family status and the patient's biopsychosocial and unique family system needs. The current health care environment and the increasing emphasis on quality initiatives demonstrated by positive patient outcomes identify the need for research and evaluation regarding the frequency and length of time the patient needs to be under care. The following is a discussion of the process and knowledge that may assist in making the best determination for frequency and length of service. Throughout this discussion, remember that all visits require orders by the physician and the nurse must maintain compliance with the Medicare Conditions of Participation, state licensure, surveyor directives, and other regulations or laws.

Much has been written about the appropriate time to admit patients to hospice. In addition, for Medicare-participating hospices, Operation Restore Trust (ORT) and other government initiatives have been developed to save the Medicare trust fund from alleged overutilization, fraud, and abuse. These efforts have heightened awareness of the types of patients and their problems and histories when admitted to hospice.

A number of considerations help in determining the appropriate frequency and length of hospice visits. This discussion provides a framework to assist hospice clinicians in making these decisions appropriately; however, it is not meant to take the place of ongoing meetings with the hospice manager or IDG to determine patients' unique frequency and duration needs. Rather, this discussion is designed to help hospice clinicians become aware of the many factors that go into making this determination.

The introduction of diagnosis-related groups (DRGs) and other prospective payment systems (PPSs) in inpatient settings has increased the scrutiny of admission to and frequency and duration of home health and hospice services. Nurses practicing in the community are acutely aware of the decreased lengths of stay in hospitals and the increased patient acuity in both the hospital and the home care setting. The increasing complexity of patient needs is demonstrated in the changing case mix of the nurse's caseload.

Forms of PPSs, such as the Medicare hospice benefit, will continue to expand to other areas of health care, including home health care. The Medicare Home Care Prospective Payment Demonstration, which is continuing to collate needed information on this significant change in payment to home care programs, is expected to be operationalized nationally by October 1, 1999.

Experienced hospice and community health nurses know that they are in an important position for identifying the patient's specific service and visit frequency needs. The objective findings in comprehensive hospice assessments are the basis for the recommendations that are made by the team member and communicated to the physician. Some patients may be seen infrequently by their physician after discharge because they lack adequate transportation to the physician's office or, in some instances, the physician does not or will not make needed home visits. The professional nurse's judgment skills can help in making these important visit frequency decisions.

In hospice, because the Medicare program is a prospective payment or "managed care" system, the decisions may be more problematic. Box 3-1 lists some factors that are considered in determining frequency and duration of care.

BOX 3-1

PATIENT-RELATED CONSIDERATIONS

The following is a list of the most common patient-related considerations that the nurse evaluates when formulating plans and beginning care. This alphabetical list is not all-inclusive; other considerations may apply, such as the hospice patient caseload and availability of services or other resources. In addition, many of these factors are interrelated.

Absence of caregiver
Activities of daily living (ADLs) limitations
Adaptive or assistive devices
Affect (e.g., depression)
Behavioral or mental disorders
Belief systems
Caregiver support
Chemical or drug problems (e.g., alcoholism)
Chronic illness(es)
Cognitive function
Communication
Competency (patient/family)
Compliance/noncompliance
Coping skills
Cultural status
Directives
Disabilities
Discharge plan
Drug considerations (number, type, interactions, etc.)
Educational level/barriers
Environment
Family
Fatigue
Fire safety
Functional limitations
Goals/expected outcomes
Handicaps
History
Home medical equipment
Home setting
Independence
Instrumental activities of daily living (IADLs)
Knowledge of emergency procedures
Language
Learning needs
Loneliness
Loss of significant other(s)
Medical equipment or supply needs
Medications
Mobility
Motivation

BOX 3-1

PATIENT-RELATED CONSIDERATIONS—cont'd

Motivation
Nursing assessment and reassessment findings
Nursing diagnoses
Nutritional status
Orthotic needs
Other considerations, based on patient's/family's unique needs
Pain
Parenting
Pathology
Physical assessment findings
Physical setting for care
Polypharmacy
Probability of further complications
Prognosis
Psychopathology
Psychosocial needs
Reason for prior hospitalization, for referral to hospice
Rehabilitative needs
Resources (e.g., financial, human)
Rights
Risk factors
Safety
Self-care status
Skin integrity
Social factors
Social supports
Socioeconomic condition
Spiritual needs
Stability
Support systems
Swallowing
Values
Voice

The nurse's rationale, experience, and sometimes intuition contribute to the decision-making process related to frequency and length of stay. According to Benner, "Intuitive judgment is what distinguishes expert human judgment from the decisions that might be made by a beginner or by a machine."[1] Home health and hospice are two settings in which experienced professional nurses use their broad knowledge base to make effective patient care decisions, such as those determining frequency and level of stay (LOS), that can have a direct impact on patient and family outcomes. The nurse also can look to the manager for specific information, feedback, and standards of the hospice organization or program.

Health care reform is primarily addressing three of the greatest problems within the U.S. health care system—access, cost, and quality. Cost is the issue that hospice programs address daily when a case management company questions or limits needed visits, services, or hours of care. As hospice experts, nurses, managers, and administrators must articulate to a case manager or third-party payor the objective rationale and plan for projected care. Nurses must be able to communicate objectively the skills used during care and explain why those visits may vary even though patients may have the same general diagnoses or problems. Nurses and other hospice clinicians can do their jobs because of their education and experience.

Payment is for the professional nurse's judgment and observational and other skills. Only nurses can compare one wound with others seen in their practice experience, make a judgment regarding healing or infection, identify dehiscence, evaluate the wound in relation to other pathological conditions, obtain a baseline assessment, teach the patient and caregivers, and apply a myriad of other skills to patients daily in homes. The role and responsibility of home care and hospice professionals are to educate others, including case managers, payors, consumers, and families, about the cost effectiveness, quality, and demonstrated positive outcomes experienced by the patients. As performance improvement focuses on the consumer of services, the industry must move toward standardizing processes, continually looking at methods to improve results (positive patient outcomes), and objectively measuring performance and demonstrated outcomes.

Research-based practice guidelines, outcome measures, and standards of care are important because of the increased emphasis on cost-effective high-quality care. These practice parameters assist clinicians in determining patient needs and care frequency and better projecting length of service.

Standardized care plans are based on North American Nursing Diagnosis Association (NANDA) nursing diagnoses and nurses' experience with particular patient problems. Other organizations have developed or purchased automated systems that help them track and define objective findings and demonstrate outcome achievement based on outcome criteria. Nurses in practice are aware of the ongoing concern regarding provision of adequate patient care in a climate of tighter reimbursement, more limited resources, frequent ethical dilemmas, and heightened emphasis on both quality and effectiveness. This cost/quality equation must balance out for the maintenance of patient and family satisfaction and success, productivity, viability of organizations, and nurses' satisfaction in their ability to meet patient and family needs.

Managers and nurses need to be adept in articulating and quantifying patient care needs based on objective evidence and supporting documentation. As nurses identify the need to streamline and more effectively provide and demonstrate care, use of such systems will help in creating and maintaining cost- and time-effective operations and quality improvement. The use of standardized care plans as the basis for individualizing hospice care helps nurses teaching patients and family members with new or multiple health needs to prioritize those needs.

HOSPICE CARE EXAMPLES

The following are examples of some patients and patient problems seen in hospice. They are just examples, and the hospice nurse's professional judgment, recognized standards of care, and information gathered from all aspects of the assessment process are still the basis for identifying patient and family services, visit frequency, and service duration needs. All hospice documentation must clearly show the disease progression of the terminally ill patient.

The answers to the following questions may help the hospice nurse determine the frequency and intensity of hospice services. Determinations must be based on the patient's and family's unique findings, situation, and supports. Generally, hospice patients may have more intensive needs toward the end of care than at the beginning. This situation is the opposite of the typical home care scenario, in which the patient is working toward independence and the team pulls back toward discharge. Keep in mind, however, that some patients are admitted to hospice appropriately for intensive services at the onset for hospice's specialty skills of support and pain and symptom management.

- What symptomatology or clinical information supports the need for hospice?
- What is the patient's current activity level, how has it changed, and how rapidly has it changed?
- What information has the doctor, patient, or others provided that supports the statement that the patient has a limited life expectancy?
- What are the expectations related to hospice care and support, and how can we best meet them?
- If this is a new diagnosis, what services are identified during the assessment and how do these services support fulfillment of the patient and family needs?
- What are the special skills and services that hospice will bring to this patient and family?
- If the patient has Alzheimer's, cardiac, or lung disease or another illness that may have long-term or chronic disease implications, what occurrences or symptoms lead the physician and clinicians to believe that the patient is dying?
- Are symptoms or side effects from therapy emerging in the history and physical assessment?
- Why were the patient and family referred to hospice? Can hospice meet their unique needs?
- What are the patient and family expressing/identifying as their needs?
  1. The patient is 82 and was recently diagnosed with cancer of the prostate. He moved into his daughter's home after his last hospitalization, hoping to return to his own home "after he was stronger." The patient had a suprapubic catheter and complained of lower back pain. After several weeks of care, it is apparent that he will not get any stronger, and he continually asks his daughter to let him go home—especially if he is dying. Understandably upset, his daughter has had multiple discussions with the physician, and hospice was called for an assessment. Because of her work schedule, the daughter frequently is not home.

     In an effort to address the patient's stated desire to return to his home, the hospice admitting nurse assesses the patient at his daughter's home. The patient clearly states that the next visit will be at his home, mentioning that he thinks his niece will move in with him if necessary. Because the patient is a widower who lives alone, the hospice team initially focuses efforts on the need for a primary caregiver. The effective use of care conferencing assists the patient and his daughter in the decision-making process and assessment of the appropriate time to make the transition to hospice and for the patient to return home.

     This patient does return to his own home, with his daughter (when available) and niece as his primary caregivers. Volunteer support, chaplain services, and other hospice support services contribute to the patient's ability to return home. His death occurs some 3 weeks later, and bereavement support assists his daughter and niece (who was identified as at risk for a difficult bereavement) during the period following his death.

Visit frequency for this patient was daily at the onset as the patient experienced continued discomfort with the catheter and was concerned about possible dislodgment. The certified nursing assistant (CNA) assisted with personal care, activities of daily living, and meal preparation. The CNA noted increasing discomfort on standing or turning in certain positions and reported this to the hospice nurse, who reassessed the patient and called the physician for a change in the medication regimen and plan of care. The niece, who at another time had moved in with and assisted another family member who had later died, was very concerned about the patient's dying at home and her being alone. The social worker visited once a week and discussed a system of communication with her to try to decrease this possibility and her anxiety. Because of this history, all team members were very clear in their communications with the niece when she daily asked, "Is he near?" or "Is it close?" The catheter was finally removed, which made the patient more comfortable and mobile. The patient died at home pain-free, and the niece was not alone; both the patient's daughter and the hospice nurse were there, and the niece and daughter had uncomplicated bereavement periods.

2. The patient is a 46-year-old woman with an aggressive metastatic breast cancer and a history of bilateral mastectomies, chemotherapy, radiation, and alternative therapies over a span of 6 years. She was initially referred to hospice by her physician for pain control and support to the patient, her husband, and their three children, aged 6, 8, and 14. On admission, the hospice nurse notes that her pain was assessed as a 2 on a scale of 1-10, and the patient notes that it worsens with movement or any activity. The hospice team contacts the physician and the pharmacist, and changes are made in her medication regimen that cause the pain to decrease to 0 with activity. Massage therapy, which the patient identifies as most effectively assisting her comfort level, is integrated into her plan of care.

Hospice volunteers assist with support for the family, and the patient dies at home, according to her request, with her symptoms fairly well controlled. At the bereavement visits, her husband verbalizes the importance of the care and support they all received from hospice. In this example the frequency of visits is intense on admission for pain assessments and reassessment and management, stabilizes as the patient's symptoms are controlled, and then increases significantly as the patient and family needs increase just before death.

3. The patient is a 47-year-old woman with cancer of the liver who is admitted for hospice care. The hospice nurse clinical specialist who admits the patient and family to the program explains the hospice philosophy and proposes a care regimen based on the needs identified. Nursing care, home health aide care, and other components of the hospice team are explained, and care is scheduled to begin. The frequency issue is sometimes more complex in patients with clearly shortened life spans. Generally, patients with a terminal illness receive more care toward the end of their lives, whereas patients with a fair or better prognosis receive more services at the

start of care; these services taper down as function and independence increase.

Depending on the patient's and family's unique needs, it can be very appropriate for the same amount of care to be provided throughout the hospice admission. Keep in mind that many patients are admitted to hospice at the end stages of their disease process after high-technology interventions and cure-oriented therapies have been exhausted. As the focus changes from cure to care, the hospice takes a holistic approach to care, with the frequency determined solely by patient and family needs. For such a patient, services could consist of 3-times-weekly RN visits with home care aides and volunteer support or any combination of services provided by the interdisciplinary hospice team. The goals/outcomes identified in this case are symptom-controlled death at home with hospice support and family presence.

SUMMARY

Nurses working in hospice must be flexible and able to explain objective reasons for frequency related to the plan of care. These decisions and the underlying rationale must be communicated clearly to the nurse's manager or third-party payor representatives who are responsible for tracking, approving, or denying visits or care. As payors try to decrease the number of patient visits, we must be able to articulate the clinical and other needs of the patient. This advocacy role will ensure quality care while the patient remains at home. Those who can explain needs based on objective information and patient findings to numerous reimbursement gatekeepers will be successful as advocates for patients and families who elect hospice care. The increasing complexity of caring for patients sent home with limited resource and coverage demands these skills for safe, effective patient care.

REVIEW EXERCISES

1. List five factors that are taken into account when projecting care needs for hospice patients and families.
2. Describe a hospice patient example and the rationale that supports the frequency and the interventions planned.
3. Explain three reasons that support admitting a patient to hospice (assume, of course, that the patient and family desire hospice).
4. What is Operation Restore Trust (ORT), and why was it developed?
5. Support the following statement: "We should use standardized care plans as the basis for individualizing patient/family hospice care."

Reference

1. Benner P, Tanner C: Clinical judgment: how expert nurses use intuition, *AJN*, January:23, 1987.

PART FOUR

MEDICAL-SURGICAL CARE GUIDELINES
Special Patients and Families

OUTLINE FOR CARE GUIDELINES

1. **General Considerations**

2. **Needs for Visit**

3. **Safety Considerations**

4. **Potential Diagnoses and Codes**

5. **Associated Nursing Diagnoses**

6. **Skills and Services Identified**
   - Hospice Nursing
     a. Comfort and Symptom Control
     b. Safety and Mobility Considerations
     c. Emotional/Spiritual Considerations
     d. Skin Care
     e. Elimination Considerations
     f. Hydration/Nutrition
     g. Therapeutic/Medication Regimens
     h. Other Considerations
   - Home Health Aide or Certified Nursing Assistant
   - Hospice Social Worker
   - Volunteer(s)
   - Spiritual Counselor
   - Dietitian/Nutritional Counseling
   - Occupational Therapist
   - Physical Therapist
   - Speech-Language Pathologist
   - Bereavement Counselor
   - Pharmacist (for some diagnoses)
   - Music, Massage, Art, or Other Therapies or Services

7. **Outcomes for Care**

8. **Patient, Family, and Caregiver Educational Needs**

9. **Specific Tips for Quality and Reimbursement**

10. **Resources for Hospice Care and Practice**

ACQUIRED IMMUNE DEFICIENCY SYNDROME (AIDS) CARE

1. **General considerations**

   Home continues to be the care setting for most patients with acquired immune deficiency syndrome (AIDS). Care is directed toward palliation of opportunistic infections and other HIV-related conditions and prevention of further problems. *Pneumocystis carinii* pneumonia continues to be one of the most serious processes in the adult patient with AIDS. The provision of comfort, support, education, and palliative care to patients and their caregivers is key to effective hospice care in the community.

   Please refer to "Cancer Care," "Pain Care," "Infusion Care," and "Bedbound Care" should these sections also pertain to your hospice patient.

2. **Needs for visit**

   Physician order for hospice care, specific to the hospice program's admission criteria and policies

   Standard precautions supplies

   Vital signs equipment for baseline assessment

   Other supplies or equipment, based on physician orders

3. **Safety considerations**

   Infection control/standard precautions

   Night-light

   Extra caution on slippery surfaces

   Removal of scatter rugs

   Tub rail, grab bars for bathroom safety

   Supportive and nonskid shoes

   Handrail on stairs

   Fall precautions

   Protective skin measures

   Identification and report of any skin problems

   Smoke detector and fire evacuation plan

   Assistance with ambulation

   Municipal water source/safety

   Pet care (e.g., mobility, infection control)

   Others, based on the patient's unique condition and environment

4. **Potential diagnoses and codes**

AIDS (general)	042
Anemia	042 and 285.9
Anorexia	042 and 783.0
Bacterial infections, recurrent	042
Burkitt's lymphoma	042 and 200.20
Cancer, cervical	042 and 195
Candidiasis	042 and 112.9
Candidiasis, esophageal	042 and 112.84

Candidiasis, oral	042 and 112.0
Candidiasis, vaginal	042 and 112.1
Cervical cancer	042 and 180.9
Chorioretinitis	042 and 363.20
Colitis	042 and 558.9
Cryptococcus	042 and 117.5
Cytomegalovirus	042 and 078.5
Cytomegalovirus retinitis	078.5, 363.20, and 042
Dementia	042 and 294.1
Diarrhea	042 and 008.69
Encephalitis	042 and 323.0
Encephalopathy, AIDS	042 and 348.3
Endocarditis	042 and 424.90
Esophagitis	042 and 530.1
Herpes simplex	042 and 054.79
Herpes zoster	042 and 053.79
Histoplasmosis	042 and 115.99
HTLV III	042
Hyperalimentation	99.15
Kaposi's sarcoma	042 and 176.9
Lymphocytic interstitial pneumonia	042 and 516.8
Lymphoma	042 and 202.80
Lymphoma, non-Hodgkin's	042 and 202.80
Lymphoma of the brain	042 and 202.80
Malaise and fatigue	780.7
Meningitis	042 and 047.8
Mycobacterium avium intracellulare	042 and 031.0
Mycobacterium tuberculosis	042 and 011.90
Myocarditis	042 and 422.99
Neuropathy, peripheral	042 and 357.4
Neutropenia	042 and 288.0
Paraplegia	042 and 344.1
Pelvic inflammatory disease (PID) (acute)	042 and 614.3
Pelvic inflammatory disease (PID) (chronic)	042 and 614.4
Peripheral neuropathy	042 and 357.4
Pneumocystis carinii pneumonia	042 and 136.3
Pneumonia (bacterial)	042 and 482.9
Pneumonia (NOS)	042 and 486
Pneumonia (viral)	042 and 480.9
Polymyositis	042 and 710.4
Polyradiculoneuropathy	042 and 357.4
Protein-caloric malnutrition	263.9
Quadriplegia	042 and 344.00
Retinal detachment	042 and 361.9
Retinal hemorrhage	042 and 362.81
Salmonella	042 and 003.9
Salmonella septicemia	042 and 003.1
Seizures	042 and 780.3
Sepsis	042 and 038.9

Shigella	042 and 004.9
Shigella dysentery	042 and 004.9
Thrombocytopenia	042 and 287.5
Total parenteral nutrition (TPN)	99.15
Toxoplasmosis	042 and 130.9
Tuberculosis (pulmonary)	042 and 011.9
Varicella	042 and 052.9
Wasting syndrome	042 and 799.4
Zoster virus	042 and 053.9

5. **Associated nursing diagnoses**
   Activity intolerance
   Activity intolerance, risk for
   Airway clearance, ineffective
   Anxiety
   Aspiration, high risk for
   Body image disturbance
   Body temperature, altered, risk for
   Bowel incontinence
   Breathing pattern, ineffective
   Cardiac output, decreased
   Caregiver role strain
   Caregiver role strain, risk for
   Communication, impaired verbal
   Confusion, acute
   Constipation
   Coping, ineffective family: compromised
   Coping, ineffective family: disabling
   Coping, ineffective individual
   Diarrhea
   Family processes, altered
   Fatigue
   Fear
   Fluid volume deficit
   Fluid volume deficit, risk for
   Gas exchange, impaired
   Grieving, anticipatory
   Health maintenance, altered
   Home maintenance management, impaired
   Hopelessness
   Incontinence, functional
   Incontinence, total
   Infection, risk for
   Injury, potential for
   Knowledge deficit (disease process and management)
   Loneliness, risk for
   Memory, impaired
   Mobility, impaired physical
   Noncompliance (specify)

Nutrition, altered: less than body requirements
Oral mucous membrane, altered
Pain
Pain, chronic
Parenting, altered
Parenting, altered, risk for
Peripheral neurovascular dysfunction, risk for
Powerlessness
Protection, altered
Role performance, altered
Self-care deficit, bathing/hygiene
Self-care deficit, dressing/grooming
Self-care deficit, feeding
Self-care deficit, toileting
Sensory/perceptual alterations (specify) (visual, auditory, kinesthetic, gustatory, tactile, olfactory)
Sexual dysfunction
Sexuality patterns, altered
Skin integrity, impaired
Skin integrity, impaired, risk for
Sleep pattern disturbance
Social interaction, impaired
Social isolation
Spiritual distress (distress of the human spirit)
Spiritual well-being, potential for enhanced
Swallowing, impaired
Thought processes, altered
Tissue integrity, impaired
Tissue perfusion, altered (specify type) (renal, cerebral, cardiopulmonary, gastrointestinal, peripheral)
Urinary elimination, altered
Urinary retention

6. **Skills and services identified**

   • *Hospice nursing*

      a. *Comfort and symptom control*
         Complete initial assessment of all systems of patient with AIDS admitted to hospice for _____ (specify problem necessitating care)
         Presentation of hospice philosophy and services
         Explain patient rights and responsibilities
         Assess patient, family, and caregiver wishes and expectations regarding care
         Assess patient, family, and caregiver resources available for care
         Teach family or caregiver physical care of patient
         Provision of volunteer support to patient and family
         Assess pain and other symptoms, including site, duration, characteristics, and relief measures

Assess patient q visit for change (increase) in levels of fatigue, weakness, or malaise

Assess and observe all systems and symptoms q visit, and report changes and new symptoms to physician

Instruct patient and caregiver to notify RN or physician for new symptoms, including fever, vomiting, diarrhea, cough, and other changes

Teach pain and symptom management regimen to caregiver

RN to instruct in pain control measures and medications

Teach caregiver or family about care of weak, terminally ill patient

Instruct in the need for elevation of edematous extremities and elevation of head of bed for comfort

Evaluate pain in relation to other symptoms, such as fatigue, confusion, diarrhea, nausea and vomiting, depression, and shortness of breath

RN to assess patient's pain or other symptoms q visit to identify need for change, addition or other plan, or dose adjustment

Measure vital signs, including pain, q visit

Assess cardiovascular, pulmonary, and respiratory status

Teach caregivers symptom control and relief measures

Oxygen at _____ liters per _____ (specific physician orders)

Identify and monitor pain, symptom, and relief measures

Nonpharmacological interventions for pain, such as progressive muscle relaxation, imagery, positive visualization, music, and humor therapy of patient's choice implemented

Comfort measures of backrub and hand or other therapeutic massage

RN to provide and teach effective oral care and comfort measures

Teach patient and family about realistic expectations of disease process

Teach care of dying and signs/symptoms of impending death

Presence and support

Other interventions, based on patient/family needs

b. *Safety and mobility considerations*

Provide patient with home safety information and instruction related to _____ and documented in the clinical record

Instruct patient regarding pet care and avoidance of cross contamination, and check with physician about certain types of pets

Teach patient and caregiver care needed for safe, effective management at home

Teach caregivers care of the bedridden patient

Instruct patient and family regarding safety and standard precautions in the home

Teach patient and family regarding planning and pacing activities

Teach patient and family regarding energy conservation techniques

Instruct caregiver regarding need to maintain activity as tolerated, range of motion (ROM) exercises to prevent loss or decrease in mobility, and need to report changes to physician

Other interventions, based on patient/family needs

c. *Emotional/spiritual considerations*

Psychosocial assessment of patient and family regarding disease and prognosis

Discuss need for guardianship or power of attorney

Discuss concepts of "living will," other advance directives, status regarding resuscitation, other medical/technical interventions, and patient's wishes

Assist with funeral plans, if appropriate

Inform patient/family/caregiver of available volunteer support

Assess patient's spiritual needs and address plan

Assess patient and caregiver coping skills

Provide emotional support to patient/family with chronic and/or terminal illness and associated implications

Assess patient for mental status and sleep disturbance problems or changes

Assist with emotional support concerning care of children and children's future

RN to provide emotional support to patient and family

Other interventions, based on patient/family needs

d. *Skin care*

Teach patient and caregiver all aspects of wound care, including safe disposal of dressing supplies

Care for and assess Kaposi lesions, cleanse with _____ (specify physician orders)

Teach caregiver regarding patient's skin care needs, including the need for frequent position changes, appropriate pressure pads and mattresses, and the prevention of breakdown

Assess skin integrity

Observation and evaluation of wound and surrounding skin

Evaluate patient's need for equipment, supplies to decrease pressure, alternating pressure mattress, gel foam seat cushion, and heel and elbow protectors

Teach family to perform dressing between RN visits, _____ (specify)

Teach patient, family, or caregiver about proper body alignment and positioning in bed to prevent skin tears from shearing skin

Observe and apply skilled assessment of areas for possible breakdown, including heels, hips, elbows, and ankles

RN to teach patient regarding care of irradiated skin sites

Assess patient's skin and mucous membranes for problems, including bacterial infection, thrush, rashes, and other changes

Other interventions, based on patient/family needs

e. *Elimination considerations*

Assess bowel regimen, and implement program as needed

Instruct patient and caregiver to report increase in diarrhea (frequency, amount) to physician

RN to teach caregiver daily catheter care

RN to evaluate the patient's bowel patterns, need for stool softeners, laxatives, and dietary adjustments and develop bowel management plan

Check for and remove impaction as needed

Condom catheter or indwelling catheter as indicated

Teach catheter care to caregiver

Assess amount and frequency of urinary output

Observation and complete systems assessment of the patient with an
   indwelling catheter

Other interventions, based on patient/family needs

f. *Hydration/nutrition*

Instruct patient about specified diet _____ (specify according
   to physician orders)

Teach food preparation and handling techniques, particularly hand
   washing, handling of uncooked foods, and the need to cook all eggs,
   meat, fish, and poultry products

Weigh patient q visit and review food intake diary and use of herbs,
   vitamins/mineral supplements, and alternative nutrition therapies

Encourage patient to eat small, more frequent meals of choice

Closely monitor parenteral feeding catheter and IV therapy site for infection or other problems/complications

Monitor patient on enteral nutrition therapy

Nutrition/hydration to be maintained by offering patient high-protein
   diet and foods of choice as tolerated

Assess nutrition and hydration status

Counsel patient with anorexia about diet and nutrition

Teach feeding-tube care to family

Encourage use of commercially prepared nutrition supplements (e.g.,
   Ensure)

Teach patient and family to expect decreased nutritional and fluid intake
   as disease progresses

Other interventions based on patient/family needs

g. *Therapeutic/medication regimens*

Monitor patient for side effects of drugs and food/drug and drug/drug
   interactions

Teach site care of Hickman catheter or other venous access device

Obtain blood samples as ordered for necessary monitoring

Implement nonpharmacological interventions with medication schedule,
   possibly including therapeutic massage, distraction, imagery, progressive muscle relaxation, humor, biofeedback, and music therapies

Medication management of patient on complex and numerous drug
   therapies

Teach regarding antiretroviral therapy medication

Teach patient and caregiver all aspects of medications, including routes,
   schedules, functions, and side effects

Teach new pain and symptom control medication regimen

Assess weight as ordered

Measure abdominal girth for ascites and edema; document sites, amount

Obtain venipuncture as ordered q _____ (specify ordered
   frequency)

Teach new medications and effects

Assess for electrolyte imbalance

Teach new medications and effects

Teach patient and caregiver use of PCA pump

Observe for side effects of palliative chemotherapy, including constipation, anemia, and fatigue, and teach patient relief measures

Venipuncture _____ (specify ordered frequency) for monitoring platelet count, other values

Demonstrate and teach use of multiple medications to caregiver

Monitor patient's level of anemia and other lab values

Assess the patient's unique response to treatments or interventions, and instruct patient/family to report changes or unfavorable responses or reactions to the physician

Other interventions, based on patient/family needs

h. *Other considerations*

Instruct patient and caregivers in all aspects of effective hand-washing techniques and proper care of bodily fluids and excretions

Address sexuality concerns and implications for safer sexual expression, including the use of latex condoms, abstinence, the use of dental dams during oral sex, and other information

Assess progression of disease process

RN to assess the patient's response to treatments and interventions and to report to the physician any changes, unfavorable responses, and reactions

Teach patient and caregiver regarding waterborne infections

Other interventions, based on patient/family needs

- **Home health aide or certified nursing assistant**
  Effective and safe personal care
  ADL assistance and support and ambulation and transfer assist
  Observation and reporting
  Respite care and active listening skills
  Meal preparation
  Homemaker services
  Comfort care
  Other duties

- **Hospice social worker**
  Psychosocial assessment of patient and family/caregiver, including adjustment to illness and its implications, and the need for care
  Identification of optimal coping strategies
  Financial assessment and counseling regarding food acquisition, ability to prepare, and costs of needed medications
  Intervention/support related to terminal illness and loss
  Identification of caregiver role strain necessitating respite/relief measures or support
  Emotional/spiritual support
  Facilitate communication among patient, family, and hospice team
  Referral/linkage to community services and resources as indicated
  Grief counseling and intervention/support related to illness/loss
  Patient/caregiver counseling and support
  For patients who live alone with no support system (e.g., able, available, willing caregiver[s]): obtain linkage with necessary community resources to allow patient to stay in the home

Identification of illness-related psychiatric condition necessitating support and care/intervention

Evaluation of situation related to patient's child(ren) and future wishes for children and pets

Depression and fears assessed

- *Volunteer(s)*

  Support, friendship, companionship, and presence

  Comfort and dignity maintained/provided for patient and family

  Errands and transportation

  Other services, based on interdisciplinary team recommendations and patient/caregiver needs

- *Spiritual counselor*

  Spiritual assessment and care

  Counseling, intervention, and support related to that dimension of life related to life's meaning (consistent with patient's/family's beliefs)

  Support, listening, and presence

  Participation in sacred or spiritual rituals or practices

  Other supportive care, based on the patient's/family's needs and belief systems

- *Dietitian/nutritional counseling*

  Assessment of patient with decreased intake, weight loss, anorexia, diarrhea, nausea, and skin breakdown

  Assessment and recommendations for swallowing difficulties

  Support and care with food and nourishment as desired by patient

  Encourage patient to ingest nutritional supplements and snacks to increase protein and caloric intake

  Counsel and instruct family regarding patient's decreased appetite and possible inability to eat

  Food and dietary recommendations incorporating patient choice and wishes

  Teach regarding proper food preparation and handling, especially hand washing, handling of uncooked foods, and need to cook eggs, meat, fish, poultry, and dairy products

  Assess and teach regarding use of alternative nutrition therapies, such as herbs, vitamin/mineral supplements, and macrobiotic diets

- *Occupational therapist*

  Evaluation

  Energy conservation techniques

  Evaluation of ADL and functional mobility

  Assess for need for adaptive equipment and assistive devices

  Safety assessment of patient's environment and ADL

- *Physical therapist*

  Evaluation

  Assessment of patient's environment for safety

  Safe transfer training

  Strengthening exercises/program

  Assessment of gait safety

Instruct/supervise caregiver and volunteers with regard to home exercise program for conditioning and strength

Assistive, adaptive devices of equipment and teaching

- *Speech-language pathologist*
Evaluation for swallowing problems

- *Bereavement counselor*
Assessment of the needs of the bereaved family and friends
Support and intervention, based on assessment and ongoing findings
Presence and counseling
Supportive visits and follow-up and other interventions (e.g., mailings, calls)
Other services related to bereavement work and support

- *Pharmacist*
Evaluation of hospice patient on multiple medications for possible food/drug, drug/drug interactions
Medication monitoring regarding therapeutic levels and dosages
Pain consult and input into interdisciplinary plan of care related to pain control, palliation, and symptom management

- *Music, massage, art, or other therapies or services*
Evaluation and intervention based on patient's and caregiver's unique wishes and needs that support care and death in the setting of the patient's choice
Pet therapy (including patient's pet, if available) and therapeutic intervention
Assessment plan to engage patient and support comfort, quality, enjoyment, and dignity

7. **Outcomes for care**

- *Hospice nursing*
Patient and caregiver verbalize satisfaction with care
Educational tools/plans incorporated in daily care, and patient/caregiver verbalizes understanding of safe, needed care
Patient will decide on care, interventions, and evaluation
Caregiver is effective in care management and knows whom to call for questions/concerns
Patient will express satisfaction with hospice support received and will experience increased comfort
Patient will be made comfortable at home through death in accordance with the patient's wishes
Patient verbalizes the effectiveness of pain and symptom control
Patient verbalizes understanding of and adheres to care and medication regimens
Patient and caregiver supported through patient's death
Comfort maintained throughout course of care
The patient and family receive hospice support and care, and family members and friends are able to spend quality time with the patient

Caregiver able and verbalizes comfort with role and lists when to call
hospice team members

Patient supported through and receives the maximum benefit from palliative chemotherapy and radiation with minimal complications

Patient/caregiver lists adverse reactions, potential complications, signs/
symptoms of infection (e.g., sputum change, chest congestion)

Comfort maintained through death with dignity

Pain effectively managed, and patient verbalizes comfort at
_____ on 0-10 scale

Patient has stable respiratory status with patent airway (e.g., no dyspnea,
infection free)

Patient protected from injury, stable respiratory status, and compliant with
medication, safety, and care regimens

Comfort and individualized intervention of patient with immobility/
bed-bound status (e.g., skin, urinary, musculature, vascular)

Spiritual and psychosocial needs met (specify) as defined by patient and
caregiver throughout course of care

Successful pain and symptom management as verbalized by patient/
caregiver

Patient will demonstrate adequate breathing patterns as evidenced by a lack
of respiratory distress symptoms

Patient will be comfortable through illness

Patient/caregiver will demonstrate _____ % compliance with
instructions related to care

Patient and caregiver demonstrate and practice effective hand washing and
other infection-control measures (specify: e.g., disposal of waste, cleaning of linens)

Adherence to POC by patient and caregivers, and able to demonstrate safe
and supportive care

Planned and effective bowel program, as evidenced by regular bowel
movements and patient/family report of comfort

Death with dignity, and symptoms controlled in setting of patient/family
choice

Optimal comfort, support, and dignity provided throughout illness

Death with maximum comfort through effective symptom control with specialized hospice support

Patient and caregiver able to list adverse drug reactions/problems with
medication regimen and whom to call for follow-up and resolution

Pain and symptoms managed/controlled in setting of patient/family choice
(e.g., patient/family report ability to eat, sleep, speak more clearly with
pacing, other intervention)

Patient's/family's privacy, independence, and choices supported with
respect and maintained through death

Enhancement and support of quality of life

Effective symptom relief and control (e.g., a peaceful and comfortable
death at home, some enjoyment of life)

Maximizing the patient's quality of life (e.g., alert and pain free/or as
patient wishes)

Pharmacological and nonpharmacological interventions such as localized
heat application, positioning, relaxation methods, and music

Patient cared for and family supported through death with physical, psychosocial, spiritual, and other concerns/needs acknowledged/addressed

Patient and family-centered hospice care provided based on the patient's/family's unique situation and needs

Infection control and palliation through death

Grief/bereavement expression and support provided

Caregiver demonstrates ability to manage pain, where applicable

Patient maintains comfort and dignity throughout illness

Patient rates pain as _____ to _____ on pain scale by next visit 0-10

Patient's catheter will remain patent and infection free

Patient and caregiver adhere to/demonstrate compliance with multiple medication regimens (e.g., times, storage, refrigeration)

Patient's and family's educational and support needs met as verbalized by caregiver and adherence to plan

Death with maximum comfort through effective symptom control and specialized hospice support

Symptoms controlled in setting of patient/family choice

Effective pain relief and control (e.g., a peaceful and comfortable death)

Patient cared for and family supported through death with physical, psychosocial, spiritual, and other needs acknowledged/addressed

Patient- and family-centered hospice care provided based on the patient/family's unique situation and needs

Infection control and palliation

- *Home health aide or certified nursing assistant*
  Effective and safe personal care and hygiene maintained
  Safe ADL assistance and ambulation
  Safe environment maintained
  Hygiene and comfort maintained
  Adequate nutritional support and sleep

- *Hospice social worker*
  Patient/caregiver able to cope adaptively with illness and death
  Identification and addressing/resolution of problems impeding the successful implementation of the POC
  Adaptive adjustment to changed body and body image
  Psychosocial support and counseling offered/initiated to patient and caregivers experiencing grieving process
  Resources identified, community linkage to appropriate patient/family

- *Volunteer(s)*
  Comfort, companionship, and friendship extended to patient/family
  Patient and caregiver support provided as defined by needs of patient and caregiver
  Support and respite provided as defined by the patient/caregiver

- *Spiritual counselor*
  Spiritual support offered and provided to patient, family, and caregivers
  Patient and family express a relief of symptom of spiritual suffering
  Provision of spiritual support and care as based on the assessed and ongoing needs of the patient and family

Intervention and support provided related to that dimension of life related to life's meaning (consistent with patient's beliefs)

Participation in sacred or spiritual rituals or practices

Others, based on the patient's/family's unique beliefs and needs

- *Dietitian/nutritional counseling*

  Caregiver integrating recommendations into daily meal planning and prepares safe meals

  Nutrition and hydration optimal for patient with difficulty eating and lack of smell contributing to anorexia

  Nutrition and hydration optimal for patient

  Patient eating foods and supplements of recommended consistency

  Patient and caregiver know whom to call for nutrition-related questions/concerns

  Patient and family verbalize comprehension of changing nutritional needs

- *Occupational therapist*

  ADL level maintained at patient's optimal level

  Optimal functional, safe mobility maintained

  Patient using adaptive devices

  Quality of life improved through assistive/adaptive devices and energy-conservation techniques

  Patient and caregiver demonstrate ADL program for maximum safety and independence

  Patient and caregiver apply principles of energy conservation to daily activities and mobility

  Patient and caregiver demonstrate safe and effective use of assistive devices to increase functioning

  Patient and caregiver demonstrate effective use of energy conservation

  Verbalization/demonstration of improved functional activity level and enhanced quality of life

  Patient and caregiver demonstrate effective use of diaphragmatic breathing to reduce shortness of breath and relaxation techniques to help in pain/symptom management

- *Physical therapist*

  Patient performs home exercise regimen taught and has _____ % increase in mobility/function/strength

  Maintenance of balance, mobility, and endurance as verbalized and demonstrated by patient

  Prevention of complications

  Safety in mobility and transfers

- *Speech-language pathologist*

  Safe swallowing and functional communication

  Swallowing improved as verbalized by patient or caregiver

  Recommended food textures list for safety and patient choice

- *Bereavement counselor*

  Support services related to grief provided to patient and family

  Well-being and resolution process of grief initiated and followed through bereavement services

- *Pharmacist*

  Multiple medication regimens reviewed for food/drug and drug/drug interactions and problems

  Infusion medications and blood-level lab reports reviewed for therapeutic dosage and safe, effective patient response and reported to physician

  Stability and safety in complex multiple medication regimens

  Effective pain control and symptom management as reported by patient or caregiver

- *Music, massage, art, or other therapies or other services*

  Therapeutic massage/touch effective for patient as self-reported or observed by caregivers/family

  Improve muscle tone, relaxation, and/or sleep

  Patient comfortable and relaxed (e.g., sleeping) after massage

  Music therapy intervention based on assessment to decrease pain perception, provide emotional expression and support

  Maintenance of comfort and physical, psychosocial, and spiritual health

  Holistic health maintained and comfort achieved through _____ (specify modality)

  Patient has pet's presence as desired—in all care sites, when possible

8. **Patient, family, and caregiver educational needs**

   Educational needs are the care regimens that contribute to safe and effective care at home between the hospice team's visits. These include the following:

   The basic tenets of hospice and the availability of support 24 hours a day, 7 days a week

   Home safety assessment and counseling

   The patient's medication regimen

   Safe and proper body mechanics to promote patient comfort and prevent caregiver safety problems

   Other teaching specific to the patient's and family's unique needs

   Support groups available to patient's family, such as the hospice program's "Caregiver Support Group" meetings for family members and friends of the patient

   Anticipated disease progression

   Symptom management

   The importance of optimal nutrition and hydration

   Standard precautions protocol

   Home safety concerns, issues, and teaching

   The avoidance of infection, whenever possible

   The importance of medical follow-up

   Support groups in the community available to the patient, caregiver, and family

   Other information based on the patient's/family's unique needs

9. **Specific tips for quality and reimbursement**

   Unless the patient is in a hospice insurance program, some insurers will not pay for a skilled nurse visit that is made at death if the patient is dead when the nurse arrives at the home. From a Medicare home care perspective, the visit at the time of death may be covered when the orders and clinical record document assessment of the patient's status and signs of death/life or state law allows pronouncement of death by a nurse.

Document any variances to expected outcomes. Many models of hospice programs exist. Those that are home health agency based must work within the framework of the Medicare home care program. For example, sometimes a hospice patient reaches a stable period in the illness and has no further skilled needs or the patient is no longer homebound per Medicare home health care criteria. When this occurs, one option is to discharge the patient from Medicare home health agency reimbursement and maintain the patient on grant funds or other available resources. If the patient's status deteriorates and again meets the Medicare criteria, a new start of care is initiated on the HCFA form 485. Usually hospices continue volunteer support, nursing, and other services indicated during these periods of no reimbursement.

The Medicare hospice benefit does not require that the patient be home-bound or have identified skilled needs. Though it is a needed and viable program, the Medicare hospice benefit may not be indicated for all Medicare eligible beneficiaries. For further information on this benefit, please refer to HCFA Hospice Manual 21.

Should the patient's status deteriorate and necessitate increased personal care, obtain a telephone order for the increased service, noting frequency and estimating the duration.

Obtain a telephone order for all medication and treatment changes of the medical regimen and document these in the clinical record.

Document patient deterioration

Document dehydration, dehydrating

Document patient change or instability

Document pain, other symptoms not controlled

Document status after acute episode of _____ (specify)

Document positive urine, sputum, etc. culture; patient started on (specify ordered antibiotic therapy)

Document patient impacted; impaction removed manually

Document RN in frequent communication with physician regarding (specify)

Document febrile at _____, pulse change at _____, irr., irr.

Document change noted in _____

Document bony prominences red, opening

Document RN contacted physician regarding _____ (specify)

Document marked SOB

Document alteration in mental status

Document medications being adjusted, regulated, or monitored

Document unable to perform ADLs, maintain personal care

Document all interdisciplinary team meetings and communications in the POC and progress notes of the clinical record

All team members involved should have input into the hospice POC and document their interventions and goals

Document in the clinical notes the clear progression and symptomatology and interventions that demonstrate caring for a patient with terminal cancer

Document when/if the patient has respiratory changes, shortness of breath, exacerbation of conditions, dysphagia, pain, and other symptoms and that they are identified and resolved

Remember that the clinical documentation is key to measuring ongoing compliance for quality and reimbursement purposes. Care coordination, timely verbal and initial physician orders, and assessment and addressing of spiritual and psychosocial needs should be clearly documented in the patient's clinical record

The documentation should support that all hospice care supports comfort and dignity while meeting patient/family needs

The documentation should include the ongoing assessment and management of pain and other symptoms and the anticipation and prevention of secondary symptoms such as constipation

It is important to note that all team members, including nurses and social workers, should assess, identify, and "hear" spiritual needs that the patient/family want to be addressed. These spiritual issues are key to the provision of high-quality hospice care and cannot be addressed effectively and promptly by the spiritual counselor only

Document clearly symptoms, clinical changes, and assessment findings that support the end stage of the disease process.

Document patient changes, symptoms, and clinical information identified from visits and team conferences that supports hospice care and a limited life expectancy

Clearly support in the documentation the rationale that supports or explains the progression of the illness from the chronic to terminal stages

Document mentation, behavioral, and cognitive changes.

Document dysphagia, weight loss, increased shortness of breath, dyspnea, infection, sepsis, new or changed medications, etc.

Document any skin changes (e.g., inflamed, painful, weeping skin site[s])

Document when the patient is actively dying, deteriorating, or progressing toward death

Remember that the "litmus test" of care coordination rests on the quality of the clinical documentation completed by all team members. Review one of your patient's clinical records, and ask yourself the following: "If I was unable to give a verbal report/update on this patient, would a peer be able to pick up and provide the same level of care and know (from the documentation) the current orders, including specific medications and other details that contribute to effective hospice care?"

Document/report any variance to expected outcomes

Obtain a telephone order for any change in the POC, including changes in the frequency of the visits, medications, services provided, and concurrence of other team members

Document your care and the patient's response to your care interventions

Document the patient's problems or changes in status, especially an exacerbation of symptoms

Document increased sputum production, coughing, SOB, pain, diarrhea, or any change in the patient's mental status

Document patient deterioration and improvements

Document blood results, cultures, and treatments

Consider patient for case management or clinical path protocol

Consider AIDS nurse or clinical specialist for consultation and review of POC

Document any increase in temperature or other objective signs that could
signal a pending infection

Document the specific teaching provided and response to teaching

Document coordination of services or consultation with other members of the
IDG

For this and other noncancer diagnoses, document clearly the symptoms and
clinical and assessment findings that support the end stage of the chronic
illness process.

Document patient changes, symptoms, and clinical information identified
from visits and team conferences that support hospice care and limited
life expectancy

10. **Resources for hospice care and practice**
    - Nutrition in AIDS Care (American Dietetic Association) 1-800-366-1655
    - People with AIDS Coalition 1-800-828-3280
    - The CDC National AIDS Clearinghouse has a free resource catalog and a
      35-page booklet entitled *Caring for Someone with AIDS at Home,* which
      has sections about symptoms in the final stages, hospice care, final ar-
      rangements, and dying at home. This can be ordered free by calling
      1-800-458-5231.
    - Another helpful resource is the NHO's second edition of *Medical Guide-
      lines for Determining Prognoses in Selected Non-Cancer Diseases.* Call
      NHO at 1-800-646-6460 for more information.
    - A helpful drug resource is *Pharmacological Treatment of AIDS,* by Kirk
      Ryan, Pharm.D. It can be accessed at www.creative.net/~Kirkryan.
    - *Positively Aware* is a publication that provides information and support to
      anyone concerned with AIDS and HIV issues. For information, call (773)
      404-8726.

ALZHEIMER'S DISEASE AND OTHER DEMENTIAS CARE

1. General considerations

As increasing numbers of elderly patients are cared for by their families or other caregivers in the home, the presence of Alzheimer's disease and other problems characterized by confusion has risen dramatically. According to the National Institute on Aging, Alzheimer's disease alone currently affects an estimated 4 million Americans. The skills of the hospice team are important to the safety and care of these patients and their families. Patients with Alzheimer's disease and other dementias may be appropriate candidates for hospice care when patients and their families face the final stages. Compassion and care are then directed toward comfort and support of the patient and family or caregivers.

2. Needs for visit

Physician order for hospice care, specific to the hospice program's admission criteria and policies
Standard precautions supplies
Vital signs equipment for baseline assessment
Other supplies or equipment, based on physician orders

3. Safety considerations

Infection control/standard precautions
Night-light
Removal of scatter rugs
Tub rail, grab bars for bathroom safety
Supportive and nonskid shoes
Wandering precautions
Smoking with supervision only
Handrail on stairs
Fall precautions
Protective skin measures
Stairway precautions
Smoke detector and fire evacuation plan
Assistance with ambulation
Supervised care and medication regimen
Others, based on the patient's unique condition and environment

4. Potential diagnoses and codes

AIDS dementia	042 and 294.1
Alzheimer's disease	331.0
Amyotrophic lateral sclerosis	335.20
Anxiety state	300.00
Aphasia	784.3
Atherosclerosis	440.9
Bladder incontinence	788.30

Constipation	564.0
Creutzfeldt-Jakob disease and dementia	046.1 and 294.1
CVA	436
Dehydration	276.5
Dementia	331.0 and 294.1
Depressive disorder	311
Depressive psychosis	296.20
Huntington's chorea	333.4
Korsakoff's dementia	294.0
Multiple sclerosis	340
Nonpsychotic brain syndrome	310.9
Organic brain syndrome	310.9
Parkinson's disease	332.0
Pernicious anemia	281.0
Pneumonia	486
Presenile dementia	290.10
Pressure (decubitus) ulcer	707.0
Psychosis	294.9
Senile dementia	290.0
Subdural hematoma (nontraumatic)	432.1
Subdural hematoma (traumatic)	852.20
Transient ischemic attack (TIA)	435.9
Unipolar affective disorder	296.99
Urinary incontinence	788.30
Urinary tract infections	599.0

5. **Associated nursing diagnoses**
   Airway clearance, ineffective
   Anxiety
   Bowel incontinence
   Caregiver role strain
   Caregiver role strain, risk for
   Communication, impaired verbal
   Confusion, chronic
   Constipation
   Coping, ineffective family: compromised
   Coping, ineffective, individual
   Diarrhea
   Environmental interpretation syndrome, impaired
   Fatigue
   Fear
   Health maintenance, altered
   Home maintenance management, impaired
   Hopelessness
   Infection, risk for
   Injury, risk for
   Knowledge deficit (related to self-care management)
   Loneliness, risk for
   Memory, impaired
   Mobility, impaired physical

Nutrition, altered: less than body requirements
Personal identity disturbance
Powerlessness
Self-care deficit, bathing/hygiene
Self-care deficit, dressing/grooming
Self-care deficit, feeding
Self-care deficit, toileting
Sensory/perceptual alterations (specify)
Skin integrity, impaired, risk for
Sleep pattern disturbance
Social interaction, impaired
Spiritual distress (distress of the human spirit)
Spiritual well-being, potential for enhanced
Swallowing, impaired
Thought processes, altered
Trauma, risk for
Urinary elimination, altered
Violence, risk for: self-directed or directed at others

6. **Skills and services identified**

   • *Hospice nursing*

      a. *Comfort and symptom control*
         Complete initial assessment of all systems of patient with Alzheimer's
            admitted to hospice for _____ (specify problem necessi-
            tating care)
         Presentation of hospice philosophy and services
         Explain patient rights and responsibilities
         Assess patient, family, and caregiver wishes and expectations regarding
            care
         Assess patient, family, and caregiver resources available for care
         Provision of volunteer support to patient and family
         Teach family or caregiver physical care of patient
         Assess pain and other symptoms, including site, duration, characteris-
            tics, and relief measures
         Skilled assessment of the patient with dementia and support/coping
            skills of family and caregiver
         Skilled observation and assessment of all systems
         Teach family and caregivers about disease and management
         Comfort measures of backrub and hand or other therapeutic massage
         Assess pain or other problems/complaints
         Assess pain, and evaluate the pain management's effectiveness
         Measure vital signs, including pain, q visit
         Assess cardiovascular, pulmonary, and respiratory status
         Teach new pain and symptom control medication regimen
         Teach caregivers symptom control and relief measures
         RN to assess patient's pain or other symptoms q visit to identify need
            for change, addition, or other plan or dose adjustment
         RN to provide and teach effective oral care and comfort measures
         Identify and monitor pain, symptoms, and relief measures

Teach caregiver or family care of weak, terminally ill patient

RN to instruct in pain control measures and medications

Teach patient and family about realistic expectations of disease process

Teach care of dying and identification of signs/symptoms of impending death

Presence and support

Other interventions, based on patient/family needs

b. *Safety and mobility considerations*

Provide caregiver with home safety information and instruction related to _____ and documented in the clinical record

Teach family regarding importance of observation of patient's safety

Teach family regarding safety of patient in home

Teach family regarding energy conservation techniques

Other interventions, based on patient/family needs

c. *Emotional/spiritual considerations*

Psychosocial assessment of patient and family regarding disease and prognosis

Provide emotional support to patient and family

Spiritual counseling/support offered to patients and caregivers who are verbalizing the reason for or meaning of suffering

Assess mental status and sleep disturbance changes

Other interventions, based on patient/family needs

d. *Skin care*

Observation of skin and patient's physical status

Teach caregiver regarding skin care needs, including the need for frequent position changes, appropriate pressure pads and mattresses, and the prevention of breakdown

Pressure ulcer care as indicated

Assess skin integrity

Observation and evaluation of wound and surrounding skin

Evaluate patient's need for equipment, supplies to decrease pressure, alternating pressure mattress, gel foam seat cushion, and heel and elbow protectors

Teach family to perform dressing between RN visits, specifically

Teach patient, family, or caregiver about proper body alignment and positioning in bed to prevent skin tears from shearing skin

Observe and apply skilled assessment of areas for possible breakdown, including heels, hips, elbows, ankles, and other pressure-prone areas

Other interventions, based on patient/family needs

e. *Elimination considerations*

Assess bowel regimen, and implement program as needed

Implement and monitor bowel regimen, and teach program to family

Observation and evaluation of bladder elimination habits and management of incontinence, and assess need for indwelling catheter

Check for and remove impaction as needed

Condom catheter or indwelling catheter as indicated

Teach catheter care to caregiver

RN to teach caregiver daily catheter care

RN to evaluate the patient's bowel patterns and need for stool softeners, laxatives, and dietary adjustments and develop bowel management plan

Assess amount and frequency of urinary output

Other interventions, based on patient/family needs

f. *Hydration/nutrition*

Encourage hand-held foods to encourage self-feeding (e.g., sandwiches, cookies)

Monitor hydration and nutrition intake

Assess nutrition and hydration status

Diet counseling for patient with anorexia

Nutrition/hydration supported by offering patient's choice of favorite or desired foods or liquids

Nutrition/hydration to be maintained by offering patient high-protein diet and foods of choice as tolerated

Teach feeding-tube care to family

Teach patient and family to expect decreased nutritional and fluid intake as disease progresses

Other interventions, based on patient/family needs

g. *Therapeutic/medication regimens*

Medication management to monitor antipsychotic behavior and other effects of therapy and/or interactions

RN monitor effects of tranquilizers given for severe agitation/anxiety

Evaluate for weight loss, weigh patient q visit, and record weights

Monitor patient's BP and compliance with medication regimen

RN to assess the patient's unique response to treatments or interventions, and report changes or unfavorable responses or reactions to the physician

Medication assessment and management

Obtain venipuncture and lab results as ordered q _____ (ordered frequency)

Teach patient and family about new medications and effects

Assess for electrolyte imbalance

Nonpharmacological interventions such as progressive muscle relaxation, imagery, positive visualization, music, massage and touch, and humor therapy of patient's choice implemented

Other interventions, based on patient/family needs

h. *Other considerations*

Assist family in setting up patient-centered routine and stress the importance of adhering to the routine once established

Assess progression of disease process

RN to assess the patient's response to treatments and interventions and to report changes, unfavorable responses, and reactions to physician

Other interventions, based on patient/family needs

- *Home health aide or certified nursing assistant*
  Effective and safe personal care
  Safe ADL assistance and support, ambulation and transfers
  Respite care

Observation and reporting
Meal preparation
Homemaker services
Comfort care
Other duties

- *Hospice social worker*
  Caregiver role strain necessitating respite/relief measures/support
  Psychosocial assessment of patient and family/caregiver, including adjustment to illness and its implications and the need for care
  Identification of optimal coping strategies
  Financial assessment and counseling regarding food acquisition, ability to prepare, and costs of needed medications
  Intervention/support related to terminal illness and loss
  Emotional/spiritual support
  Facilitate communication among patient, family, and hospice team
  Identification of optimal coping strategies
  Referral/linkage to community services and resources as indicated
  Grief counseling and intervention/support related to illness/loss
  Patient/caregiver counseling and support
  Identification of illness-related psychiatric condition necessitating care

- *Volunteer(s)*
  Support, friendship, companionship, and presence
  Errands and transportation
  Other services, based on interdisciplinary team recommendations and patient/caregiver needs

- *Spiritual counselor*
  Spiritual assessment and care
  Counseling, intervention, and support related to that dimension of life related to life's meaning (consistent with patient's beliefs)
  Support, listening, and presence
  Participation in sacred or spiritual rituals or practices
  Other supportive care, based on patient/family needs and belief systems

- *Dietitian/nutritional counseling*
  Assessment of patient with decreased caloric intake, weight loss, anorexia, and nausea
  Assessment and recommendations for swallowing difficulties
  Teaching and support of family members and caregivers
  Support and care with food and nourishment as desired by patient
  Assessment of family's view of benefits/burdens of tube feeding to prolong life

- *Occupational therapist*
  Evaluation of ADL and functional mobility
  Assess for need for adaptive equipment and assistive devices
  Safety assessment of patient's environment and ADL
  Assessment for energy conservation training
  Assessment of upper extremity function, retraining motor skills and/or splinting for contracture(s)

- *Physical therapy*

    Evaluation

    Safety assessment of patient's environment

    Instruct and supervise caregivers and volunteers on home exercise program/
    ROM and safe transfers

- *Bereavement counselor*

    Assessment of the needs of the bereaved family and friends

    Support and intervention, based on assessment and ongoing findings

    Presence and counseling

    Supportive visits and follow-up, other interventions (e.g., mailings, calls,
    etc.)

    Services related to bereavement work and support

- *Music, massage, art, or other therapies or services*

    Evaluation and intervention based on patient's and caregiver's unique
    wishes and needs that support care, comfort, and death in the setting of
    the patient's choice

    Pet therapy (including patient's pet, if available) and therapeutic interven-
    tion

    Assessment plan to engage patient and support comfort, quality, enjoyment,
    and dignity

7. **Outcomes for care**

- *Hospice nursing*

    Patient/caregiver verbalizes satisfaction with care

    Educational tools/plans incorporated in daily care, and patient/caregiver
    verbalizes understanding of safe, needed care

    Patient will decide on care, interventions, and evaluation

    Caregiver effective in care management and knows whom to call for
    questions/concerns

    Patient will express satisfaction with hospice support received and will ex-
    perience increased comfort

    Patient will be made comfortable at home through death in accordance
    with the patient's wishes

    Effective pain control and symptom control verbalized by patient

    Patient verbalizes understanding of and adheres to care and medication
    regimens

    Patient and caregiver supported through patient's death

    Comfort maintained through course of care

    The patient and family receive hospice support and care, and family
    members and friends are able to spend quality time with the patient

    Caregiver able and verbalizes comfort with role and lists when to call
    hospice team members

    Patient supported through and receives the maximum benefit from pallia-
    tive chemotherapy and radiation with minimal complications

    Patient and caregiver list adverse reactions, potential complications, signs/
    symptoms of infection (e.g., sputum change, chest congestion)

    Comfort maintained through death with dignity

Pain effectively managed, and patient verbalizes comfort

Patient has stable respiratory status with patent airway (e.g., no dyspnea, infection free)

Comfort and individualized intervention of patient with immobility/bedbound status (e.g., skin, urinary, musculature, vascular)

Spiritual and psychosocial needs met (specify) as defined by patient and caregiver throughout course of care

Teaching program related to the prevention of infection and injuries demonstrated by caregivers

Family and caregivers taught and supported regarding the need for a safe, consistent, and nurturing physical environment

Caregivers demonstrate information taught, including the role of reassurance and consistency in activities and schedules

Patient will be comfortable; caregiver reports no or decreased fear, anxiety, and frustration

Patient and caregiver will demonstrate _____ % compliance with instructions related to care

Patient and caregiver demonstrate and practice effective hand washing and other infection control measures (specify, e.g., disposal of waste, cleaning linens)

Adherence to POC by patient and caregivers, and able to demonstrate safe and supportive care

Nutritional needs maintained/addressed as evidenced by patient's weight maintained/increased by _____ lbs.

Patient will be maintained in home with caregiver stating/demonstrating adherence to POC

Adherence to medication regimen

Caregiver and family taught to care for patient as demonstrated by observation/interviews

Patient's daily, consistent routine maintained as noted in caregiver log/notes

Family and caregiver integrate information and care regarding implications of disease and terminal nature

Death with dignity and symptoms controlled in setting of patient/family choice

Death with maximum comfort through effective symptom control with specialized hospice support

Symptoms controlled in setting of patient/family choice

Effective pain relief and control (e.g., a peaceful and comfortable death)

Maximizing the patient's quality of life (e.g., patient is alert and pain free)

Pharmacological and nonpharmacological interventions such as localized heat application, positioning, relaxation methods, music and others

Patient cared for and family supported through death with physical, psychosocial, spiritual, and other needs acknowledged/addressed

Patient and family-centered hospice care provided based on the patient/family unique situation and needs

Infection control and palliation through death

Patient states pain is at _____ on 0-10 scale by next visit

- *Home health aide or certified nursing assistant*
  Effective and safe hygiene, personal care, and comfort
  ADL assistance
  Safe environment maintained

- *Hospice social worker*
  Psychosocial support and counseling provided
  Financial/access problems addressed, resources identified as demonstrated
    by food in the refrigerator and medication availability to patient per
    POC
  Linkage with community services, support groups, and other resources
  Referral of patient and caregiver to _____ (specify)
  Adjustment to long-term implications of disease as stated in plan for con-
    tinued care by RN and MSS
  Caregiver able to demonstrate/verbalize effective coping skills
  Resources identified, community linkage as appropriate for patient/family

- *Volunteer(s)*
  Patient and caregiver support provided as defined by needs of patient and
    caregiver
  Support, friendship, companionship, presence
  Comfort and dignity maintained/provided to patient and family

- *Spiritual counselor*
  Intervention and support provided related to that dimension of life related
    to life's meaning (consistent with patient's beliefs)
  Spiritual support offered and provided as defined by needs of patient/
    caregiver
  Provision of spiritual support and care as based on the assessed and
    ongoing needs of the patient and family
  Support, listening, and presence
  Spiritual support offered, and patient and family needs met
  Participation in sacred or spiritual rituals or practices
  Patient/family express a relief of symptoms of spiritual suffering
  Other outcomes, based on the patient's/family's unique beliefs and needs

- *Dietitian/nutritional counseling*
  Family and caregiver integrate recommendations into nutrition teaching
    (where appropriate)
  Patient and caregiver know whom to call for nutrition- and hydration-
    related questions/concerns
  Patient and family verbalize comprehension of nutritional needs

- *Occupational therapist*
  Maximize independence in ADLs for patient/caregiver
  Optimal function maintained/attained
  Patient and caregiver demonstrates ADL program for maximum safety

- *Physical therapist*
  Safe ambulation, transfers
  Home exercise program supports optimal function/mobility

- *Bereavement counselor*
  Grief support services provided to patient and family
  Well-being and resolution process of grief initiated and followed through
    bereavement services

- *Music, massage, art, or other therapies or services*
  Therapeutic massage/touch effective for patient as self-reported or observed
    by caregivers/family
  Improved muscle tone, relaxation, and/or sleep
  Patient comfortable and relaxed (e.g., sleeping) after massage
  Music therapy intervention based on assessment to decrease pain percep-
    tion, provide emotional expression and support
  Maintenance of comfort, physical, psychosocial, and spiritual health
  Patient has pet's presence as desired—in all care sites, when possible
  Holistic health maintained and comfort achieved through _____
    (specify modality)

8. **Patient, family and caregiver educational needs**
   Educational needs are the care regimens that contribute to safe and effec-
   tive care at home between the hospice team's visits. These include the fol-
   lowing:
   The basic tenets of hospice and the availability of support 24 hours a day, 7
     days a week
   Home safety assessment and counseling
   The patient's medication regimen
   Safe and proper body mechanics to promote patient comfort and prevent
     caregiver safety problems
   Other teaching specific to the patient's and family's unique needs
   Support groups available to patient's family, such as the hospice program's
     "Caregiver Support Group" meetings for family members and friends of
     the patient
   Home safety concerns, issues, and teaching
   The prevention of infection/skin problems by regularly inspecting patient's
     skin
   Multiple medications and their relationship to each other
   The importance of maintaining the patient's daily, consistent routines, when
     possible
   Anticipated disease progression

9. **Specific tips for quality and reimbursement**
   For this and other noncancer diagnoses, document clearly the symptoms and
     clinical and assessment findings that support the end stage of the chronic
     illness process
   Document patient changes, symptoms, and clinical information identified
     from visits and team conferences that supports hospice care and limited
     life expectancy
   Clearly support in the documentation the rationale that supports/explains the
     progression of the illness from the chronic to terminal stages
   Document mentation, behavioral, and cognitive changes

Document dysphagia, weight loss, increased shortness of breath, dyspnea, infection, sepsis, and new or changed medications, etc.

Document skin changes (e.g., inflamed, painful, weeping skin site[s])

Document coordination of services and consultation with other members of the IDG

Unless the patient is in a hospice insurance program, some insurers will not pay for a skilled nurse visit that is made at death if the patient is dead when the nurse arrives at the home. From a Medicare home care perspective, the visit at the time of death may be covered when the orders and clinical record document assessment of the patient's status and signs of death/life or state law allows pronouncement of death by a nurse.

Document any variances to expected outcomes. There are many models of hospice programs. Those that are home health agency based must work within the framework of the Medicare home care program. For example, sometimes a hospice patient reaches a stable period in the illness and has no further skilled needs or the patient is no longer homebound per Medicare home health care criteria. When this occurs, one option is to discharge the patient from Medicare home health agency reimbursement and maintain the patient on grant funds or other available resources. If the patient's status deteriorates and again meets the Medicare criteria, a new start of care is initiated on the HCFA form 485. Usually hospices continue volunteer support, nursing, and other services indicated during these periods of no reimbursement.

The Medicare hospice benefit does not require that the patient be homebound or have identified skilled needs. Though it is a needed and viable program, the Medicare hospice benefit may not be indicated for all Medicare-eligible beneficiaries. For further information on this benefit, please refer to HCFA Hospice Manual 21.

Should the patient's status deteriorate and increased personal care be needed, obtain a telephone order for the increased service, noting frequency and estimating the duration.

Obtain a telephone order for all medication and treatment changes of the medical regimen and document these in the clinical record.

Document patient deterioration

Document dehydration, dehydrating

Document patient change or instability

Document pain, other symptoms not controlled

Document status after acute episode of _____ (specify)

Document positive urine, sputum, etc. culture; patient started on _____ (specify ordered antibiotic therapy)

Document patient impacted; impaction removed manually

Document RN in frequent communication with physician regarding _____ (specify)

Document febrile at _____, pulse change at _____, irr., irr.

Document change noted in _____

Document bony prominences red, opening

Document RN contacted physician regarding _____ (specify)

Document marked SOB

Document alteration in mental status

Document medications being adjusted, regulated, or monitored

Document unable to ADLs, personal care

Document all interdisciplinary team meetings and communications in the
POC and in the progress notes of the clinical record

All team members should have input into the POC and document their interventions and goals

10. **Resources for hospice care and practice**

The book *The 36-Hour Day*, by Nancy L. Mace and Peter V. Rabins, MD,
addresses all aspects of the difficulties encountered by families and friends as
they care for their loved ones with Alzheimer's disease or other dementias.
Call 800-537-5487.

In addition, the National Institute of Health, National Institute on Aging,
has an Alzheimer's Disease Education and Referral Center. This center has
information such as home safety booklets available to both professionals and
families caring for patients with dementias. Its number is 1-800-438-4380.

Another helpful resource is the NHO's second edition of *Medical Guidelines for Determining Prognoses in Selected Non-Cancer Diseases.* Call NHO
at 800-646-6460 for more information.

The American Hospice Foundation offers a pamphlet entitled *Alzheimer's
Disease and Hospice* that can be obtained by calling (202) 223-0204 or
writing to American Hospice Foundation, 1130 Connecticut Avenue NW,
Suite 700, Washington, DC 20036-4101.

The Alzheimer's Association has created fact sheets entitled "Ethical Considerations" to assist with ethical questions that may occur when caring for
individuals with Alzheimer's disease. "Issues in Death and Dying" and
"Issues of Diagnostic Disclosure" are available free by calling (800) 272-
3900.

AMYOTROPHIC LATERAL SCLEROSIS (ALS) AND OTHER NEUROMUSCULAR CARE

1. **General considerations**

   Amyotrophic lateral sclerosis (ALS) is usually known as *Lou Gehrig's disease*. This rare neurological disease occurs usually between 40 and 70 years of age and affects twice as many men as women. Unfortunately, the prognosis is poor with this disease, with patients progressively degenerating toward respiratory failure.

2. **Needs for visit**

   Physician order for hospice care, specific to the hospice program's admission criteria and policies

   Standard precautions supplies

   Vital signs equipment for baseline assessment

   Other supplies or equipment based on physician orders

3. **Safety considerations**

   Infection control/standard precautions

   Night-light

   Removal of scatter rugs

   Tub rail, grab bars for bathroom safety

   Oxygen precautions (if ordered)

   Supportive and nonskid shoes

   Handrail on stairs

   Fall precautions

   Identification and reporting of any skin problems

   Smoke detector and fire evacuation plan

   Assistance with ambulation

   Others, based on the patient's unique condition and environment

4. **Potential diagnoses and codes**

Amyotrophic lateral sclerosis	335.20
Dysarthria	784.5
Dysphagia	787.2
Joint contracture	718.49
Muscular dystrophy	359.1
Multiple sclerosis	340
Parkinson's disease	332.0
Seizure disorder	780.3

5. **Associated nursing diagnoses**

   Airway clearance, ineffective

   Anxiety

   Aspiration, risk for

   Body image disturbance

   Bowel incontinence

Breathing pattern, ineffective
Caregiver role strain
Caregiver role strain, risk for
Communication, impaired verbal
Constipation
Coping, ineffective family: compromised
Coping, ineffective family: disabling
Decisional conflict (ventilator and care)
Denial, ineffective
Diarrhea
Family processes, altered
Fatigue
Fear
Fluid volume deficit, risk for
Gas exchange, impaired
Grieving, anticipatory
Hopelessness
Infection, risk for
Injury, risk for
Knowledge deficit (care and disease)
Mobility, impaired physical
Nutrition, altered: less than body requirements
Parenting, altered
Powerlessness
Role performance, altered
Self-care deficit (specify)
Social interaction, impaired
Spiritual distress (distress of the human spirit)
Spiritual well-being, potential for enhanced
Swallowing, impaired
Urinary elimination, altered
Urinary retention
Ventilation, inability to sustain spontaneous

6. **Skills and services identified**

   • *Hospice nursing*

      a. *Comfort and symptom control*
         Complete initial assessment of all systems of patient with ALS admitted
            to hospice for _____ (specify problem necessitating care)
         Presentation of hospice philosophy and services
         Explain patient rights and responsibilities
         Assess patient, family, and caregiver wishes and expectations regarding
            care
         Assess patient, family, and caregiver resources available for care
         Provision of volunteer support to patient and family
         Teach family or caregiver physical care of patient
         Assess pain and other symptoms, including site, duration, characteris-
            tics, and relief measures
         RN to provide and teach effective oral care and comfort measures

RN to assess and observe all systems and symptoms q visit and report changes, new symptoms to physician

Care coordination, teaching related to mechanical/respiratory support devices, ventilator, suction, etc.

Observation with assessment of pain and other symptoms to be managed within parameters of disease process

Comfort measure provided to patient who is essentially bedbound and alert, including backrub, hand massage, and music of choice

Teach family and caregiver signs, changes to report to nurse and physician

Assess pain, and evaluate the pain management's effectiveness

Teach care of the bedridden patient

Measure vital signs, including pain, q visit

Assess cardiovascular, pulmonary, and respiratory status

Teach caregivers symptom control and relief measures

Teach caregiver or family care of weak, terminally ill patient

RN to assess patient's pain or other symptoms q visit to identify need for change, addition, or other plan or dose adjustment

Oxygen at _____ liters per _____ (specific physician orders)

RN to instruct in pain control measures and medications

Teach patient and family about realistic expectations of disease process

Teach care of dying, signs/symptoms of impending death

Presence and support

Other interventions, based on patient/family needs

b. *Safety and mobility considerations*

Provide patient with home safety information and instruction related to _____ and documented in the clinical record

Rehabilitation management related to safe bed mobility and transfers

Teach family regarding safety of patient in home

Teach patient and family regarding energy conservation techniques

Teach caregiver to observe for increased secretions, and teach safe suctioning when needed

Other interventions, based on patient/family needs

c. *Emotional/spiritual considerations*

Psychosocial assessment of patient and family regarding disease and prognosis

Provide emotional support to patient and family

Spiritual counseling/support offered to patients and caregivers who are verbalizing the reason for or meaning of suffering

Patient and family assisted through grieving process

Other interventions, based on patient/family needs

d. *Skin care*

Teaching and training of family and caregivers about skin care, positioning, and feeding regimens

Observation and evaluation of wound and surrounding skin

Assess skin and pressure-prone areas

Evaluate patient's need for equipment, supplies to decrease pressure, alternating pressure mattress, gel foam seat cushion, and heel and elbow protectors

Teach family to perform dressing between RN visits, specifically

_____

Teach patient and family or caregiver about proper body alignment and positioning in bed to prevent skin tears from shearing skin

Observe and apply skilled assessment of areas for possible breakdown, including heels, hips, elbows, ankles, and other pressure-prone areas

Teach caregiver about skin care needs, including the need for frequent position changes, pressure pads, appropriate mattresses, and the prevention of breakdown

Other interventions, based on patient/family needs

e. *Elimination considerations*

Assess bowel regimen, and implement program as needed

RN to change catheter every 4 weeks and 3 prn visits for catheter problems, including patient complaints, signs and symptoms of infection, and other factors necessitating evaluation and possible catheter change

Observation and complete systems assessment of the patient with an indwelling catheter

RN to monitor bowel and bladder function

Check for and remove impaction as needed

Condom catheter or indwelling catheter as indicated

RN to teach caregiver daily catheter care

RN to evaluate the patient's bowel patterns, need for stool softeners, laxatives, and dietary adjustments and develop bowel management plan

Other interventions, based on patient/family needs

f. *Hydration/nutrition*

Monitor patient who has nutritional supplements and water via NG/G tube daily

Assess nutrition and hydration status

Diet counseling for patient with anorexia

Nutrition/hydration provided by offering patient's choice of favorite or desired foods or liquids

Nutrition/hydration to be maintained by offering patient high-protein diet and foods of choice as tolerated

Teach feeding-tube care to family

Teach patient and family to expect decreased nutritional and fluid intake as disease progresses

Other interventions, based on patient/family needs

g. *Therapeutic/medication regimens*

Medication management of patient receiving morphine, antibiotic, muscle relaxant, and prednisone via NG/G tube

RN to assess the patient's unique response to treatments or interventions, and report changes or unfavorable responses or reactions to the physician

Teach new pain- and symptom-control medication regimen

Nonpharmacological interventions such as progressive muscle relaxation, imagery, positive visualization, music, massage and touch, and humor therapy of patient's choice implemented

Medication assessment and management

Other interventions, based on patient/family needs

h. *Other considerations*

Assess disease progression process

Comfort/safety through ongoing assessment related to swallowing and other changes

RN to assess the patient's response to treatments and interventions and to report to physician any changes, unfavorable responses, or reactions

Other interventions, based on patient/family needs

- *Home health aide or certified nursing assistant*

Effective and safe personal care

Safe ADL assistance and support

Observation and reporting

Respite care

Meal preparation

Homemaker services

Comfort care

Other duties

- *Hospice social worker*

Psychosocial assessment of patient and family/caregiver, including adjustment to illness and its implications and the need for care

Identification of optimal coping strategies

Financial assessment and counseling regarding food acquisition, ability to prepare, and costs of needed medications

Intervention/support related to terminal illness and loss

Emotional/spiritual support

Depression/fear assessed and addressed

Facilitate communication among patient, family, and hospice team

Identification of caregiver role strain necessitating respite/relief measures and support

Referral/linkage to community services and resources as indicated

Grief counseling and intervention/support related to illness/loss

Assessment/intervention related to depression and fear

Patient/caregiver counseling and support

For patients who live alone with no support system (e.g., able, available, willing caregiver[s]), obtain linkage with community resources to allow patient to remain in the home

Identification of illness-related psychiatric condition necessitating care

- *Volunteer(s)*

Support, friendship, companionship, and presence

Comfort and dignity maintained/provided for patient and family

Errands and transportation

Other services, based on interdisciplinary team recommendations and patient/caregiver needs

- *Spiritual counselor*
  Spiritual assessment and care
  Counseling, intervention, and support related to that dimension of life related to life's meaning (consistent with patient's beliefs)
  Support, listening, and presence
  Participation in sacred or spiritual rituals or practices
  Other supportive care, based on patient/family needs and belief systems

- *Dietitian/nutritional counseling*
  Assessment of patient with decreased intake, weight loss, anorexia, and nausea
  Assessment and recommendations for swallowing difficulties
  Teaching and support of family members and caregivers
  Support and care with soft foods and nourishment as desired by patient
  Evaluation of patient on G-tube or NG tube feedings and teach feeding safety techniques
  Monitoring and management of patient
  Teach caregiver regarding aspects of nutritional support system
  Evaluation/management of nutritional and fluid deficits and needs
  Encourage nutritional supplements and snacks to increase protein and caloric intake, as appropriate
  Food, dietary recommendations incorporating patient choice and wishes
  Care coordination with care team to decrease tube feeding near time of death to avoid choking, increased fluids, etc.

- *Occupational therapist*
  Evaluation of ADL and functional mobility
  Assess for need for adaptive equipment and assistive devices
  Safety assessment of patient's environment and ADL
  Assessment for energy conservation training
  Assessment of upper extremity function, retraining motor skills

- *Physical therapist*
  Evaluation
  Assessment of motor strength, presence of flaccidity or spasticity, contractures
  Safety assessment of patient and patient's environment
  Safe transfer training
  Strengthening exercises/program
  Assessment of gait safety
  Instruct/supervise caregiver and volunteers with regard to home exercise program for conditioning and strength
  Assistive, adaptive devices of equipment and teaching
  Assessment of upper body strength for trapeze or other methods to maintain function/bed mobility

- *Speech-language pathologist*
  Evaluation for speech/swallowing problems
  Teach communication techniques

- *Bereavement counselor*

  Assessment of the needs of the bereaved family and friends

  Support and intervention, based on assessment and ongoing findings

  Presence and counseling

  Supportive visits and follow-up and other interventions (e.g., mailings, calls)

  Services related to bereavement work and support

- *Music, massage, art, or other therapies or services*

  Evaluation and intervention based on patient's/caregiver's unique wishes and needs that support care and death in the setting of the patient's choice

  Therapeutic massage/touch effective for patient as self-reported or observed by caregivers/family

  Improved muscle tone, relaxation, and/or sleep

  Patient comfortable and relaxed (e.g., sleeping) after massage

  Music therapy intervention based on assessment to decrease pain perception, provide emotional expression and support

  Pet therapy (including patient's pet, if available) and therapeutic intervention

  Assessment plan to engage patient and support comfort, quality, enjoyment, and dignity

  Maintenance of comfort and physical, psychosocial, and spiritual health

  Holistic health maintained and comfort achieved through _____ (specify modality)

7. **Outcomes for care**

- *Hospice nursing*

  Patient will be comfortable and pain free through illness and death, and interdisciplinary team members will work together to improve/maintain patient's quality of life

  Patient/caregiver verbalizes satisfaction with care

  Educational tools/plans incorporated in daily care, and patient/caregiver verbalizes understanding of safe, needed care

  Patient will decide on care, interventions, and evaluation

  Caregiver effective in care management and knows whom to call for questions/concerns

  Patient will express satisfaction with hospice support received and will experience increased comfort

  Patient will be made comfortable at home through death in accordance with the patient's wishes

  Effective pain control and symptom control verbalized by patient

  Patient verbalizes understanding of and adheres to care and medication regimens

  Patient and caregiver supported through patient's death

  Comfort maintained through course of care

  The patient and family receive hospice support and care, and family members and friends are able to spend quality time with the patient

  Caregiver able and verbalizes comfort with role and lists when to call hospice team members

Patient or caregiver lists adverse reactions, potential complications, signs/symptoms of infection (e.g., sputum change, chest congestion)

Comfort maintained through death with dignity

Pain effectively managed, and patient verbalizes comfort

Patient has stable respiratory status with patent airway

Patient protected from injury, stable respiratory status, and compliant with medication, safety, and care regimens

Comfort and individualized intervention of patient with immobility/bedbound status (e.g., skin, urinary, musculature, vascular)

Spiritual and psychosocial needs met (specify) as defined by patient and caregiver throughout course of care

Patient states pain is at _____ on 0-10 scale by next visit

Death with dignity, and symptoms controlled in setting of patient/family choice

Death with maximum comfort through effective symptom control with specialized hospice support

Symptoms controlled in setting of patient/family choice

Effective pain relief and control (e.g., a peaceful and comfortable death)

Maximizing the patient's quality of life (e.g., patient is alert and pain free)

Pharmacological and nonpharmacological interventions such as localized heat application, positioning, relaxation methods, music, and others

Patient cared for, and family supported through death with physical, psychosocial, spiritual, and other needs acknowledged/addressed

Patient- and family-centered hospice care provided based on the patient's/family's unique situation and needs

Infection control and palliation through death

- *Home health aide or certified nursing assistant*
  Effective hygiene, personal care, and comfort
  ADL assistance
  Safe environment maintained

- *Hospice social worker*
  Psychosocial assessment and counseling of patient and family, including adjustment to illness and its implications
  Emotional support
  Facilitate communication among patient, family, and staff
  Referrals to resources as indicated
  Grief counseling
  Patient/caregiver able to cope adaptively with illness and death
  Identification and addressing/resolution of problems impeding the successful implementation of the POC
  Adaptive adjustment to changed body and body image
  Psychosocial support and counseling offered/initiated to patient and caregivers experiencing grieving process
  Resources identified, community linkage as appropriate for patient/family

- *Volunteer(s)*
  Comfort, companionship, and friendship extended to patient/family
  Support provided as defined by the needs of the patient/caregiver
  Respite support

- *Spiritual counselor*

  Spiritual support offered and provided as defined by needs of patient/ caregiver

  Provision of spiritual support and care as based on the assessed and ongoing needs of the patient and family

  Spiritual support offered and patient and family needs met

  Patient/caregiver express a relief of symptoms of spiritual suffering

  Intervention and support provided related to that dimension of life related to life's meaning (consistent with patient's beliefs)

  Participation in sacred or spiritual rituals or practices

  Support, listening, and presence

  Other outcomes, based on the patient's/family's unique beliefs and needs

- *Dietitian/nutritional counseling*

  Family and caregiver integrating recommendations into nutrition teaching (where appropriate)

  Patient and caregiver know whom to call for nutrition- and hydration-related questions/concerns

  G-tube or NG tube is patent, and patient is receiving safe and maximum nutrition as ordered; no side effects reported by patient, caregiver, or nurse

  Patient and family verbalize comprehension of changing nutritional needs

- *Occupational therapist*

  Patient and caregiver demonstrate maximum independence with ADL, adaptive techniques, and assistive devices

  Patient and caregiver demonstrate maximum safety in ADL and functional mobility

  Patient and caregiver demonstrate effective use of energy conservation techniques

  Verbalization/demonstration of improved functional activity level and enhanced quality of life

  Patient and caregiver demonstrate effective use of diaphragmatic breathing to reduce shortness of breath and relaxation techniques to help in pain/ symptom management

  Maximize independence in ADLs for patient and caregiver

  Optimal function maintained or attained

  Patient and caregiver demonstrate ADL program for maximum safety

- *Physical therapist*

  Maintenance of balance, mobility, and endurance as verbalized and demonstrated by patient

  Prevention of complications

  Safety in mobility and transfers

- *Speech-language pathologist*

  Safe swallowing and functional communication

- *Bereavement counselor*

  Grief support services provided to patient and family

  Well-being and resolution process of grief initiated and followed through bereavement services

- *Music, massage, art, or other therapies or services*
  Therapeutic massage/touch effective for patient as self-reported or observed
    by caregivers/family
  Improved muscle tone, relaxation, and/or sleep
  Patient comfortable and relaxed (e.g., sleeping) after massage
  Music therapy intervention based on assessment to decrease pain percep-
    tion, provide emotional expression and support
  Maintenance of comfort and physical, psychosocial, and spiritual health
  Holistic health maintained, and comfort achieved through _____
    (specify modality)
  Patient has pet's presence as desired—in all care sites, when possible

8. **Patient, family, and caregiver educational needs**
   Educational needs are the care regimens that contribute to safe and effective
   care at home between the hospice team's visits. These include the following:
   The basic tenets of hospice and the availability of support 24 hours a day, 7
     days a week
   Home safety assessment and counseling
   The patient's medication regimen
   Safe and proper body mechanics to promote patient comfort and prevent
     caregiver safety problems
   Other teaching specific to the patient's and family's unique needs
   Support groups available to patient's family, such as the hospice program's
     "Caregiver Support Group" meetings for family members and friends of
     the patient
   Anticipated disease progression

9. **Specific tips for quality and reimbursement**
   Document any variances to expected outcomes. There are many models of
   hospice programs. Those that are home health agency based must work
   within the framework of the Medicare home care program. For example,
   sometimes a hospice patient reaches a stable period in the illness and has no
   further skilled needs or the patient is no longer homebound per Medicare
   home health care criteria. When this occurs, one option is to discharge the
   patient from Medicare home health agency reimbursement and maintain the
   patient on grant funds or other available resources. If the patient's status deteriorates and again meets the Medicare criteria, a new start of care is initiated on the HCFA form 485. Usually hospices continue volunteer support,
   nursing, and other services indicated during these periods of no reimbursement.
      The Medicare hospice benefit does not require that the patient be home-
   bound or have identified skilled needs. Though it is a needed and viable
   program, the Medicare hospice benefit may not be indicated for all Medicare
   eligible beneficiaries. For further information on this benefit, please refer to
   HCFA Hospice Manual 21.
      Should the patient's status deteriorate and increased personal care be
   needed, obtain a telephone order for the increased service, noting frequency
   and estimating the duration.
      Obtain a telephone order for all medication and treatment changes of the
   medical regimen, and document these in the clinical record.

Unless the patient is in a hospice insurance program, some insurers will not pay for a skilled nurse visit that is made at death if the patient is dead when the nurse arrives at the home. From a Medicare home care perspective, the visit at the time of death may be covered when the orders and clinical record document assessment of the patient's status or signs of death/life or state law allows pronouncement of death by a nurse.

Document patient deterioration

Document dehydration, dehydrating

Document patient change or instability

Document pain, other symptoms not controlled

Document status after acute episode of _____ (specify)

Document positive urine, sputum, etc. culture; patient started on _____ (specify ordered antibiotic therapy)

Document patient impacted; impaction removed manually

Document RN in frequent communication with physician regarding _____ (specify)

Document febrile at _____, pulse change at _____, irr., irr.

Document change noted in _____

Document bony prominences red, opening

Document RN contacted physician regarding _____ (specify)

Document marked SOB

Document alteration in mental status

Document medications being adjusted, regulated, or monitored

Document unable to perform own ADLs, personal care

Document all interdisciplinary team meetings and communications in the POC and in the progress notes of the clinical record

All disciplines involved should have input into the POC and document their interventions and goals

Document need for G-tube feeding, inability to swallow without choking, or history of aspiration

Document coordination of services and consultation with other members of the IDG

Remember that the clinical documentation is key to measuring compliance for quality and reimbursement purposes. Care coordination, timely verbal and initial physician orders, and assessment and addressing of spiritual and psychosocial needs should be ongoing and documented in the patient's clinical record

The documentation should support that all hospice care supports comfort and dignity while meeting patient/family needs

The documentation should include ongoing assessment and management of pain and other symptoms and the anticipation and prevention of secondary symptoms such as constipation

It is important to note that all team members, including nurses and social workers, should assess, identify, and "hear" spiritual needs that the patient and family want to be addressed. These spiritual issues are key to the provision of quality hospice care and cannot be addressed effectively and promptly by the spiritual counselor only

Document clearly symptoms, clinical changes, and assessment findings related to pain and patient care

Document weight loss, increased shortness of breath, dyspnea, infection, sepsis, new or changed medications, etc.

Document any skin changes (e.g., inflamed, painful, weeping skin site[s])

Remember that the "litmus test" of care coordination rests on the quality of the clinical documentation by all team members. Review one of your patient's clinical records and ask yourself the following: "If I was unable to give a verbal report/update on this patient's/family's course of care, would a peer be able to pick up and provide the same level of care and know (from the documentation) the current orders, medications, and other details that contribute to effective hospice care?"

This patient population usually has many clinical changes that should be documented. These include weight loss, frequent upper respiratory infection(s) (URI), and multiple and changed medication regimens with varying routes. Side effects to the drug regimen should be observed, noted, documented, and reported

Your assessments, observations, and clinical findings assist in painting a picture to support coverage, accreditation, and documentation requirements for hospice care

Document any hospitalizations and changed clinical findings

Document patient changes, symptoms, and psychosocial issues impacting the patient and family and plan of care

Document coordination of care with other care providers, such as skilled nursing facility, nursing home, and hired caregiver

10. **Resources for hospice care and practice**
    The Amyotrophic Lateral Sclerosis (ALS) Association offers resources for patients, families, and health care professionals. They have local chapters throughout the U.S. and offer support groups. All the services provided to patients and family are provided at no cost. The phone number for the ALS association is (800) 782-4747.

    The Muscular Dystrophy Association has a comprehensive guide available for caregivers of people affected by amyotrophic lateral sclerosis (ALS, or Lou Gehrig's disease).

    When a Loved One Has ALS: A Caregiver's Guide is a 94-page, illustrated manual filled with practical advice for meeting the medical, emotional, financial, and everyday challenges faced by those who are primary caregivers for family members or others with ALS. *When a Loved One Has ALS* can be ordered through your local MDA office, listed in the phone directory. If you have difficulty locating the office nearest you, call MDA national headquarters at (800) 572-1717, or visit MDA's Web site, www.mdausa.org.

BEDBOUND CARE

1. **General considerations**

   Many hospice patients spend their last days in bed, depending on the diagnosis and health history of the patient. Though bedbound status is not a diagnosis, it is an important factor that affects all body systems and results in many teaching and guidance implications for family members and other caregivers.

   With more patients choosing to be cared for at home, the number of patients who are essentially bedridden continues to increase. While being bedridden is not a diagnosis, it is an important factor with implications for all body systems of patients. Caregivers and family members are the key to these patients being cared for safely and effectively in their own home setting.

   Please refer to "Acquired Immuned Deficiency Syndrome (AIDS) Care," "Cancer Care," and "Cardiac Care (End Stage)," or another specific patient problem for a more in-depth discussion for these possible patient care needs.

2. **Needs for visit**

   Physician order for hospice care, specific to the hospice program's admission criteria and policies

   Standard precautions supplies

   Vital signs equipment for baseline assessment

   Other supplies or equipment, based on physician orders

3. **Safety considerations**

   Infection control/standard precautions

   Side rail use and position

   Supervised medication administration

   Wheelchair/fall precautions

   Prevention of injury related to proper positioning

   The need for meticulous skin care and observation

   Disposal of soiled dressings

   Multiple medications (e.g., side effects, interactions, safe storage)

   Night-light

   Safety for home medical equipment (e.g., bed, lift)

   Symptoms that necessitate immediate reporting/assistance

   Smoke detector and fire evacuation plan

   Extra caution on slippery surfaces

   Removal of scatter rugs

   Tub rail, grab bars for bathroom safety

   Supportive and nonskid shoes

   Handrail on stairs

   Fall precautions

   Protective skin measures

   Identify and report any skin problems

   Assistance with ambulation

   Others, based on the patient's unique condition and environment

4. **Potential diagnoses and codes**

Acute myocardial infarction	410.92
Adenocarcinoma, metastatic	199.1
Adrenal cancer	194.0
AIDS	042
ALS	335.20
Alzheimer's	331.0
Anorexia	783.0
Aphasia	784.3
Ascites, malignant	197.6
Bladder atony	496.4
Bladder cancer	188.9
Bone metastases	198.5
Brain, cancer of	191.9
Brain tumor	239.2
Breast cancer	174.9
Cancer of the head or neck	195.0
Cardiomyopathy	425.4
Cerebral vascular accident	436
Cervix, cancer of the	180.9
Cirrhosis of the liver	571.5
CHF	428.0
Colon, cancer	153.9
Colon lymphoma	202.83
Colostomy, attention to	V55.3
Constipation	564.0
COPD	496
Cor pulmonale	416.9
Coronary artery disease (CAD)	414.00
CVA	436
Decubitus (pressure) ulcer	707.0
Dehydration	276.5
Depression	311
Diabetes mellitus (NIDDM)	250.90
Diabetes mellitus (IDDM)	250.91
Dysphagia and CVA	436.0 and 787.2
Esophagus, cancer of the	150.9
Fracture, pathological	733.10
Gastric cancer, metastatic	197.8
Gastric leiomyosarcoma with metastasis	151.9 and 199.1
Gastrostomy, attention to	V55.1
Heart disease, end stage	429.9
Heart failure	428.9
Hemiplegia	342.9
Huntington's disease	333.4
Hyperalimentation	99.15
Hypertension	401.9
Ileostomy, attention to	V55.2
Ileus	560.1

Impaction	560.39
Incontinence of feces	787.6
Incontinence of urine	788.30
Kaposi's sarcoma	176.9
Kaposi's sarcoma with AIDS	042 and 176.9
Kidney, cancer of the (renal)	189.0
Laryngectomy	30.4
Larynx, cancer of the	161.9
Leukemia, acute	208.0
Leukopenia	288.0
Liver, end-stage disease	571.8
Lou Gehrig's disease (ALS)	335.20
Lung cancer, squamous cell	162.9
Lupus	710.0
Lymphoma with bone metastases	202.8
Mastectomy, radical	88.45
Mastectomy, simple	85.41
Metastases, general	199.1
Multiple myeloma	203.0
Multiple sclerosis	340
Myocardial infarction	410.92
Nasopharyngeal cancer	147.9
Oropharyngeal cancer	146.9
Osteoporosis	733.00
Ovarian cancer	183.0
Pain, low back	724.2
Pancreas, cancer of the	157.9
Paralysis	344.9
Paraplegia	344.1
Parkinson's disease	332.0
Pathological fracture	733.10
Peripheral vascular disease	443.9
Pharynx, cancer of the	149.0
Pleural effusion	197.2
Pneumocystis carinii	136.3
Pneumonia	486
Pneumonia, aspiration	507.0
Pressure (decubitus) ulcer	707.0
Prostate, cancer of	185
Protein-caloric malnutrition	263.9
Pulmonary edema	514
Pulmonary edema with cardiac disease	428.1
Pulmonary fibrosis	515
Quadriplegia	344.0
Radiation enteritis	558.1
Radiation myelitis	990 and 323.8
Rectosigmoid, cancer of	154.0
Rectum, cancer of the	154.1
Renal cell cancer, metastatic	198.0

Renal failure, chronic	585
Respirator, dependence on	V46.1
Respiratory failure	518.81
Respiratory insufficiency (acute)	518.82
Seizure disorder	780.3
Septicemia	038.9
Skin cancer	173.9
Spinal cord tumor	239.7
Squamous cell carcinoma	199.1
Stomach, cancer of the	151.9
TIAs	435.9
Tongue, cancer of the	141.9
TPN	99.15
Trachea, cancer of	162.0
Tracheostomy, attention to	V55.0
Urinary incontinence	788.30
Urinary retention	788.20
Urinary tract infection	599.0
Uterine sarcoma, metastatic	198.82
Uterus, cancer of the	179.0

5. **Associated nursing diagnoses**
   Activity intolerance, risk for
   Anxiety
   Aspiration, risk for
   Body image disturbance
   Body temperature, altered, risk for
   Bowel incontinence
   Breathing pattern, ineffective
   Cardiac output, decreased
   Caregiver role strain
   Caregiver role strain, risk for
   Communication, impaired verbal
   Constipation
   Coping, ineffective family: compromised
   Coping, ineffective family: disabling
   Coping, ineffective individual
   Diarrhea
   Disuse syndrome, risk for
   Diversional activity deficit
   Family processes, altered
   Fatigue
   Fear
   Fluid volume deficit, risk for
   Fluid volume excess
   Gas exchange, impaired
   Grieving, anticipatory
   Growth and development, altered
   Home maintenance management, impaired

Hyperthermia
Hypothermia
Incontinence, functional
Incontinence, total
Infection, risk for
Injury, risk for
Knowledge deficit (specify)
Memory, impaired
Mobility, impaired physical
Noncompliance (specify)
Nutrition, altered: less than body requirements
Oral mucous membrane, altered
Pain
Pain, chronic
Parenting, altered
Peripheral neurovascular dysfunction, risk for
Powerlessness
Protection, altered
Role performance, altered
Self-care deficit, bathing/hygiene
Self-care deficit, dressing/grooming
Self-care deficit, feeding
Self-care deficit, toileting
Sensory/perceptual alterations (specify) (visual, auditory, kinesthetic, gustatory, tactile, olfactory)
Sexual dysfunction
Sexuality patterns, altered
Skin integrity, impaired
Skin integrity, impaired, risk for
Sleep pattern disturbance
Social interaction, impaired
Spiritual distress (distress of the human spirit)
Spiritual well-being, potential for enhanced
Swallowing, impaired
Thought processes, altered
Tissue integrity, impaired
Tissue perfusion, altered (specify type) (renal, cerebral, cardiopulmonary, gastrointestinal, peripheral)
Trauma, potential for
Urinary elimination, altered
Urinary retention
Ventilation, inability to sustain spontaneous

6. Skills and services identified

- *Hospice nursing*

    a. *Comfort and symptom control*
    Complete initial assessment of all systems of patient who is bedbound admitted to hospice for _____ (specify problem)
    Presentation of hospice philosophy and services

Explain patient rights and responsibilities

Assess patient, family, and caregiver wishes and expectations regarding care

Assess patient, family, and caregiver resources available for care

Provision of volunteer support to patient and family

Teach family or caregiver physical care of patient

Assess pain and other symptoms, including site, duration, characteristics, and relief measures

Teach caregiver aspects of care and management

Comprehensive assessment and observation of cardiovascular and other systems in bedridden patient with _____

RN to instruct on all aspects of care of the immobilized patient

Observation and assessment of blood pressure and other vital signs

Comfort measures provided to patient for pain and other symptom relief, including backrub, hand massage, and soothing music of patient's choice, when possible

Assess pain, and evaluate the pain management's effectiveness

Measure vital signs, including pain, q visit

Assess cardiovascular, pulmonary, and respiratory status

Teach caregivers symptom control and relief measures

Oxygen on at _____ liter per _____ (specify physician orders)

RN to provide and teach effective oral care and comfort measures

Identify and monitor pain, symptoms, and relief measures

Teach caregiver or family care of weak, terminally ill patient

RN to instruct in pain control measures and medications

RN to assess patient's pain or other symptoms q visit to identify need for change, addition, or other plan or dose adjustment

RN to observe and assess patient for signs, symptoms of infection

Antiembolus hose applied and application method taught to caregiver

Teach patient and family about realistic expectations of disease process

Teach care of dying, signs/symptoms of impending death

Presence and support

Other interventions, based on patient/family needs

b. *Safety and mobility considerations*

Teach safe PO intake (especially liquids)

Monitor for choking/aspiration if PO intake possible

Provide caregiver with home safety information and instruction related to _____ and documented in the clinical record

Teach caregiver effective and safe suctioning of patient

Teach family regarding safety of patient in home

Teach family regarding energy conservation techniques

Safety related to safe bed mobility and transfers

Other interventions, based on patient/family needs

c. *Emotional/spiritual considerations*

Psychosocial assessment of patient and family regarding disease and prognosis

RN to provide emotional support to patient and family with _____, an illness of a terminal nature

Assess mental status and sleep disturbance changes

Spiritual counseling/support offered to patients and caregiver who are verbalizing to nurse and aide team members the reason or meaning of suffering

Provide support to patient and family-member caregivers

Other interventions, based on patient/family needs

d. *Skin care*

Teach proper positioning and techniques for turning

Teach caregiver effective use of turn/pull sheet to avoid friction, skin tears, and burns

RN to change dressing at wound site bid using aseptic technique of (define ordered care)

Observation of the wound site and healing

Teach family and caregiver proper, safe wound care and signs and symptoms of infection to watch for and report to RN or physician

Teach caregiver importance of and all aspects of effective skin care regimens to prevent (further) breakdown. Include the need for position changes every 1 to 2 hours, pressure pads or mattresses, and other measures for prevention

RN to culture wound and urine for C and S and send to lab

RN enterostomal therapist to visit patient and evaluate wound for specific care needs

Pressure ulcer care as indicated

Assess skin integrity

Evaluate patient's need for equipment and supplies to decrease pressure, including alternating pressure mattress, gel foam seat cushion, and heel and elbow protectors

Observation and evaluation of wound and surrounding skin

Teach family to perform dressing between RN visits, specifically

Teach family or caregiver about proper body alignment and positioning in bed to prevent skin tears from shearing skin

Instruct patient and family regarding safety and standard precautions

Teach patient/caregiver all aspects of wound care, including safe disposal of soiled supplies

Observe and apply skilled assessment of areas for possible breakdown, including heels, hips, elbows, ankles, and other pressure-prone areas

Teaching and training of family caregivers about skin care, positioning, and feeding regimens

Teach caregiver regarding skin care needs, including the need for frequent position changes, appropriate pressure pads and mattresses, and the prevention of breakdown

Other interventions, based on patient/family needs

e. *Elimination considerations*

Assess bowel regimen, and implement program as needed

Monitor bowel patterns, including frequency of bowel movements, and evaluate bowel regimen (e.g., stool softeners, laxatives, and dietary changes)

Check for and remove impaction per physician orders

RN to implement bladder training program

Teach caregiver daily catheter care and equipment care and signs and symptoms that necessitate calling the RN/physician

RN to change catheter (specify type size) q (specify frequency)

Condom catheter or indwelling catheter as indicated

Assess amount and frequency of urinary output

RN to evaluate the patient's bowel patterns, need for stool softeners, laxatives, and dietary adjustments and develop bowel management plan

Other interventions, based on patient/family needs

f. *Hydration/nutrition*

RN to monitor hydration/nutrition status

Assess nutrition/hydration statuses

Diet counseling to patient with anorexia

Teach feeding-tube care to family

Nutrition/hydration supported by offering patient's choice of favorite or desired foods or liquids

Nutrition/hydration to be maintained by offering patient high-protein diet and foods of choice as tolerated

Teach patient and family to expect decreased nutritional and fluid intake as disease progresses

Other interventions, based on patient/family needs

g. *Therapeutic/medication regimens*

RN to instruct on all medications, including schedule, functions of specific drugs and their side effects

RN to monitor and assess for complications of new medication regimen

Medication management related to drug/drug, drug/food side effects

RN to monitor patient's response to medications for pain and other symptom control

RN to assess the patient's unique response to treatments or interventions, and report changes or unfavorable responses or reactions to the physician

Medication assessment and management

Teach new pain and symptom control medication regimen

Teach new medication and effects

Obtain venipuncture as ordered q _____ (ordered frequency)

Teach patient and caregiver use of PCA pump

Assess for electrolyte imbalance

Nonpharmacological interventions such as progressive muscle relaxation, imagery, positive visualization, music, massage and touch, and humor therapy of patient's choice implemented

Other interventions, based on patient/family needs

h. *Other considerations*

Teach proper positioning and techniques for turning

Teach caregiver effective use of turn/pull sheet to prevent friction, skin tears, or burns

Assess disease progression process

RN to assess the patient's response to treatments and interventions and to report to the physician any changes, unfavorable responses, or reactions.

Other interventions, based on patient/family needs

- **Home health aide or certified nursing assistant**

  Effective and safe personal care

  Safe ADL assistance and support, ambulation and transfers

  Respite care

  Observation and reporting

  Meal preparation

  Homemaker services

  Comfort care

  Other duties

- **Hospice social worker**

  Psychosocial assessment of patient and family/caregiver, including adjustment to illness and its implications

  Financial assessment and counseling regarding food acquisition, ability to prepare, and costs of needed medications

  Intervention/support related to terminal illness and loss

  Emotional/spiritual support

  Depression/fear assessed and addressed

  Facilitate communication among patient, family, and hospice team

  Identification of optimal coping strategies

  Referral/linkage to community services and resources as indicated

  Grief counseling and intervention/support related to illness/loss

  Patient/caregiver counseling and support

  For patients who live alone with no support system (e.g., able, available, willing caregiver[s]): obtain linkage to necessary community resources to allow patient to remain in the home

  Illness-related psychiatric condition necessitating care, support, and intervention

  Identification of caregiver role strain necessitating respite/relief/support

- **Volunteer(s)**

  Support, friendship, companionship, and presence

  Comfort and dignity maintained/provided for patient and family

  Errands and transportation

  Other services, based on interdisciplinary team recommendations and patient/caregiver needs

- **Spiritual counselor**

  Spiritual assessment and care

  Counseling, intervention, and support related to that dimension of life related to life's meaning (consistent with patient's beliefs)

  Support, listening, and presence

  Participation in sacred or spiritual rituals or practices

  Other supportive care, based on patient/family needs and belief systems

- *Dietitian/nutritional counseling*
    Assessment of patient with decreased intake, weight loss, anorexia, and
        nausea
    Assessment and recommendations for swallowing difficulties
    Teaching and support of family members and caregivers
    Support and care with food and nourishment as desired by patient
    Teach safe PO and tube feeding techniques to prevent choking, aspiration,
        or overhydration (if on TPN)
    Evaluation/management of nutritional deficits and needs
    Encourage nutritional supplements and snacks to increase protein and
        caloric intake
    Food, dietary recommendations incorporated into patient choice and
        wishes
    Evaluation of patient on enteral/nutritional feedings

- *Occupational therapist*
    Evaluation of ADL, functional mobility
    Assess for need for adaptive equipment and assistive devices
    Safety assessment of patient's environment and ADL
    Assessment for energy conservation training
    Assessment of upper extremity function, retraining motor skills, and/or
        splinting for contracture(s)

- *Physical therapist*
    Evaluation
    Safety assessment of patient's environment
    Safe transfer training
    Strengthening exercises/program
    Teach transfer safety/lift use
    Bed mobility exercises, as tolerated
    Instruct and supervise caregiver and volunteers on home exercise regimen

- *Speech-language pathologist*
    Evaluation for speech/swallowing problems
    Food texture recommendations
    Speech dysphagia program
    Alternate communication program

- *Bereavement counselor*
    Assessment of the needs of the bereaved family and friends
    Support and intervention, based on assessment and ongoing findings
    Presence and counseling
    Supportive visits and follow-up, other interventions (e.g., mailings, calls)
    Other services related to bereavement work and support

- *Music, massage, art, or other therapies or services*
    Evaluation and intervention based on patient's and caregiver's unique
        wishes and needs that support care, comfort, and death in the setting of
        the patient's choice
    Pet therapy (including patient's pet, if available) and therapeutic interven-
        tion

Assessment plan to engage patient and support comfort, quality, enjoyment, and dignity

7. **Outcomes for care**

- *Hospice nursing*
  Patient and caregiver verbalize satisfaction with care
  Adherence to POC as demonstrated by caregiver demonstrations and verbalizations and patient findings by _____ (specify date)
  Caregiver effective in care management and knows whom to call for questions/concerns
  Skin integrity maintained as evidenced by problem-free skin
  Patient uses catheter without complaints or signs/symptoms of infection
  Patient will exhibit a reduction in problems such as pain, SOB, clot formation, urinary infection, and decreased function caused by immobility/disease processes
  Regulated bowel program, as evidenced by regular bowel movements
  Patient will express satisfaction with hospice support received and will experience increased comfort
  Patient will be made comfortable at home through death in accordance with the patient's wishes
  Effective pain control and symptom control verbalized by patient
  Patient verbalizes understanding of and adheres to care and medication regimens
  Patient and caregiver supported through patient's death
  Comfort maintained through course of care
  The patient and family receive hospice support and care, and family members and friends are able to spend quality time with the patient
  Caregiver able and verbalizes comfort with role and lists when to call hospice team members
  Patient supported through and receives the maximum benefit from palliative chemotherapy and radiation with minimal complications
  Patient or caregiver lists adverse reactions, potential complications, signs/symptoms of infection (e.g., sputum change, chest congestion)
  Comfort maintained through death with dignity
  Pain effectively managed, and patient verbalizes comfort
  Comfort and individualized intervention of patient with immobility/bedbound status (e.g., skin, urinary, musculature, vascular)
  Spiritual and psychosocial needs met (specify) as defined by patient and caregiver throughout course of care
  Caregiver, by _____ (date), will verbalize care of patient
  Symptom relief and supportive intervention and care
  Compliance to care program as evidenced by observation and demonstration during nurse's and other team members' visits
  Patient can describe medication regimen and side effects and knows when and for what symptoms to call the nurse
  Catheter patent and infection free
  Comfort through death with dignity at home with loved ones
  Patient or caregiver will express increased patient comfort

Patient able to spend quality time with family and friends through illness and death

Death with dignity, and symptoms controlled in setting of patient/family choice

Death with maximum comfort through effective symptom control with specialized hospice support

Symptoms controlled in setting of patient/family choice

Effective pain relief and control (e.g., a peaceful and comfortable death)

Maximizing the patient's quality of life (e.g., patient is alert and pain free)

Pharmacological and nonpharmacological interventions, such as localized heat application, positioning, relaxation methods, music and others

Patient cared for, and family supported through death with physical, psychosocial, spiritual, and other needs acknowledged/addressed

Patient- and family-centered hospice care provided based on the patient's/family's unique situation and needs

Infection control and palliation through death

- ***Home health aide or certified nursing assistant***
  Effective hygiene, personal care, and comfort
  ADL assistance
  Safe environment maintained
  Safe ambulation and transfers

- ***Hospice social worker***
  Resources identified, community linkage as appropriate for patient/family
  Problems are identified and addressed, and patient and caregiver are linked with appropriate support services. Plan of care successfully implemented
  Patient and caregiver cope adaptively with illness and death
  Adaptive adjustment to changed body and body image
  Psychosocial support and counseling offered to patient and caregivers experiencing loss and grief
  Optimal care for patient in home environment

- ***Volunteer(s)***
  Comfort, companionship, and friendship extended to patient/family
  Support and respite provided as defined by the needs of the patient/caregiver

- ***Spiritual counselor***
  Spiritual support offered and provided as defined by needs of patient/caregiver
  Provision of spiritual support and care as based on the assessed and ongoing needs of the patient and family
  Spiritual support offered, and patient and family needs met
  Intervention and support provided related to that dimension of life related to life's meaning (consistent with patient's beliefs)
  Support, listening, and presence
  Participation in sacred rituals or practices
  Other outcomes, based on the patient's/family's unique beliefs and needs

- *Dietitian/nutritional counseling*
  Family and caregiver integrate dietary recommendations into nutrition-related care and intervention
  Patient and caregiver know whom to call for nutrition- and hydration-related questions/concerns
  Patient and family verbalize comprehension of changing nutritional needs

- *Occupational therapist*
  Patient and caregiver demonstrate effective use of energy conservation
  Verbalization/demonstration of improved functional activity level and enhanced quality of life
  Patient demonstrates effective use of diaphragmatic breathing to reduce shortness of breath and relaxation techniques to help in pain/symptom management
  Patient and caregiver demonstrate correct use of exercise and splints for maximum upper extremity function and joint position

- *Physical therapist*
  Prevention of complications
  Home exercise and upper extremity program taught to caregiver
  Optimal strength and mobility maintained/achieved
  Compliance with home exercise program by _____ (date)
  Safety in bed mobility

- *Speech-language pathologist*
  Communication method implemented, and patient able to be understood as self-reported or reported by family/caregivers
  Swallowing safety evaluated and maintained

- *Bereavement counselor*
  Support services related to grief provided to patient and family
  Well-being and resolution process of grief initiated and followed through bereavement services

- *Music, massage, art, or other therapies or services*
  Therapeutic massage/touch effective for patient as self-reported or observed by caregivers/family
  Improved muscle tone, relaxation, and/or sleep
  Patient comfortable and relaxed (e.g., sleeping) after massage
  Music therapy intervention based on assessment to decrease pain perception and provide emotional expression and support
  Maintenance of comfort, physical, psychosocial, and spiritual health
  Patient has pet's present as desired—in all care sites, when possible
  Holistic health maintained and comfort achieved through _____ (specify modality)

8. **Patient, family, and caregiver educational needs**
   Educational needs are the care regimens that contribute to safe and effective care at home between the hospice team's visits. These include the following:
   The basic tenets of hospice and the availability of support 24 hours a day, 7 days a week
   Home safety assessment and counseling

Safe and proper body mechanics to promote patient comfort and prevent
  caregiver safety problems
Other teaching specific to the patient's and family's unique needs
Support groups available to patient's family, such as the hospice program's
  "Caregiver Support Group" meetings for family members and friends of
  the patient
Skin care regimens
Catheter and wound care programs
Effective personal hygiene habits
Home exercise program, including ROM
Safety measures in the home when the patient is immobilized
Prevention of infections
Medication program and the medications' relationships to each other
Importance of medical follow-up
When to call the hospice or the physician
Anticipated disease progression
Other information based on the patient's/family's unique needs

9. **Specific tips for quality and reimbursement**
   Document any variances to expected outcomes. There are many models of
   hospice programs. Those that are home health agency based must work
   within the framework of the Medicare home care program. For example,
   sometimes a hospice patient reaches a stable period in the illness and has no
   further skilled needs or the patient is no longer homebound per Medicare
   home health care criteria. When this occurs, one option is to discharge the
   patient from Medicare home health agency reimbursement and maintain the
   patient on grant funds or other available resources. If the patient's status deteriorates and again meets the Medicare criteria, a new start of care is initiated on the HCFA form 485. Usually hospices continue volunteer support,
   nursing, and other services indicated during these periods of no reimbursement.
   The Medicare hospice benefit does not require that the patient be homebound or have identified skilled needs. Though it is a needed and viable
   program, the Medicare hospice benefit may not be indicated for all Medicare
   eligible beneficiaries. For further information on this benefit, please refer to
   HCFA Hospice Manual 21.
   Should the patient's status deteriorate and increased personal care be
   needed, obtain a telephone order for the increased service, noting frequency
   and estimating the duration.
   Obtain a telephone order for all medication and treatment changes of the
   medical regimen and document these in the clinical record.
   Remember that nutritional solutions/supplements are usually covered by
   Medicare or other third-party payors when they are the *sole* source of nutrition. (They usually cannot be supplementary.) Also, they are generally
   covered when taken by routes other than po—for example, enteral tube feedings.
   Unless the patient is in a hospice insurance program, some insurers will
   not pay for a skilled nurse visit that is made at death if the patient is dead
   when the nurse arrives at the home. From a Medicare home care perspective,
   the visit at the time of death may be covered when the orders and clinical

record document assessment of the patient's status or signs of death/life or state law allows pronouncement of death by a nurse.

Document patient deterioration

Document dehydration, dehydrating

Document patient change or instability

Document pain, other symptoms not controlled

Document status after acute episode of _____ (specify)

Document positive urine, sputum, etc. culture; patient started on _____ (specify ordered antibiotic therapy)

Document patient impacted; impaction removed manually

Document RN in frequent communication with physician regarding _____ (specify)

Document febrile at _____, pulse change at _____, irr., irr.

Document change noted in _____

Document bony prominences red, opening

Document RN contacted physician regarding _____ (specify)

Document marked SOB

Document alteration in mental status

Document medications being adjusted, regulated, or monitored

Remember that the clinical documentation is key to measuring compliance for quality and reimbursement purposes. Care coordination, timely verbal and initial physician orders, and assessment and addressing of spiritual and psychosocial needs should be ongoing and documented in the patient's clinical record

The documentation should support that all hospice care supports comfort and dignity while meeting patient/family needs

The documentation should include ongoing assessment and management of pain and other symptoms and the anticipation and prevention of secondary symptoms such as constipation

It is important to note that all team members, including nurses and social workers, should assess, identify, and "hear" spiritual needs that the patient and family want to be addressed. These spiritual issues are key to the provision of quality hospice care and cannot be addressed effectively and promptly by the spiritual counselor only

Document clearly symptoms, clinical changes, and assessment findings related to pain and patient care

Document weight loss, increased shortness of breath, dyspnea, infection, sepsis, new or changed medications and the patient's response, etc.

Document any skin changes (e.g., inflamed, painful, weeping skin site[s])

Remember that the "litmus test" of care coordination rests on the quality of the clinical documentation by all team members. Review one of your patient's clinical records and ask yourself the following: "If I was unable to give a verbal report/update on this child/family's course of care, would a peer be able to pick up and provide the same level of care and know (from the documentation) the current orders, including specific medications, and other details that contribute to effective hospice care?"

This patient population usually has many clinical changes that should be documented. These include weight loss and multiple and changed medica-

tion regimens with varying routes. Side effects to the drug regimen should
be observed, noted, documented, and reported

Your assessments, observations, and clinical findings assist in painting a
picture to support coverage and documentation requirements for hospice
care

Document any hospitalizations and changed clinical findings

Document patient changes, symptoms, and psychosocial issues impacting the
patient and family and plan of care

Document coordination of services or consultation with other members of the
IDG

10. **Resources for hospice care and practice**
    Available free from the Agency for Health Care Policy and Research
    (AHCPR) are *Clinical Practice Guideline Number 3: Preventing Pressure
    Ulcers: Patient Guide, Pressure Ulcers in Adults: Prediction and Prevention,
    and Pressure Ulcers in Adults: Prediction and Prevention. Treating Pressure
    Sores: Consumer Guide Number 15* and *Pressure Ulcer Treatment: Quick
    Reference Guide for Clinicians Number 15* are also available. The patient
    guides are available in English and Spanish, and all can be ordered by calling
    1-800-358-9295.

    Reference Guide for Clinicians: Management of Cancer Pain: Adults, and
    Consumer's Guide: Management of Cancer Pain are patient guides available
    in English and Spanish, and all can be ordered by calling 1-800-358-9295.

    The pamphlet *Get Relief From Cancer Pain* is available from the National
    Cancer Institute's Cancer Information Service. Call 1-800-4-CANCER
    (1-800-422-6237).

    The 76-page booklet *Questions and Answers About Pain Control* is avail-
    able free from the National Cancer Institute's Cancer Information Service.
    Call 1-800-4-CANCER (1-800-422-6237).

BRAIN TUMOR CARE

1. **General considerations**

   Hospice nurses use all their skills in the care of patients with brain tumors and family members. The many symptoms and problems may be overwhelming to the family and caregivers. The patient's care needs vary depending on the tumor site and specific type. The support and assurance provided to these patients and families may be as important as control of seizures or other symptoms that can be difficult to manage at home.

   Please refer also to "Cancer Care," "Bedbound Care," or "Pain Care" should these sections also pertain to your patient.

2. **Needs for visit**

   Physician order for hospice care, specific to the hospice program's admission
       criteria and policies
   Standard precautions supplies
   Vital signs equipment for baseline assessment
   Other supplies or equipment, based on physician orders

3. **Safety considerations**

   Infection control/standard precautions
   Side rail use and position
   Supervised medication administration
   Wheelchair/fall/seizure precautions and postseizure actions to take
   Prevention of injury related to proper position
   Need for meticulous skin care and observation
   Multiple medications (e.g., side effects, interactions, safe storage)
   Night-light
   Safety for home medical equipment (e.g., bed, lift)
   Symptoms that necessitate immediate reporting/assistance
   Smoke detector and fire evacuation plan
   Extra caution on slippery surfaces
   Removal of scatter rugs
   Tub rail, grab bars for bathroom safety
   Supportive and nonskid shoes
   Handrail on stairs
   Fall precautions
   Protective skin measures
   Identification and report of any skin problems
   Phone number of whom to call with a care problem
   Smoke detector and fire evacuation plan
   Assistance with ambulation
   Others, based on the patient's unique condition and environment

4. **Potential diagnoses and codes**

Acoustic neuroma	225.1
Astrocytoma	191.9
Bone marrow transplant (surgical)	41.00

Bone metastases	198.5
Brain tumor, recurrent	239.6
Cancer of the brain	191.9
Cerebrovascular accident	436
Depression, reactive	300.4
Glioblastoma	191.9
Meningitis	322.9
Metastases (general)	199.1
Metastatic brain tumor	198.3
Pathological fracture	733.10
Pneumonia	486
Seizures	780.3
Radiation enteritis	558.1
Radiation myelitis	990 and 323.8
Transient ischemic attacks	435.9
Urinary tract infection	599.0

5. **Associated nursing diagnoses**
   Activity intolerance
   Activity intolerance, risk for
   Airway clearance, ineffective
   Anxiety
   Aspiration, risk for
   Body image disturbance
   Body temperature, altered, risk for
   Bowel incontinence
   Breathing pattern, ineffective
   Caregiver role strain
   Caregiver role strain, risk for
   Communication, impaired verbal
   Constipation
   Coping, ineffective family: compromised
   Coping, ineffective family: disabling
   Coping, ineffective individual
   Decisional conflict (specify)
   Denial, ineffective
   Diarrhea
   Disuse syndrome, risk for
   Family processes, altered
   Fatigue
   Fear
   Fluid volume deficit, risk for
   Fluid volume excess
   Gas exchange, impaired
   Grieving, anticipatory
   Health maintenance, altered
   Home maintenance management, impaired
   Hopelessness
   Hyperthermia
   Hypothermia

Incontinence, total
Infection, risk for
Injury, risk for
Knowledge deficit (specify)
Memory, impaired
Mobility, impaired physical
Noncompliance (specify)
Nutrition, altered: less than body requirements
Nutrition, altered: more than body requirements
Oral mucous membrane, altered
Pain
Pain, chronic
Parenting, altered
Peripheral neurovascular dysfunction, risk for
Powerlessness
Protection, altered
Role performance, altered
Self-care deficit, bathing/hygiene
Self-care deficit, dressing/grooming
Self-care deficit, feeding
Self-care deficit, toileting
Sensory/perceptual alterations (specify) (visual, auditory, kinesthetic, gustatory, tactile, olfactory)
Sexual dysfunction
Skin integrity, impaired
Skin integrity, impaired, risk for
Sleep pattern disturbance
Social interaction, impaired
Social isolation
Spiritual distress (distress of the human spirit)
Spiritual well-being, potential for enhanced
Swallowing, impaired
Thought processes, altered
Tissue integrity, impaired
Tissue perfusion, altered (specify type) (renal, cerebral, cardiopulmonary, gastrointestinal, peripheral)
Trauma, risk for
Urinary elimination, altered
Urinary retention

6. Skills and services identified

- *Hospice nursing*

    a. *Comfort and symptom control*
    Complete initial assessment of all systems of patient with seizures admitted to hospice for _____ (specify problem)
    Skilled observation, and complete systems assessment of the patient with seizures and a brain tumor
    Presentation of hospice philosophy and services

Explain patient rights and responsibilities

Assess patient, family, and caregiver wishes and expectations regarding care

Assess patient, family, and caregiver resources available for care

Provision of volunteer support to patient and family

Teach family or caregiver physical care of patient

Assess pain and other symptoms, including site, duration, characteristics, and relief measures

Monitor for signs and symptoms of infection

Observation and assessment of patient's pain and other symptoms

RN to conduct neurological checks q visit, including levels of consciousness, pupil checks, and others as ordered

Comfort measures of backrub and hand massages

Observe for alopecia, and implement management regimen

RN to monitor blood pressure and other vital signs

RN to monitor patient for seizure activity and teach seizure and associated safety precautions

Monitor for fluid retention

Pain assessment and management

Observe oral mucosa for breakdown and other problems

Assess effectiveness of pain relief program

Comfort measures of backrub and hand or other therapeutic massage

RN to provide and teach effective oral care and comfort measures

Assess pain and evaluate the pain management's effectiveness

Teach care of bedridden patient

Measure vital signs, including pain, q visit

Assess cardiovascular, pulmonary, and respiratory status

Teach caregivers symptom control and relief measures

Oxygen on at _____ liter per _____ (specify physician orders)

Identify and monitor pain, symptoms, and relief measures

Assess neurological status

Teach patient and family seizure precautions

RN to assess patient's pain with other symptoms q visit to identify need for dose addition or other plan or dose adjustment

Teach signs and symptoms of TIA or stroke

Seizure precautions interventions

RN to assess patient's pain or other symptoms q visit to identify need for change, addition, or other plan or dose adjustment

Teach caregiver or family care of weak, terminally ill patient

Teach patient family about realistic expectations of disease process

Teach care of dying, signs/symptoms of impending death

Presence and support

Other interventions, based on patient/family needs

b. *Safety and mobility considerations*

Assess need for a personal emergency response system

Provide caregiver with home safety information and instruction related to _____ and documented in the clinical record

Teach family regarding safety of patient in home

Teach family regarding energy conservation techniques

Patient and caregiver provided with home safety information and instruction related to seizures and documented in clinical record

Other interventions, based on patient/family needs

c. *Emotional/spiritual considerations*

Psychosocial assessment of patient and family regarding disease and
prognosis

RN to provide emotional support to patient and family with
_____, an illness of a terminal nature

Assess mental status and sleep disturbance changes

Provide emotional support to patient and spouse

Provide support to patient and family-member caregivers

Other interventions, based on patient/family needs

d. *Skin care*

Teach caregiver regarding skin care needs, including the need for frequent position changes, appropriate pressure pads and mattresses,
and the prevention of breakdown

Pressure ulcer care as indicated

RN to teach patient regarding care of irradiated skin sites

Assess skin integrity

Observation and evaluation of wound and surrounding skin

Evaluate patient's need for equipment and supplies to decrease pressure,
including alternating pressure mattress, gel foam seat cushion, and
heel and elbow protectors

Observation and evaluation of wound and surrounding skin

Teach family to perform dressing between RN visits, specifically
_____

Teach patient and family or caregiver about proper body alignment and
positioning in bed to prevent skin tears from shearing skin

Observe and apply skilled assessment of areas for possible breakdown,
including heels, hips, elbows, ankles, and other pressure-prone areas

Other interventions, based on patient/family needs

e. *Elimination considerations*

Assess bowel regimen, and implement program as needed

Monitor bowel patterns, including frequency of bowel movements, and
evaluate bowel regimen (e.g., stool softeners, laxatives, and dietary
changes)

RN to teach caregiver daily care of catheter

Observation and complete systems assessment of the patient with an
indwelling catheter

Check for and remove impaction as needed

Condom catheter or indwelling catheter as indicated

Assess amount and frequency of urinary output

Teach catheter care to caregiver

RN to evaluate the patient's bowel patterns, need for stool softeners, laxatives, and dietary adjustments and develop bowel management plan

Other interventions, based on patient/family needs

f. *Hydration/nutrition*
  Assess nutrition and hydration statuses
  Diet counseling to patient with anorexia
  Teach feeding-tube care to family
  Nutrition/hydration supported by offering patient's choice of favorite or desired foods or liquids
  Teach patient and family to expect decreased nutritional and fluid intake as disease progresses
  Other interventions, based on patient/family needs

g. *Therapeutic/medication regimens*
  Teach about and observe side effects of palliative chemotherapy, including constipation, anemia, and fatigue
  Monitor weight gain caused by steroids (potential for diabetes and edema)
  RN to instruct caregiver on all aspects of medication management, including schedule, functions, and side effects
  RN to assess the patient's unique response to treatments or interventions, and report changes or unfavorable responses or reactions to the physician
  Medication assessment and management
  Teach new pain and symptom control medication regimen
  Teach about new medication and effects
  Teach new medication regimen
  Obtain venipuncture as ordered q _____ (ordered frequency)
  Teach patient and caregiver use of PCA pump
  Assess for electrolyte imbalance
  Nonpharmacological interventions such as progressive muscle relaxation, imagery, positive visualization, music, massage and touch, and humor therapy of patient's choice implemented
  Assess effectiveness and side effects of new medication regimen, including food/drug and possible drug/drug interactions
  Other interventions, based on patient/family needs

h. *Other considerations*
  Teach patient radiation therapy regimen and schedule
  Support patient/caregiver through radiation, chemotherapy, and other modalities for tumor reduction
  Teach patient and caregiver about steroid therapy and side effects to watch for
  Assess disease progression process
  RN to assess the patient's response to treatments and interventions and to report to the physician any changes, unfavorable responses, or reactions
  Other interventions, based on patient/family needs

• **Home health aide or certified nursing assistant**
  Effective and safe personal care
  Safe ADL assistance, support, ambulation, and transfer assist
  Respite care and active listening skills

Observation and reporting
Meal preparation
Homemaker services
Comfort care
Other duties

- *Hospice social worker*
  Psychosocial assessment of patient and family/caregiver, including adjustment to illness and its implications and the need for care
  Identification of optimal coping strategies
  Financial assessment and counseling regarding food acquisition, ability to prepare, and costs of needed medications
  Identification of caregiver role strain necessitating respite/relief measures or support
  Intervention/support related to terminal illness and loss
  Emotional/spiritual support
  Depression/fear assessed and addressed
  Facilitate communication among patient, family, and hospice team
  Referral/linkage to community services and resources as indicated
  Grief counseling and intervention/support related to illness/loss
  Patient/caregiver counseling and support
  For patients who live alone with no support system (e.g., able, available, willing caregiver[s]), linkage to necessary community resources to allow patient to remain in home.
  Illness-related psychiatric condition necessitating care/support/intervention
  Counseling support to patient/family regarding patient's behavioral changes
  Assessment of depression, fears, or anxiety

- *Volunteer(s)*
  Support, friendship, companionship, and presence
  Comfort and dignity maintained/provided for patient and family
  Errands and transportation
  Other services, based on interdisciplinary team recommendations and patient/caregiver needs

- *Spiritual counselor*
  Spiritual assessment and care
  Counseling, intervention, and support related to that dimension of life related to life's meaning (consistent with patient's beliefs)
  Support, listening, and presence
  Participation in sacred or spiritual rituals or practices
  Other supportive care, based on patient/family needs and belief systems

- *Dietitian/nutritional counseling*
  Assessment of patient with decreased intake, weight loss, anorexia, weight gain or loss caused by steroids, and nausea
  Assessment and recommendations for swallowing difficulties
  Teaching and support of family members and caregivers
  Support and care with food and nourishment as desired by patient

- *Occupational therapist*
  Evaluation of ADL and functional mobility
  Assess for need for adaptive equipment and assistive devices

Safety assessment of patient's environment and ADL

Assessment for energy conservation training

Assessment of upper extremity function, retraining motor skills, and/or splinting for contracture(s)

- *Physical therapist*

  Evaluation

  Assessment of patient's environment for safety

  Safe transfer training

  Strengthening exercises/program

  Assessment of gait safety

  Instruct and supervise caregiver and volunteers on home exercise program for conditioning and strength

  Assistive, adaptive devices or equipment and teaching

- *Speech-language pathologist*

  Evaluation for speech/swallowing problems

- *Bereavement counselor*

  Assessment of the needs of the bereaved family and friends

  Support and intervention, based on assessment and ongoing findings

  Presence and counseling

  Supportive visits and follow-up, other interventions (e.g., mailings, calls)

  Other services related to bereavement work and support

- *Pharmacist*

  Evaluation of hospice patient on multiple medications for possible food/drug, drug/drug interactions

  Medication monitoring regarding therapeutic levels and dosages

  Pain consult and input into interdisciplinary plan of care related to pain control, palliation, and symptom management

  Assessment of medication regimen and plan for safety and compliance

- *Music, massage, art, or other therapies or services*

  Evaluation and intervention based on patient's and caregiver's unique wishes and needs that support care, comfort, and death in the setting of the patient's choice

  Pet therapy (including patient's pet, if available) and therapeutic intervention

  Assessment plan to engage patient and support comfort, quality, enjoyment, and dignity

7. **Outcomes for care**

- *Hospice nursing*

  Seizures controlled through illness and death

  Death with dignity, and symptoms controlled in setting of patient/family choice

  Death with maximum comfort through effective symptom control with specialized hospice support

  Symptoms controlled in setting of patient/family choice

  Effective pain relief and control (e.g., a peaceful and comfortable death)

  Maximizing the patient's quality of life (e.g., patient is alert and pain free)

Pharmacological and nonpharmacological interventions, such as localized heat application, positioning, relaxation methods, and music

Patient cared for, and family supported through death with physical, psychosocial, spiritual, and other needs acknowledged/addressed

Patient- and family-centered hospice care provided based on the patient's/family's unique situation and needs

Infection control and palliation

Patient states pain is at _____ on 0-10 scale by next visit

Patient and caregiver verbalize satisfaction with care

Educational tools/plans incorporated in daily care, and patient and caregiver verbalize understanding of safe, needed care

Patient will decide on care, interventions, and evaluation

Caregiver effective in care management and knows whom to call for questions/concerns

Patient will express satisfaction with hospice support received and will experience increased comfort

Patient will be made comfortable at home through death in accordance with the patient's wishes

Effective pain control and symptom control verbalized by patient

Patient verbalizes understanding of and adheres to care and medication regimens

Patient and caregiver supported through patient's death

Comfort maintained through course of care

The patient and family receive hospice support and care, and family members and friends are able to spend quality time with the patient

Caregiver able and verbalizes comfort with role and knows when to call hospice team members

Patient supported through and receives the maximum benefit from palliative chemotherapy and radiation with minimal complications

Patient and caregiver list adverse reactions, potential complications, signs/symptoms of infection (e.g., sputum change, chest congestion)

Comfort maintained through death with dignity

Pain effectively managed and patient verbalizes comfort

Patient protected from injury, stable respiratory status, and compliant with medication, safety, and care regimens

Comfort and individualized intervention of patient with immobility/bed-bound status (e.g., skin, urinary, musculature, vascular)

Spiritual and psychosocial needs met (specify) as defined by patient and caregiver throughout course of care

Injury protection related to patient with seizures

Seizures controlled, protected from injury, stable neurological status, and compliance with medication and care regimens (e.g., steroids)

Patient and caregiver knowledgeable about side effects (e.g., constipation) and interventions needed

Patient and caregiver knowledgeable about and compliant with seizure care regimen and care for optimal control, when possible

Early detection and intervention of problems related to patients with immobility/bedbound status (e.g., skin, urinary, musculature, vascular)

Patient will be comfortable and pain free through illness and death, and interdisciplinary team will work together to improve/maintain the patient's quality of life

Caregiver and patient, when able, express satisfaction with care

Caregiver, by _____ (date), will verbalize specific care of patient

Compliance to care program as evidenced by observation and demonstration during visits by nurse and other team members

- *Home health aide or certified nursing assistant*
  Effective hygiene, personal care, and comfort
  Safe ADL assistance and ambulation
  Safe environment maintained

- *Hospice social worker*
  Problems are identified and addressed with patient and caregiver, and they are linked with appropriate support services. Plan of care successfully implemented
  Patient and caregiver cope adaptively with illness and death
  Adaptive adjustment to changed body and body image
  Psychosocial support and counseling offered to patients and caregivers experiencing loss and grief
  Resources identified, and community linkage is provided as appropriate for patient and family

- *Volunteer(s)*
  Comfort, companionship, and friendship extended to patient/family
  Support provided as defined by the needs of the patient/caregiver

- *Spiritual counselor*
  Spiritual assessment and care
  Counseling, intervention, and support related to that dimension of life related to life's meaning (consistent with patient's beliefs)
  Support, listening, and presence
  Intervention and support provided related to that dimension of life related to life's meaning (consistent with patient's beliefs)
  Participation in sacred or spiritual rituals or practices
  Other supportive care, based on patient/family needs and belief systems
  Spiritual support offered and provided as defined by needs of patient/caregiver
  Provision of spiritual support and care as based on the assessed and ongoing needs of the patient and family
  Spiritual support offered and patient and family needs met

- *Dietitian/nutritional counseling*
  Family and caregiver integrating dietary recommendations into nutrition teaching (where appropriate)
  Patient and caregiver know whom to call for nutrition- and hydration-related questions/concerns
  Nutrition and hydration per patient's choices
  Caregiver integrating dietary recommendations into daily meal planning
  Patient and family verbalize comprehension of changing nutritional needs

- *Occupational therapist*
  Optimal functional and safe mobility maintained or enhanced
  Patient demonstrates maximum independence with ADL, adaptive techniques, and assistive devices

Patient and caregiver demonstrate maximum safety in ADL and functional mobility

Patient demonstrates effective use of energy conservation

Verbalization/demonstration of improved functional activity level and enhanced quality of life

Patient demonstrates effective use of diaphragmatic breathing to reduce shortness of breath and relaxation techniques to help in pain/symptom management

Patient and caregiver demonstrate correct use of exercise and splints for maximum upper extremity function and joint position

- **Physical therapist**
  Prevention of complications
  Home exercise and upper extremity program taught to caregiver
  Optimal strength and mobility maintained or achieved
  Compliance with home exercise program by _____ (date)
  Safety in mobility and transfers

- **Speech-language pathologist**
  Communication method implemented, and patient able to be understood as self-reported or reported by family/caregivers
  Safe swallowing and functional communication
  Recommended lists of foods/textures for safety and patient choice

- **Bereavement counselor**
  Support services related to grief provided to patient and family
  Well-being and resolution process of grief initiated and followed through bereavement services

- **Pharmacist**
  Multiple-drug regimen reviewed for food/drug and drug/drug interactions in patient on steroids and other medications
  Stability and safety in complex medication regimen
  Effective pain and symptom control and symptom management as reported by patient/caregiver

- **Music, massage, art, or other therapies or other services**
  Therapeutic massage/touch effective for patient as self-reported or observed by caregivers/family
  Improved muscle tone, relaxation, and/or sleep
  Patient comfortable and relaxed (e.g., sleeping) after massage
  Music therapy intervention based on assessment to decrease pain perception, provide emotional expression and support
  Maintenance of comfort and physical, psychosocial, and spiritual health
  Patient has pet's presence as desired—in all care sites, when possible
  Holistic health maintained and comfort achieved through _____ (specify modality)

8. **Patient, family, and caregiver educational needs**
   Educational needs are the care regimens that contribute to safe and effective care at home between the hospice team's visits. These include the following:
   The basic tenets of hospice and the availability of support 24 hours a day, 7 days a week

Home safety assessment and counseling

The patient's medication regimen

Safe and proper body mechanics to promote patient comfort and prevent caregiver safety problems

Other teaching specific to the patient's and family's unique needs

Support groups available to the patient's family, such as the hospice program's "Caregiver Support Group" meetings for family members and friends of the patient

Effective personal hygiene habits

Avoidance of infections

Pain and other symptom control measures and management

Patient's medications and their relationship to each other

Information about the disease process and seizure activity care

Importance of taking the prescribed seizure medications

Need to report new symptoms to the physician immediately

Home safety related to mental status, stairs in home, ambulation

Importance of steroids and other medications

Catheter care

Anticipated disease progression

Other information based on the patient's pathology from the tumor and the patient's unique needs

9. **Specific tips for quality and reimbursement**

For this and other diagnoses, document clearly the symptoms and clinical and assessment findings that support the end stage of the chronic illness process

Document patient changes, symptoms, and clinical information identified from visits and team conferences that support hospice care and limited life expectancy

Clearly support in the documentation the rationale that supports/explains the progression of the illness from the chronic to terminal stages

Document mentation, behavioral, and cognitive changes

Document dysphagia, weight loss, increased shortness of breath, dyspnea, infection, sepsis, new or changed medications, etc.

Document skin changes (e.g., inflamed, painful, weeping skin site[s])

Unless the patient is in a hospice insurance program, some insurers will not pay for a skilled nurse visit that is made at death if the patient is dead when the nurse arrives at the home. From a Medicare home care perspective, the visit at the time of death may be covered when the orders and clinical record document assessment of the patient's status or signs of death/life or state law allows pronouncement of death by a nurse.

Document any variances to expected outcomes. There are many models of hospice programs. Those that are home health agency–based must work within the framework of the Medicare home care program. For example, sometimes a hospice patient reaches a stable period in the illness and has no further skilled needs or the patient is no longer homebound per Medicare home health care criteria. When this occurs, one option is to discharge the patient from Medicare home health agency reimbursement and maintain the patient on grant funds or other available resources. If the patient's status deteriorates and again meets the Medicare criteria, a new start of care is initiated on the HCFA form 485. Usually hospices continue volunteer support,

nursing, and other services indicated during these periods of no reimbursement.

The Medicare hospice benefit does not require that the patient be homebound or have identified skilled needs. Though it is a needed and viable program, the Medicare hospice benefit may not be indicated for all Medicare-eligible beneficiaries. For further information on this benefit, please refer to HCFA Hospice Manual 21.

Should the patient's status deteriorate and increased personal care be needed, obtain a telephone order for the increased service, noting frequency and estimating the duration.

Obtain a telephone order for all medication and treatment changes of the medical regimen and document these in the clinical record.

Document patient deterioration

Document dehydration, dehydrating

Document patient change or instability

Document pain, other symptoms not controlled

Document status after acute episode of _____ (specify)

Document positive urine, sputum, etc. culture; patient started on _____ (specify ordered antibiotic therapy)

Document patient impacted; impaction removed manually

Document RN in frequent communication with physician regarding _____ (specify)

Document febrile at _____, pulse change at _____, irr., irr.

Document change noted in _____

Document bony prominences red, opening

Document RN contacted physician regarding _____ (specify)

Document marked SOB

Document alteration in mental status

Document medications being adjusted, regulated, or monitored

Document unable to perform own ADLs, personal care

Document all interdisciplinary team meetings and communications in the POC and in the progress notes of the clinical record

Document coordination of services and consultation with other members of the IDG

10. **Resources for hospice care and practice**

The Epilepsy Foundation offers *Seizure Recognition and First Aid,* which can be ordered by calling 1-800-332-1000.

The American Cancer Society has support groups such as "I Can Cope" and other programs. To locate the chapter nearest your patient, call 1-800-ACS-2345.

The American Cancer Society also has a "Look Good . . . Feel Better Program" for women undergoing chemotherapy or radiation. They can be reached at 1-800-395-LOOK.

The Brain Tumor Association can be reached at 1-800-886-2282. The National Brain Tumor Foundation can be reached at 1-800-934-CURE (2873).

BREAST CANCER AND MASTECTOMY CARE

1. **General considerations**

   The high incidence of breast cancer is appropriately alarming to all women. Patients with breast cancer need physical care and psychosocial support from the hospice team.

   Please refer to "Cancer Care" or "Pain Care" should these sections also pertain to your patient.

2. **Needs for visit**

   Physician order for hospice care, specific to the hospice program's admission criteria and policies

   Standard precautions supplies

   Vital signs equipment for baseline assessment

   Other supplies or equipment, based on physician orders

3. **Safety considerations**

   Infection control/standard precautions

   Supervised medication administration

   Multiple medications (e.g., side effects, interactions, safe storage)

   Night-light

   Safety for home medical equipment (e.g., bed, lift)

   Symptoms that necessitate immediate reporting/assistance

   Smoke detector and fire evacuation plan

   Extra caution on slippery surfaces

   Removal of scatter rugs

   Tub rail, grab bars for bathroom safety

   Supportive and nonskid shoes

   Handrail on stairs

   Fall precautions

   Protective skin measures

   Identification and report of any skin problems

   Others, based on the patient's unique condition and environment

4. **Potential diagnoses and codes**

Bone marrow transplant (surgical)	41.00
Bone metastases	198.5
Breast cancer	174.9
Cancer of the breast	174.9
Fibrocystic disease	610.1
Fracture (pathological)	733.10
Lumpectomy (partial mastectomy)	85.21
Lymphedema (postmastectomy)	457.0
Malignant neoplasms of the breast	174.9
Mastectomy (radical)	85.45
Mastectomy (simple)	85.41
Metastatic lung cancer	197.0
Paget's disease	731.0

Pneumonia	486
Radiation enteritis	558.1
Radiation myelitis	990 and 323.8
Secondary malignant neoplasm breast	198.81
Wound dehiscence	998.3
Wound infection	998.5

5. **Associated nursing diagnoses**
   Activity intolerance
   Activity intolerance, risk for
   Aspiration, risk for
   Anxiety
   Body image disturbance
   Body temperature, altered, risk for
   Bowel incontinence
   Breathing pattern, ineffective
   Cardiac output, decreased
   Caregiver role strain
   Caregiver role strain, risk for
   Communication, impaired verbal
   Constipation
   Coping, ineffective family: compromised
   Coping, ineffective family: disabling
   Coping, ineffective individual
   Decisional conflict (e.g., treatment options)
   Diarrhea
   Disuse syndrome, risk for
   Family processes, altered
   Fatigue
   Fear
   Fluid volume deficit, risk for
   Fluid volume excess
   Gas exchange, impaired
   Grieving, anticipatory
   Growth and development, altered
   Home maintenance management, impaired
   Hyperthermia
   Hypothermia
   Incontinence, total
   Infection, risk for
   Injury, risk for
   Knowledge deficit (specify)
   Mobility, impaired physical
   Noncompliance (specify)
   Nutrition, altered: less than body requirements
   Nutrition, altered: more than body requirements
   Oral mucous membrane, altered
   Pain
   Pain, chronic

Parenting, altered

Protection, altered

Role performance, altered

Self-care deficit, bathing/hygiene

Self-care deficit, feeding

Self-care deficit, toileting

Sensory/perceptual alterations (specify) (visual, auditory, kinesthetic, gustatory, tactile, olfactory)

Sexual dysfunction

Sexuality patterns, altered

Skin integrity, impaired

Skin integrity, impaired, risk for

Sleep pattern disturbance

Social interaction, impaired

Spiritual distress (distress of the human spirit)

Spiritual well-being, potential for enhanced

Swallowing, impaired

Thought processes, altered

Tissue integrity, impaired

Tissue integrity, impaired, risk for

Tissue perfusion, altered (specify type) (renal, cerebral, cardiopulmonary, gastrointestinal, peripheral)

Trauma, potential for

Urinary elimination, altered

Urinary retention

6. **Skills and services identified**

   • *Hospice nursing*

      a. *Comfort and symptom control*

         Complete initial assessment of all systems of patient with breast cancer admitted to hospice for _____ (specify problem necessitating care)

         Skilled observation and complete systems assessment of the patient with breast cancer, including nutrition, hydration, pain and other symptoms, and patient and family coping skills

         Comprehensive assessment of the patient after mastectomy with diagnoses of cancer

         Presentation of hospice philosophy and services

         Explain patient rights and responsibilities

         Assess patient, family, and caregiver wishes and expectations regarding care

         Assess patient, family, and caregiver resources available for care

         Provision of volunteer support to patient and family

         Teach family or caregiver physical care of patient

         Assess pain and other symptoms, including site, duration, characteristics, and relief measures

         RN to provide and teach effective oral care and comfort measures

         Pain assessment and management q visit

         RN to teach about and observe for signs, symptoms of infection

RN to evaluate amount and type of drainage in hemovac at home

Teach about pain regimen, including care for phantom sensations such as itching, tingling, and pain, and relief of these sensations

Patient to elevate affected arm

Check affected arm for edema or circulatory problems

Teach use/care of Hemovac

RN to assess and monitor pain after reconstructive surgery and patient's response to interventions and effective pain and other symptom relief measures

RN to assess blood pressure, other vital signs, including pain, q visit

Comfort measures of backrub and hand or other therapeutic massage

Teach about and observe side effects of palliative chemotherapy, including constipation, anemia, and fatigue

Assess weight as ordered

Assess pain and evaluate the pain management's effectiveness

Teach care of bedridden patient

RN to instruct in pain control measures and medication

Measure vital signs, including pain, q visit

Assess cardiovascular, pulmonary, and respiratory status

Teach caregivers symptom control and relief measures

Oxygen on at _____ liter per _____ (specify physician orders)

Identify and monitor pain, symptoms, and relief measures

RN to assess patient's pain or other symptoms q visit to identify need for change, addition, or other plan or dose adjustment

RN to teach about compression garments or pneumatic pumping

Effective management of pain and prevention of secondary symptoms

Interventions of symptoms directed toward comfort and palliation

Teach caregiver or family care of weak, terminally ill patient

Teach patient and family about realistic expectations of disease process

Teach care of dying, signs/symptoms of impending death

Presence and support

Other interventions, based on patient/family needs

b. *Safety and mobility considerations*

Provide caregiver with home safety information and instruction related to _____ and documented in the clinical record

Teach family about safety of patient in home

Teach family about energy conservation techniques

Instruct patient and caregiver to protect arm from infection and injury

RN to teach patient to avoid venipunctures, blood pressure readings, etc, in affected arm

Other interventions, based on patient/family needs

c. *Emotional/spiritual considerations*

Psychosocial assessment of patient and family regarding disease and prognosis

RN to provide emotional support to patient with significant body image change

Assess mental status and sleep disturbance changes

RN to provide emotional support to patient and family

Ongoing acknowledgment of spirituality and related concerns of patient/
family

Other interventions, based on patient/family needs

d. *Skin care*

RN to evaluate for deterrents to wound healing (e.g., radiation, poor
nutrition)

Teach patient and caregiver wound care, including infection control
measures

RN to provide skilled observation and assessment of surgical site

RN to teach patient about care of irradiated skin sites

RN to assess healing in reconstruction of breast site

Pressure ulcer care as indicated

Assess skin integrity

Observation and evaluation of wound and surrounding skin

Evaluate patient's need for equipment and supplies to decrease pressure,
including alternating pressure mattress, gel foam seat cushion, and
heel and elbow protectors

Teach family to perform dressing between RN visits, specifically

_____

Teach patient and family or caregiver about proper body alignment and
positioning in bed to prevent skin tears from shearing skin

Observe and apply skilled assessment of areas for possible breakdown,
including heels, hips, elbows, ankles, and other pressure-prone areas

Teach caregiver about skin care needs, including the need for frequent
position changes, appropriate pressure pads and mattresses, and the
prevention of breakdown

Other interventions, based on patient/family needs

e. *Elimination considerations*

Assess bowel regimen, and implement program as needed

Monitor bowel patterns, including frequency of bowel movements, and
evaluate bowel regimen (e.g., stool softeners, laxatives, dietary
changes)

RN to teach caregiver daily care of catheter

Observation and complete systems assessment of the patient with an
indwelling catheter

Check for and remove impaction as needed

Condom catheter or indwelling catheter as indicated

Assess amount and frequency of urinary output

Teach catheter care to caregiver

RN to evaluate the patient's bowel patterns, need for stool softeners,
laxatives, and dietary adjustments, and develop bowel management
plan

Other interventions, based on patient/family needs

f. *Hydration/nutrition*

RN to instruct patient and spouse in importance of adequate hydration
and nutrition needed for effective postoperative healing

Assess nutrition/hydration status

Diet counseling to patient with anorexia

Teach feeding-tube care to family

Nutrition/hydration supported by offering patient's choice of favorite or desired foods or liquids

Nutrition/hydration to be maintained by offering patient high-protein diet and foods of choice as tolerated

Teach patient and family to expect decreased nutritional and fluid intake as disease progresses

Other interventions, based on patient/family needs

g. *Therapeutic/medication regimens*

Teach about chemotherapy regimen, if appropriate

RN to instruct caregiver on all aspects of medications, including schedule, functions, possible side effects, and drug/drug and drug/food interactions

RN to assess the patient's unique response to treatments or interventions, and report changes or unfavorable responses or reactions to the physician

Medication assessment and management

Measure abdominal girth for ascites and edema, and document sites and amount

Obtain venipuncture as ordered q _____ (ordered frequency)

Teach new medication and effects

Teach new pain and symptom control medication regimen

Assess for electrolyte imbalance

Teach patient and caregiver use of PCA pump

Nonpharmacological interventions such as progressive muscle relaxation, imagery, positive visualization, music, massage and touch, and humor therapy of patient's choice implemented

Other interventions, based on patient/family needs

h. *Other considerations*

Instruct patient in increased risk of infection and lymphedema in affected arm, including signs and symptoms of cellulitis

Teach importance of Medic Alert bracelet and the need to avoid venipunctures, blood tests, and other procedures on affected arm

RN to assess the patient's response to treatments and interventions and to report to physician any changes, unfavorable responses, or reactions

Assess disease process progression

Other interventions, based on patient/family needs

- **Home health aide or certified nursing assistant**
Effective and safe personal care
Safe ADL assistance and support
Observation and reporting
Respite care and active listening skills
Meal preparation
Homemaker services
Comfort care
Other duties

- **Hospice social worker**
Psychosocial assessment of patient and family/caregiver, including adjustment to illness and its implications

Identification of optimal coping strategies

Financial assessment and counseling regarding food acquisition, ability to prepare, and costs of needed medications

Identification of caregiver role strain necessitating respite/relief measures or support

Intervention/support related to terminal illness and loss

Emotional/spiritual support

Depression/fear assessed and addressed

Facilitate communication among patient, family, and hospice team

Referral/linkage to community services and resources as indicated

Grief counseling and intervention/support related to illness/loss

Patient/caregiver counseling and support

For patients who live alone with no support system (e.g., able, available, willing caregiver[s], linkage to community resources to enable patient to remain in the home

Identification of illness-related psychiatric condition necessitating care, support, and intervention

Counseling regarding body image changes

- *Volunteer(s)*

  Support, friendship, companionship, and presence

  Comfort and dignity maintained/provided for patient and family

  Errands and transportation

  Other services, based on interdisciplinary team recommendations and patient/caregiver needs

- *Spiritual counselor*

  Spiritual assessment and care

  Counseling, intervention, support related to that dimension of life related to life's meaning (consistent with patient's beliefs)

  Support, listening, and presence

  Participation in sacred or spiritual rituals or practices

  Other supportive care, based on patient's/family's needs and belief

- *Dietitian/nutritional counseling*

  Assessment of patient with decreased intake, weight loss, anorexia, and nausea

  Teaching and support of family members and caregivers

  Support and care with food and nourishment as desired by patient

  Evaluation/management of nutritional deficits and needs

  Encouragement of nutritional supplements and snacks to increase protein and caloric intake

  Food, dietary recommendations incorporating patient choice and wishes (If patient on tube feeding, teach safe tube feeding techniques)

  Assessment of and instruction in use of alternative nutritional therapies, such as herbs, vitamin/mineral supplements, and macrobiotic diets

- *Occupational therapist*

  Evaluation of ADL and functional mobility

  Assess for need for adaptive equipment and assistive devices

  Safety assessment of patient's environment and ADL

  Assessment for energy conservation training

  Assessment of upper extremity function, retraining motor skills

Measures to improve function and problems with body image, such as the breast prosthesis and altered upper extremity function

- *Physical therapist*
  Evaluation
  Assessment of patient's environment for safety
  Safe transfer training
  Strengthening exercises/program
  Assessment of gait safety
  Instruct/supervise caregiver and volunteers on home exercise program for conditioning and strength
  Assistive, adaptive devices of equipment and teaching

- *Bereavement counselor*
  Assessment of the needs of the bereaved family and friends
  Support and intervention, based on an assessment and ongoing findings
  Presence and counseling
  Supportive visits, follow-up, and other interventions (e.g., mailings, calls)
  Other services related to bereavement work and support

- *Music, massage, art, or other therapies or services*
  Evaluation and intervention based on patient's and caregiver's unique wishes and needs that support care, comfort, and death in the setting of the patient's choice
  Pet therapy (including patient's pet, if available) and therapeutic intervention
  Assessment plan to engage patient and support comfort, quality, enjoyment, and dignity

7. **Outcomes for care**

- *Hospice nursing*
  Death with dignity and symptoms controlled in setting of patient/family choice
  Death with maximum comfort through effective symptom control with specialized hospice support
  Symptoms controlled in setting of patient/family choice
  Effective pain relief and control (e.g., a peaceful and comfortable death)
  Maximizing the patient's quality of life (e.g., patient is alert and pain free/or as patient wishes)
  Pharmacological and nonpharmacological interventions, such as localized heat application, positioning, relaxation methods, and music
  Patient cared for and family supported through death with physical, psychosocial, spiritual, and other needs acknowledged/addressed
  Patient- and family-centered hospice care provided based on the patient's/family's unique situation and needs
  Infection control and palliation
  Patient states pain is at _____ on a scale of 0-10 by next visit
  Patient/caregiver verbalizes satisfaction with care
  Adherence to POC as demonstrated by caregiver demonstrations and verbalizations and patient findings by _____ (specify date)

Caregiver effective in care management and knows whom to call for questions/concerns

Skin integrity maintained as evidenced by problem-free skin

Pain controlled, and comfort needs met throughout POC

IV access site remains patent, and flushing/dressing care is provided per protocol without signs/symptoms of infection

Patient's weight will be maintained/increased/decreased by

_____

Regulated bowel program, as evidenced by regular bowel movements

Wound site healing tracked through measurements of site and amount and type of drainage. Date projected for healing is _____ (specify date).

Patient will report being comfortable _____ % of the day (comfortable defined as pain free)

Complications/side effects of chemotherapy/radiation, including infection, bleeding, dehydration, nausea, and vomiting, controlled by _____ as reported by patient/caregiver

Compliance with and adherence to interdisciplinary care plan as demonstrated by observation and reporting by caregiver/patient

Caregiver demonstrates ability to manage pain, where applicable

Patient maintains comfort and dignity throughout illness

Patient protected from injury, stable respiratory status, and compliant with medication, safety, and care regimens

Comfort and individualized intervention of patient with immobility/bedbound status (e.g., skin, urinary, musculature, vascular)

Spiritual and psychosocial needs met (specify) as defined by patient and caregiver throughout course of care

Educational tools/plans incorporated in daily care and patient/caregiver verbalizes understanding of safe, needed care

Patient will decide on care, interventions, and evaluation

Caregiver effective in care management and knows whom to call for questions/concerns

Patient will express satisfaction with hospice support received and will experience increased comfort

Patient will be made comfortable at home through death in accordance with the patient's wishes

Effective pain control and symptom relief verbalized by patient

Patient verbalizes understanding of and adheres to care and medication regimens

Patient and caregiver supported through patient's death

Comfort maintained through course of care

The patient and family receive hospice support and care, and family members and friends are able to spend quality time with the patient

Caregiver able and verbalizes comfort with role and lists when to call hospice team members

Patient supported through and receives the maximum benefit from palliative chemotherapy and radiation with minimal complications

Patient/caregiver lists adverse reactions, potential complications, signs/symptoms of infection (e.g., sputum change, chest congestion)

Comfort maintained through death with dignity

Pain effectively managed, and patient verbalizes comfort

Patient has stable respiratory status with patent airway (e.g., no dyspnea, infection free)

Patient has reduction in complications resulting from chemotherapy and radiation therapy

Patient and caregiver demonstrate compliance with care instructions

Patient is able to maintain comfort and dignity throughout illness

Patient verbalizes self-care regimen and comfort level

Patient verbalizes and demonstrates care identified on plan, including medication regimen, exercise program, and diet instructions

Other goals/outcomes based on the patient's unique needs and problems

- *Home health aide or certified nursing assistant*

  Effective hygiene, personal care, and comfort

  ADL assistance

  Safe environment maintained

- *Hospice social worker*

  Problem identified and addressed with patient/caregiver and linked with appropriate support services and plan of care successfully implemented

  Patient and caregiver cope adaptively with illness and death

  Adaptive adjustment to changed body and body image

  Psychosocial support and counseling offered to patient/caregivers experiencing loss and grief

  Needs of minor children assessed and incorporated into plan

  Resources identified, community linkage obtained as appropriate for patient/family

- *Volunteer(s)*

  Comfort, companionship, and friendship extended to patient/family

  Support provided as defined by the needs of the patient/caregiver

  Support and respite provided as defined by patient/caregiver

- *Spiritual counseling*

  Spiritual support offered and provided as defined by needs of patient/caregiver

  Provision of spiritual support and care as based on the assessed and ongoing needs of the patient and family

  Intervention and support provided related to that dimension of life related to life's meaning (consistent with patient's beliefs)

  Spiritual support offered, and patient and family needs met

  Patient/family express a relief of symptoms of spiritual suffering

  Support, listening, and presence

  Participation in sacred or spiritual rituals or practices

  Other outcomes, based on the patient's/family's unique beliefs and needs

- *Dietitian/nutritional counseling*

  Family and caregiver integrating recommendations into nutrition teaching (where appropriate)

  Patient and caregiver know whom to call for nutrition- and hydration-related questions/concerns

  Nutrition and hydration per patient's choices

  Caregiver integrating dietary recommendations into daily meal planning

Patient and family verbalize comprehension of decreasing nutritional needs as disease progresses

- **Occupational therapist**
  Patient and caregiver demonstrate maximum independence with ADL, adaptive techniques, and assistive devices
  Patient and caregiver demonstrate maximum safety in ADL and enhanced functional mobility
  Patient and caregiver demonstrate effective use of energy conservation
  Verbalization/demonstration of improved functional activity level and enhanced quality of life
  Patient and caregiver demonstrate effective use of diaphragmatic breathing to reduce shortness of breath and relaxation techniques to help in pain/ symptom management
  Patient and caregiver demonstrate correct use of exercise
  Patient and caregiver will be independent in prosthesis and upper extremity exercise programs, and patient will verbalize improved body image

- **Physical therapist**
  Prevention of complications
  Home exercise and upper extremity program taught to caregiver
  Optimal strength and mobility maintained/achieved
  Compliance with home exercise program by _____ (date)

- **Bereavement counselor**
  Support services related to grief provided to patient and family
  Well-being and resolution process of grief initiated and followed through bereavement services

- **Music, massage, art, or other therapies or services**
  Therapeutic massage/touch effective for patient as self-reported or observed by caregivers/family
  Improved muscle tone, relaxation, and/or sleep
  Patient comfortable and relaxed (e.g., sleeping) after massage
  Music therapy intervention based on assessment to decrease pain perception and provide emotional expression and support
  Maintenance of comfort and physical, psychosocial and spiritual health
  Patient has pet's presence as desired—in all care sites, when possible
  Holistic health maintained and comfort achieved through _____ (specify modality)

8. **Patient, family and caregiver educational needs**
   Educational needs are the regimens that the caregiver will be managing with the patient. These include the following:
   The basic tenets of hospice and the availability of support 24 hours a day, 7 days a week
   Home safety assessment and counseling
   The patient's medication regimen
   Safe and proper body mechanics to promote patient comfort and prevent caregiver safety problems
   Other teaching specific to the patient's and family's unique needs
   Support groups available to patient's family, such as the hospice program's

"Caregiver Support Group" meetings for family members and friends of the patient

Home safety assessment and teaching

Effective personal hygiene habits

The avoidance of infections

Multiple medications and their relationship to one other

The importance of medical follow-up

Self-care observational aspects of care, particularly the postoperative wound site

Support groups in the community that are available to your patients and their caregivers

The importance of wearing a Medic Alert™ bracelet

Anticipated disease progression

Other information based on patient's unique needs

9. **Specific tips for quality and reimbursement**

Document in the clinical notes the clear progression and symptomatology and interventions that demonstrate caring for a patient with terminal cancer

Document when/if the patient has respiratory changes, shortness of breath, exacerbation of conditions, dysphagia, pain, and other symptoms and that they are identified and resolved.

Remember that the clinical documentation is key to measuring ongoing compliance for quality and reimbursement purposes. Care coordination, timely verbal and initial physician orders, and assessment and addressing of spiritual and psychosocial needs should be clearly documented in the patient's clinical record

The documentation should support that all hospice care supports comfort and dignity while meeting patient/family needs

The documentation should include the ongoing assessment and management of pain and other symptoms and the anticipation and prevention of secondary symptoms such as constipation

It is important to note that all team members, including nurses and social workers, should assess, identify, and "hear" spiritual needs that the patient/family want to be addressed. These spiritual issues are key to the provision of high-quality hospice care and cannot be addressed effectively and promptly by the spiritual counselor only

Document clearly symptoms, clinical changes, and assessment findings that support the end stage of the disease process.

Document patient changes, symptoms, and clinical information identified from visits and team conferences that supports hospice care and a limited life expectancy

Clearly support in the documentation the rationale that supports or explains the progression of the illness from the chronic to terminal stages

Document mentation, behavioral, and cognitive changes.

Document dysphagia, weight loss, increased shortness of breath, dyspnea, infection, sepsis, new or changed medications, etc.

Document any skin changes (e.g., inflamed, painful, weeping skin site[s])

Document when the patient is actively dying, deteriorating, or progressing toward death

Remember that the "litmus test" of care coordination rests on the quality of
the clinical documentation completed by all team members. Review one
of your patient's clinical records, and ask yourself the following: "If I
was unable to give a verbal report/update on this patient, would a peer be
able to pick up and provide the same level of care and know (from the
documentation) the current orders, including specific medications and
other details that contribute to effective hospice care?"
Document any variances to expected outcomes. Although these patients have
appropriate psychosocial needs, make sure that your documentation reflects
what the particular third-party payor or insurer perceives as "skilled,"
hands-on nursing care. Be sure that in addition to the needed professional
support you provide, the wound care, observation and assessment, or pain
management is reflected in your notes.

There are many models of hospice programs. Those that are home health
agency–based must work within the framework of the Medicare home care
program. For example, sometimes a hospice patient reaches a stable period in
the illness and has no further skilled needs or the patient is no longer homebound per Medicare home health care criteria. When this occurs, one option
is to discharge the patient from Medicare home health agency reimbursement
and maintain the patient on grant funds or other available resources. If the
patient's status deteriorates and again meets the Medicare criteria, a new start
of care is initiated on the HCFA form 485. Usually hospices continue volunteer support, nursing, and other services indicated during these periods of no
reimbursement.

The Medicare hospice benefit does not require that the patient be homebound or have identified skilled needs. Though it is a needed and viable
program, the Medicare hospice benefit may not be indicated for all Medicare-
eligible beneficiaries. For further information on this benefit, please refer to
HCFA Hospice Manual 21.

Should the patient's status deteriorate and increased personal care be
needed, obtain a telephone order for the increased service, noting frequency
and estimating the duration.

Obtain a telephone order for all medication and treatment changes of the
medical regimen, and document these in the clinical record.
Document coordination of services and consultation with other members of
the IDG
Obtain orders for any change in the POC and concurrence of other team
members

10. **Resources for hospice care and practice**
The American Cancer Society (ACS) has a "Look Good . . . Feel Better
Program" that offers support and make-over services by cosmetologists for
women undergoing chemotherapy or radiation therapy. Call 1-800-395-LOOK
for more information.

"tlc" is a magazine/catalog available through the ACS. Items include
bathing suits, wigs, hair pieces, mesh hair caps to catch hair lost at night
from chemotherapy, and other specifically designed products to help women
feel and look dignified and attractive after loss and change. Call the ACS at
(800) 850-9445 to obtain a free catalogue.

The Y-ME National Breast Cancer Organization provides information, support, and referrals. Whenever possible, trained breast cancer survivors are matched to callers by background and experience, (800) 221-2141. Spanish language services available, (800) 986-9505.

Contact the American Cancer Society (ACS) to learn about *Reach to Recovery,* a visitation program offered by trained breast cancer survivors for women and their families, (800) ACS-2345. Spanish language services are available.

Contact Y-ME's Wig and Prosthesis Bank for women with financial need, (800) 221-2141. Spanish language services are available, (800) 986-9505.

CANCER CARE

1. **General considerations**

   Cancer care and the generalized care of patients with cancer are characterized by frequent contact with health care providers over a long period of time.

   Please refer to "Breast Cancer and Mastectomy Care," "Brain Tumor Care," "Constipation Care," "Infusion Care," and "Head and Neck Cancer Care" should these sections also pertain to your patient.

2. **Needs for visit**

   Physician order for hospice care, specific to the hospice program's admission criteria and policies

   Standard precautions supplies

   Vital signs equipment for baseline assessment

   Other supplies or equipment, based on physician orders

3. **Safety considerations**

   Infection control/standard precautions

   Night-light

   Extra caution on slippery surfaces

   Removal of scatter rugs

   Tub rail, grab bars for bathroom safety

   Supportive and nonskid shoes

   Handrail on stairs

   Fall precautions

   Protective skin measures

   Identification and report of any skin problems

   Smoke detector and fire evacuation plan

   Assistance with ambulation

   Disposal of soiled dressing/sharps, intravenous (IV)/infusion administration supplies

   Symptoms that necessitate immediate reporting/assistance

   Safety for home medical equipment (e.g., bed, lift)

   Supervised medication administration

   Multiple medications (e.g., side effects, interactions, safe storage)

   Smoke detector and fire evacuation plan

   Others, based on the patient's unique condition and environment

4. **Potential diagnoses and codes**

Attention to ileostomy	V55.2
Bladder cancer	188.9
Bone marrow transplant (surgical)	41.00
Bone metastases	198.5
Bowel obstruction	560.9
Brain cancer	191.9
Breast cancer	174.9
Cervix, cancer of	180.9
Colon cancer	153.9

Colon lymphoma	202.83
Colostomy, attention to	V55.3
Colostomy (surgical)	46.10
Debility	799.3
Endometrial cancer	182.0
Esophagus, cancer of the	150.9
Ewing's sarcoma	170.9
Fitting and adjustment of urinary devices	V53.6
Fracture, pathological	733.10
Gastric cancer, metastatic	197.8
Gastrostomy, attention to	V55.1
Gastrostomy, temporary	43.19
Glioma	191.9
Head or neck, cancer of the	195.0
Hickman catheter insertion	38.93
Hodgkin's disease	201.90
Ileostomy, attention to	V55.2
Intestinal obstruction	560.9
Kaposi's sarcoma	042 and 176.9
Kidney cancer	189.0
Laryngectomy, complete (surgical)	30.3
Leukemia, acute	208.0
Leukopenia	288.0
Liver cancer	155.2
Liver, metastatic cancer of	197.7
Lung, adenocarcinoma	162.9
Lung cancer, squamous cell	162.9
Lung resection, segmental (surgical)	32.3
Lymphoma (non-Hodgkin's)	202.80
Malaise and fatigue	780.7
Mastectomy, radical	85.46
Mastectomy, simple	85.42
Melanoma, malignant	172.9
Metastases, general	199.1
Multiple myeloma	203.0
Nasopharyngeal	147.9
Nausea with vomiting	787.01
Neuroblastoma	194.0
Obstruction, intestinal	560.9
Oropharyngeal	146.9
Osteosarcoma	170.9
Ovarian cancer	183.0
Pancreatectomy (surgical)	52.6
Pancreatic cancer	157.9
Pharynx cancer	149.0
Pleural effusion, right or left	197.2
Pneumonia	486
Pressure wound	707.0
Prostate, cancer of	185

Protein-caloric malnutrition	263.9
Radiation enteritis	558.1
Radiation myelitis	990 and 323.8
Rectosigmoid	154.0
Rectum, cancer of the	154.1
Renal (cancer of the kidney)	189.0
Renal cell cancer, metastatic	198.0
Sarcoma	171.9
Secondary malignant neoplasm breast	198.81
Septicemia	038.9
Skin carcinoma	173.9
Spinal cord compression	151.9
Spinal cord tumor	239.7
Stomach, cancer of the	151.9
Testis, cancer of	186.9
Tongue, cancer of the	141.9
Tracheostomy, attention to	V55.0
Urinary tract infection	599.0
Uterine sarcoma, metastatic	198.82
Uterus, cancer of the	179
Vulvar cancer	184.4
Wound dehiscence	998.3

5. **Associated nursing diagnoses**
   Activity intolerance
   Activity intolerance, risk for
   Adjustment, impaired
   Airway clearance, ineffective
   Anxiety
   Aspiration, risk for
   Body image disturbance
   Body temperature, altered, risk for
   Bowel incontinence
   Breathing pattern, ineffective
   Cardiac output, decreased
   Caregiver role strain
   Caregiver role strain, risk for
   Constipation
   Coping, ineffective family: compromised
   Decisional conflict (treatment choices)
   Denial, ineffective
   Diarrhea
   Family processes, altered
   Fatigue
   Fear
   Grieving, anticipatory
   Home maintenance management, impaired
   Incontinence, total
   Infection, risk for

Injury, risk for
Knowledge deficit (disease and management)
Mobility, impaired physical
Nutrition, altered: less than body requirements
Oral mucous membrane, altered
Pain
Pain, chronic
Parenting, altered
Protection, altered
Role performance, altered
Self-care deficit (specify)
Sensory/perceptual alterations (specify) (visual, auditory, kinesthetic, gustatory, tactile, olfactory)
Sexual dysfunction
Skin integrity, impaired
Skin integrity, impaired, risk for
Sleep pattern disturbance
Social interaction, impaired
Social isolation
Spiritual distress (distress of the human spirit)
Spiritual well-being, potential for enhanced
Swallowing, impaired
Thought processes, altered
Tissue integrity, impaired
Urinary elimination, altered
Urinary retention

6. **Skills and services identified**

   • *Hospice nursing*

      a. *Comfort and symptom control*
         Complete initial assessment of all systems of patient with cancer admitted to hospice for _____ (specify problem necessitating care)
         Observation and complete assessment of the patient with cancer of _____ (specify site/type)
         Presentation of hospice philosophy and services
         Explain patient rights and responsibilities
         Assess patient, family, and caregiver wishes and expectations regarding care
         Assess patient, family, and caregiver resources available for care
         Assess pain and other symptoms including site, duration, characteristics, and relief measures (see Part Seven)
         Provision of volunteer support to patient and family
         Teach family or caregiver physical care of patient
         Assess pain and other symptoms
         RN to provide and teach effective oral care and comfort measures
         Teach care of bedridden patient
         Measure vital signs, including pain, q visit
         Assess cardiovascular, pulmonary, and respiratory status

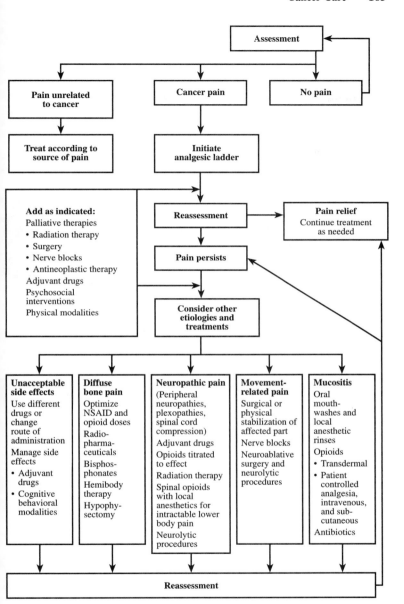

Figure 4-1 Continuing pain management in patients with cancer. (From Cancer Pain Management Guideline Panel: *Management of cancer pain. Clinical practice guideline,* AHCPR Publication No. 94-0592, Rockville, Md, 1994, Agency for Health Care Policy and Research Public Health Service, U.S. Department of Health and Human Services, p 13.)

Teach new pain- or symptom-control medication regimen

Teach caregivers symptom control and relief measures

Assess weight as ordered

Oxygen on at _____ liter per _____ (specific physician orders)

Teach caregiver or family care of weak, terminally ill patient

RN to instruct in pain control measures and medications

RN to assess patient's pain or other symptoms q visit to identify need for change, addition, or other plan or dose adjustment

RN to teach patient and caregiver about disease process and management

Comfort measures of backrub and hand or other therapeutic massage

Assess pain, and evaluate the pain management's effectiveness q visit

Effective management of pain and prevention of secondary symptoms

Interventions of symptoms directed toward comfort and palliation

Teach caregiver/patient use of pain assessment tool/scale and reporting mechanism(s)

Observation and assessment of patient with nausea and vomiting who is receiving palliative radiation and chemotherapy

Teach patient and family about realistic expectations of disease process

Teach care of dying and signs/symptoms of impending death

Presence and support

Other interventions, based on patient/family needs

b. *Safety and mobility considerations*

Provide caregiver with home safety information and instruction related to _____ and documented in the clinical record

Notify Fire Department (with permission from patient) of ventilator-dependent/tracheostomy patient

Teach family about safety

Teach family about energy conservation techniques

Teach patient and caregiver care needed for safe, effective management at home

Other interventions, based on patient/family needs

c. *Emotional/spiritual considerations*

Psychosocial assessment of patient and family regarding disease and prognosis

Assess patient's and family's coping skills

Assess mental status, sleep disturbance changes

Inform patient/family/caregiver of available volunteer support

RN to provide emotional support to patient and family

Psychosocial aspects of pain control (e.g., depression) with team support/intervention

Ongoing acknowledgment of spirituality and related concerns of patient/family

Other interventions, based on patient/family needs

d. *Skin care*

Pressure ulcer care as indicated

RN to teach patient regarding care of irradiated skin sites

RN to assess skin site after radiation therapy and teach skin care regimen

Observation and evaluation of wound and surrounding skin

Evaluate patient's need for equipment and supplies to decrease pressure, including alternating pressure mattress, gel foam seat cushion, and heel and elbow protectors

Teach family to perform dressing between RN visits, specifically

_____

Teach patient and family or caregiver about proper body alignment and positioning in bed to prevent skin tears from shearing skin

Observe and apply skilled assessment of areas for possible breakdown, including heels, hips, elbows, ankles, and other pressure-prone areas

Teach caregiver about skin care needs, including the need for frequent position changes, appropriate pressure pads and mattresses, and the prevention of breakdown

Other interventions, based on patient/family needs

e. *Elimination considerations*

Assess bowel regimen, and implement program as needed

Rectal tube for increased flatulence/gas pain

Check for and remove impaction as needed

Condom catheter or indwelling catheter as indicated

Assess amount and frequency of urinary output

Teach catheter care to caregiver

RN to teach caregiver daily care of catheter

RN to evaluate bowel patterns and need for stool softeners, laxatives, and dietary adjustments and develop bowel management plan

Other interventions, based on patient/family needs

f. *Hydration/nutrition*

Instruct patient about specific diet _____ (specify physician orders)

Assess nutrition/hydration status

Diet counseling for patient with anorexia

Teach feeding-tube care to family

Nutrition/hydration supported by offering patient's choice of favorite or desired foods or liquids

Nutrition/hydration to be maintained by offering patient high-protein diet and foods of choice as tolerated

RN to teach family regarding patient's need for small, high-calorie, and frequent meals of patient's choice

Teach patient and family to expect decreased nutritional and fluid intake as disease progresses

Other interventions, based on patient/family needs

g. *Therapeutic/medication regimens*

Medication review and management (e.g., drug/drug, drug/food interactions)

Measure abdominal girth for ascites and edema, and document sites and amount

Obtain venipuncture as ordered q _____ (ordered frequency)

Teach new medication and effects

Teach new pain and symptom control medication regimen

Assess for fluid and electrolyte imbalance

Administer IM or sq injection for pain control

Nonpharmacological interventions such as progressive muscle relaxation, imagery, positive visualization, music, massage and touch, and humor therapy of patient's choice implemented

Assess the patient's unique response to treatments or interventions, and report changes or unfavorable responses or reactions to the physician

Teach about and observe side effects of chemotherapy, including constipation, anemia, and fatigue

Teach patient and caregiver use of PCA pump

Other interventions, based on patient/family needs

h. *Other considerations*

RN to assess the patient's response to treatments and interventions and to report to the physician changes, unfavorable responses, or reactions

Teach family or caregiver signs of bleeding, including hematuria and bruising

Observation and assessment, communication with physician related to signs and symptoms of oncologic emergencies (e.g., spinal cord compression, superior vena cava syndrome, hypercalcemia) and symptom treatment

Assess disease process progression

Other interventions, based on patient/family needs

- **Home health aide or certified nursing assistant**

Effective and safe personal care

Safe ADL assistance and support and ambulation and transfer assist

Observation and reporting

Respite care

Active listening skills

Meal preparation

Homemaker services

Comfort care

Other duties

- **Hospice social worker**

Psychosocial assessment of patient and family/caregiver, including adjustment to illness and its implications

Identification of optimal coping strategies

Financial assessment and counseling regarding food acquisition, ability to prepare, and costs of needed medications

Intervention/support related to terminal illness and loss

Emotional/spiritual support

Depression/fear assessed and addressed

Facilitation of communication among patient, family, and hospice team

Identification of optimal coping strategies

Referral/linkage to community services and resources as indicated

Grief counseling and intervention/support related to illness/loss

Patient/caregiver counseling and support

For patients who live alone with no support system (e.g., able, available, willing caregiver[s]): obtain linkage with necessary community resources to allow patient to stay in the home

Identification of illness-related psychiatric condition necessitating care

Facilitation of completion of will and arrangements for funeral

- *Volunteer(s)*

  Support, friendship, companionship, and presence

  Comfort and dignity maintained/provided for patient and family

  Errands and transportation

  Other services, based on interdisciplinary team recommendations and patient/caregiver needs

- *Spiritual counselor*

  Spiritual assessment and care

  Counseling, intervention, and support related to that dimension of life related to life's meaning (consistent with patient's beliefs)

  Support, listening, and presence

  Participation in sacred or spiritual rituals or practices

  Other supportive care, based on patient's/family's needs and belief systems

- *Dietitian/nutritional counseling*

  Assessment of patient with decreased intake, weight loss, anorexia, and nausea

  Assessment and recommendations for swallowing difficulties

  Teaching and support of family members and caregivers

  Support and care with food and nourishment as desired by patient

  Evaluation/management of nutritional deficits and needs

  Encourage nutritional supplements and snacks to increase protein and caloric intake

  Food and dietary recommendations incorporating patient choice and wishes

  Counseling and instruction of family regarding patient's decreased appetite and possible eventual inability to eat

  Assessment of and instruction in use of alternative nutritional therapies such as herbs, vitamin/mineral supplements, and macrobiotic diets

- *Occupational therapist*

  Evaluation of ADL and functional mobility

  Energy conservation techniques

  Adaptive, assistive, safety supports/devices and training

  ADL training

  Measures to improve function and body image (e.g., breast prosthesis), as patient requests

  Assess need for adaptive/equipment devices

  Teach compensatory techniques

  Safety assessment of patient's environment and ADL measures to improve function and body image, such as breast or other prosthesis and extremity function

- *Physical therapist*
  Evaluation
  Safety assessment of patient's environment
  Safe transfer training or bed mobility exercises
  Pain assessment/reduction factors
  Strengthening exercises/program
  Assessment of gait safety and home safety measures
  Instruct/supervise caregiver and volunteers on home exercise program for conditioning and strength
  Evaluation of equipment (e.g., assistive, adaptive devices) and teaching

- *Speech-language pathologist*
  Evaluation for speech/swallowing problems
  Food texture recommendations
  Alternate functional communication

- *Bereavement counselor*
  Assessment of the needs of the bereaved family and friends
  Support and intervention, based on assessment and ongoing findings
  Presence and counseling
  Supportive visits and follow-up, other interventions (e.g., mailings, calls)
  Other services related to bereavement work and support

- *Pharmacist*
  Evaluation of hospice patient on multiple medications for possible food/drug, drug/drug interactions
  Medication monitoring regarding therapeutic levels and dosages
  Pain consult and input into interdisciplinary plan of care related to pain control, palliation, and symptom management
  Assessment of medication regimen and plan for safety and compliance

- *Music, massage, art, or other therapies or services*
  Evaluation and intervention based on patient's and caregiver's unique wishes and needs that support care, comfort, and death in the setting of the patient's choice
  Assessment plan to engage patient and support comfort, quality, enjoyment, and dignity
  Pet therapy (including patient's pet, if available) and therapeutic intervention

7. **Outcomes for care**

- *Hospice nursing*
  Death with dignity, and symptoms controlled in setting of patient/family choice
  Optimal comfort, support, and dignity provided throughout illness
  Death with maximum comfort through effective symptom control with specialized hospice support
  Patient and caregiver able to list adverse drug/chemotherapy/radiation reactions and know whom to call for follow-up and resolution
  Pain and symptoms managed/controlled in setting of patient/family choice (e.g., patient and family report ability to eat, sleep, perform other activities)

BOX 4-1

BARRIERS TO CANCER PAIN MANAGEMENT

Problems Related to Health Care Professionals
Inadequate knowledge of pain management
Poor assessment of pain
Concern about regulation of controlled substances
Fear of patient addiction
Concern about side effects of analgesics
Concern about patients becoming tolerant to analgesics

Problems Related to Patients
Reluctance to report pain
    Concern about distracting physicians from treatment of underlying disease
    Fear that pain means disease is worse
    Concern about not being a "good" patient
Reluctance to take pain medications
    Fear of addiction or of being thought of as an addict
    Worries about unmanageable side effects
    Concern about becoming tolerant to pain medications

Problems Related to the Health Care System
Low priority given to cancer pain treatment
Inadequate reimbursement
    The most appropriate treatment may not be reimbursed or may be too costly for patients and families
Restrictive regulation of controlled substances
Problems of availability of treatment or access to it

Modified from Cancer Pain Management Guideline Panel: *Management of cancer pain. Clinical practice guideline,* AHCPR Publication No. 94-0592, Rockville, Md, 1994, Agency for Health Care Policy and Research, Public Health Service, U.S. Department of Health and Human Services.

Patient's and family's privacy, independence, and choices supported with respect and maintained through death
Enhancement and support of quality of life
Effective pain relief and symptom control (e.g., a peaceful and comfortable death at home, some enjoyment of life) (see Box 4-1)
Maximizing the patient's quality of life (e.g., alert and pain free/or as patient wishes)
Pharmacological and nonpharmacological interventions, such as localized heat application, positioning, relaxation methods, and music
Patient cared for and family supported through death with physical, psychosocial, spiritual, and other concerns/needs acknowledged/addressed
Patient- and family-centered hospice care provided based on the patient's/family's unique situation and needs
Infection control and palliation
Grief/bereavement expression and support provided
Caregiver demonstrates ability to manage pain, where applicable

Patient maintains comfort and dignity throughout illness

Patient will report being comfortable _____% of the day (*comfortable* defined as pain free by patient)

Complications/side effects of chemotherapy/radiation, including infection, bleeding, dehydration, nausea, and vomiting, controlled by _____, as reported by patient/caregiver

Planned and effective bowel program, as evidenced by regular bowel movement and patient/family report of comfort

Compliance with and adherence to interdisciplinary care plan as demonstrated by observation and reporting by caregiver/patient

Patient states pain is at _____ on a scale of 1-10 by next visit

Other goals/outcomes based on the patient's unique needs and problems

- ***Home health aide or certified nursing assistant***
  Effective hygiene, personal care, and comfort
  Safe ADL assistance and ambulation
  Safe environment maintained

- ***Hospice social worker***
  Problems identified and addressed, with patient/caregiver linked with appropriate support services and plan of care successfully implemented
  Patient and caregiver cope adaptively with illness and death
  Adaptive adjustment to changed body and body image
  Psychosocial support and counseling offered to patient/caregivers experiencing loss and grief
  Facilitation of will and funeral arrangements

- ***Volunteer(s)***
  Comfort, companionship, and friendship extended to patient/family
  Support provided as defined by the needs of the patient/caregiver
  Patient and family supported by team with care, comfort, and companionship

- ***Spiritual counseling***
  Spiritual support offered and provided as defined by needs of patient/caregiver
  Provision of spiritual support and care as based on the assessed and ongoing needs of the patient and family
  Spiritual support offered and patient and family needs met
  Patient and family express relief of symptoms of spiritual suffering
  Support, listening, and presence
  Participation in sacred or spiritual rituals or practices
  Intervention and support provided related to that dimension of life related to life's meaning (consistent with patient's beliefs)

- ***Dietitian/nutritional counseling***
  Family/caregiver integrating recommendations into nutrition teaching (where appropriate)
  Patient and family verbalize understanding of changing nutritional needs
  Patient/caregiver know whom to call for nutrition- and hydration-related questions/concerns

Nutrition/hydration per patient's choices
Caregiver integrating recommendations into daily meal planning

- *Occupational therapist*
    Patient and caregiver demonstrate maximum independence with ADL, adaptive techniques, and assistive devices
    Patient and caregiver demonstrate maximum safety in ADL and functional mobility
    Patient and caregiver demonstrate effective use of energy conservation
    Verbalization/demonstration of improved functional activity level and enhanced quality of life
    Patient and caregiver demonstrate effective use of diaphragmatic breathing to reduce shortness of breath and relaxation techniques to help in pain/symptom management
    Patient and caregiver will be independent in prosthesis and upper extremity exercise programs, and will verbalize improved body image

- *Physical therapist*
    Prevention of complications
    Home exercise and upper extremity program taught to caregiver
    Optimal strength and mobility maintained/achieved
    Compliance with home exercise program by _____ (date)

- *Speech-language pathologist*
    Communication method implemented, and patient able to be understood as self-reported or reported by family/caregivers
    Safe swallowing and functional communication
    Recommended list of food textures for safety and patient choice

- *Bereavement counselor*
    Grief support services provided to patient and family
    Well-being and resolution process of grief initiated and followed through bereavement services

- *Pharmacist*
    Multiple drug regimen reviewed for food/drug and drug/drug interactions in patient on steroids and other medications
    Stability and safety in complex medication regimen
    Effective pain and symptom control and symptom management as reported by patient/caregiver

- *Music, massage, art, or other therapies or services*
    Therapeutic massage/touch effective for patient as self-reported or observed by caregivers/family
    Improved muscle tone, relaxation, and/or sleep
    Patient comfortable and relaxed (e.g., sleeping) after massage
    Music therapy intervention based on assessment to decrease pain perception and provide emotional expression and support
    Maintenance of comfort and physical, psychosocial, and spiritual health
    Holistic health maintained and comfort achieved through _____ (specify modality)
    Patient has pet's presence as desired—in all care sites, when possible

8. **Patient, family, and caregiver educational needs**

Educational needs are the care regimens that contribute to safe and effective care at home between the hospice team's visits. These include the following:

The basic tenets of hospice and the availability of support 24 hours a day, 7 days a week

Home safety assessment and counseling

The patient's medication regimen

Safe and proper body mechanics to promote patient comfort and prevent caregiver safety problems

Anticipated disease progression

Support groups available to patient's family, such as the hospice program's "Caregiver Support Group" meetings for family members and friends of the patient

9. **Specific tips for quality and reimbursement**

Other teaching specific to the patient's and family's unique needs

Document any variances to expected outcomes. There are many models of hospice programs. Those that are home health agency–based must work within the framework of the Medicare home care program. For example, sometimes a hospice patient reaches a stable period in the illness and has no further skilled needs or the patient is no longer homebound per Medicare home health care criteria. When this occurs, one option is to discharge the patient from Medicare home health agency reimbursement and maintain the patient on grant funds or other available resources. If the patient's status deteriorates and again meets the Medicare criteria, a new start of care is initiated on the HCFA form 485. Usually hospices continue volunteer support, nursing, and other services indicated during these periods of no reimbursement.

The Medicare hospice benefit does not require that the patient be homebound or have identified skilled needs. Though it is a needed and viable program, the Medicare hospice benefit may not be indicated for all Medicare eligible beneficiaries. For further information on this benefit, please refer to HCFA Hospice Manual 21.

Should the patient's status deteriorate and increased personal care be needed, obtain a telephone order for the increased service, noting frequency and estimating the duration.

Obtain a telephone order for all medication and treatment changes of the medical regimen and document these in the clinical record.

Document in the clinical notes the clear progression and symptomatology of the disease process and interventions that demonstrate caring for a patient with terminal cancer

Document when/if the patient has respiratory changes, shortness of breath, exacerbation of conditions, dysphagia, pain, and other symptoms and that they are identified and resolved

Remember that the clinical documentation is key to measuring compliance for quality and reimbursement purposes. Care coordination, timely verbal and initial physician orders, and assessment and addressing of spiritual and psychosocial needs should be clearly documented in the patient's clinical record.

The documentation should support that all hospice care supports comfort and dignity while meeting patient/family needs

The documentation should include the ongoing assessment and management of pain and other symptoms and the anticipation and prevention of secondary symptoms such as constipation

It is important to note that all team members, including nurses and social workers, should assess, identify, and "hear" spiritual needs that the patient/family want to be addressed. These spiritual issues are key to the provision of high-quality hospice care and cannot be addressed effectively and promptly by the spiritual counselor only

Document clearly symptoms, clinical changes, and assessment findings that support the end stage of the cancer process

Document patient changes, symptoms, and clinical information identified from visits and team conferences that support hospice care and a limited life expectancy

Clearly support in the documentation the rationale that supports/explains the progression of the illness from the chronic to terminal stages

Document mentation, behavioral, and/or cognitive changes

Document dysphagia, weight loss, increased shortness of breath, dyspnea, infection, sepsis, new or changed medications, etc.

Document any skin changes (e.g., inflamed, painful, weeping skin site[s])

Document when the patient is actively dying, deteriorating, and progressing toward death

Remember that the "litmus test" of care coordination rests on the quality of the clinical documentation by all team members. Review one of your patient's clinical records, and ask yourself, "If I was unable to give a verbal report/update on this patient, would a peer be able to pick up and provide the same level of care and know (from the documentation) the current orders, medications, and other details that contribute to effective hospice care?"

Documentation of coordination of services and consultation with the other members of the IDG

Unless the patient is in a hospice insurance program, some insurers will not pay for a skilled nurse visit that is made at death if the patient is dead when the nurse arrives at the home. From a Medicare home care perspective, the visit at the time of death may be covered when the orders and clinical record document assessment of the patient's status or signs of death/life or state law allows pronouncement of death by a nurse.

Document patient deterioration

Document dehydration, dehydrating

Document patient change or instability

Document pain, other symptoms not controlled

Document status after acute episode of _____ (specify)

Document positive urine, sputum, etc. culture; patient started on _____ (specify ordered antibiotic therapy)

Document patient impacted; impaction removed manually

Document RN in frequent communication with physician regarding _____ (specify)

Document febrile at _____, pulse change at _____, irr., irr.

Document change noted in _____

Document bony prominences red, opening

Document RN contacted physician regarding _____ (specify)

Document marked SOB

Document alteration in mental status

Document medications being adjusted, regulated, or monitored

Document unable to ADLs, personal care

Document all interdisciplinary team meetings and communications in the
   POC and in the progress notes of the clinical record

All disciplines involved should have input into the POC and document their
   interventions and goals

10. **Resources for hospice care and practice**

The National Cancer Institute (NCI) offers a 37-page free publication entitled
Advanced Cancer: Living Each Day, which can be ordered by calling 1-800-
4-CANCER. The NCI and the American Cancer Society (ACS) offer a publication called *Caring for the Patient with Cancer at Home: A Guide for
Patients and Families.* This 90-page publication covers many symptoms and
problems associated with cancer and cancer therapy. This booklet can be
ordered by calling the ACS at 1-800-ACS-2345 or the NCI at 1-800-4-
CANCER.

The American Cancer Society has support groups such as "I Can Cope"
and other programs. To locate the chapter nearest your patient, call 1-800-
ACS-2345.

The American Cancer Society also has a "Look Good . . . Feel Better
Program" for women undergoing chemotherapy or radiation. It can be
reached at 1-800-395-LOOK.

Available free from the Agency for Health Care Policy and Research
(AHCPR) are three resources: *Clinical Practice Guideline Number 9: Management of Cancer Pain; Quick Reference Guide for Clinicians: Management
of Cancer Pain—Adults;* and *Patient Guide: Managing Cancer Pain.* The
patient guides are available in English and Spanish, and all can be ordered by
calling 1-800-358-9295.

A pamphlet entitled *Get Relief from Cancer Pain* is available from
the National Cancer Institute's Cancer Information Service by calling
1-800-4-CANCER (1-800-422-6237).

Questions and Answers about Pain Control, a 76-page booklet, is available free from the Cancer Information Service by calling the toll-free
number.

Helping Hand: The Resource Guide for People with Cancer is a comprehensive listing of resources and services available to patients with cancer and
their families. This book is available free by calling 800-813-4673 (HOPE)
or 212-221-3300.

CARDIAC CARE (END STAGE)

1. **General considerations**

   Patients and families may be referred to hospice for progressive and cardiac myopathies, severe congestive heart failure, angina, post myocardial infarctions, and many other cardiac problems. These patients and their families have usually had a long history of curative and aggressive treatment directed toward the cardiac pathology. Supportive and skillful care is directed toward comfort and symptomatic relief of chest pain, shortness of breath, and other problems.

2. **Needs for visit**

   Physician order for hospice care, specific to the hospice program's admission criteria and policies

   Standard precautions supplies

   Vital signs equipment for baseline assessment

   Other supplies or equipment, based on physician orders

3. **Safety considerations**

   Infection control/standard precautions

   Disposal of soiled dressings, sharps, intravenous (IV) infusion administration supplies

   Supervised medication administration

   Tub rail, grab bars, shower seat for bathroom safety

   Supportive and nonskid shoes

   Fall precautions

   Oxygen precautions

   Identification and report of any skin problems/changes

   Multiple medications (e.g., side effects, heparin precautions, interactions, safe storage)

   Night-light

   Safety for home medical equipment (e.g., bed, lift)

   Cardiac or other symptoms that necessitate reporting/assistance

   Smoke detector and fire evacuation plan

   Pace activities

   Change positions slowly

   Protective skin measures

   Others, based on the patient's unique condition and environment

4. **Potential diagnoses and codes**

Abdominal aortic aneurysm	441.02
AMI	410.92
Anemia	285.9
Aneurysm repair (surgical)	39.52
Angina	413.9
Angina, unstable	411.1
Angioplasty (percutaneous) (surgical)	39.50
Aortic stenosis	424.1

Aortic valve disorder	424.1
Aortocoronary bypass (1 vessel) (surgical)	36.11
Aortocoronary bypass (4 vessels) (surgical)	36.14
Atherosclerosis (coronary)	414.00
Atrial fibrillation	427.31
Atrial flutter	427.32
Bacterial endocarditis	421.0
Cardiac dysrhythmia	427.9
Cardiac murmurs	785.2
Cardiomegaly	429.3
Cardiomyopathy	425.4
Chronic ischemic heart disease	414.9
Congestive heart failure	428.0
COPD	496
Cor pulmonale	416.9
Coronary artherosclerosis (coronary artery disease)	414.00
Coronary artery bypass graft surgery	
two coronary arteries (surgical)	36.12
three coronary arteries (surgical)	36.13
four coronary arteries (surgical)	36.14
Coronary bypass syndrome	411.1
CVA	436
Depressive disorder	311
Diabetes (Type I) juvenile, with complications	250.91
Diabetes (Type II) adult, with complications	250.90
Digoxin toxicity	995.2 and E942.1
Electrolyte and fluid imbalance	276.9
Endocarditis	424.90
HCVD with CHF	402.91
Heart block	426.9
Heart disease, end stage	429.9
Heart transplant (surgical)	37.5
Hypertension with heart involvement	402.90
Ischemic heart disease	414.9
Left heart failure	428.1
Mediastinitis	519.2
Mitral valve disease	394.9
Mitral valve disorder	424.0
Myocardial infarction	410.92
Obesity	278.00
Other aftercare following surgery	V58.4
Pacemaker (S/P)	V45.00
Pericardial disease	423.9
Peripheral vascular disease	443.9
Pleural effusion	511.9
Pneumonia	486
Postsurgical status, aortocoronary bypass status	V45.81
Postsurgical status, presence of neuropacemaker or other electronic device (implanted automatic cardiac defibrillator)	V45.89

Pulmonary edema with cardiac disease	428.1
Respiratory arrest (S/P)	799.1
Respiratory failure	518.81
Substernal wound infection	998.5
Transplant, heart (surgical)	37.5
Venous thrombosis	453.9
Wound dehiscence	998.3
Wound infection	998.5

5. **Associated nursing diagnoses**
   Activity intolerance
   Activity intolerance, risk for
   Anxiety
   Body image disturbance
   Breathing pattern, ineffective
   Cardiac output, decreased
   Caregiver role strain, risk for
   Communication, impaired verbal
   Constipation
   Coping, ineffective family: compromised
   Decisional conflict (treatments)
   Denial, ineffective
   Diversional activity deficit
   Family processes, altered
   Fatigue
   Fear
   Fluid volume excess
   Gas exchange, impaired
   Grieving, anticipatory
   Home maintenance management, impaired
   Infection, risk for
   Injury, risk for
   Knowledge deficit (disease process and management)
   Mobility, impaired physical
   Nutrition, altered: less than body requirements
   Nutrition, altered: more than body requirements
   Pain
   Pain, chronic
   Self-care deficit, bathing/hygiene
   Self-care deficit, dressing/grooming
   Self-care deficit, feeding
   Self-care deficit, toileting
   Sexual dysfunction
   Sexuality patterns, altered
   Skin integrity, impaired, risk for
   Sleep pattern disturbance
   Spiritual distress (distress of the human spirit)
   Spiritual well-being, potential for enhanced

Tissue perfusion, altered (cardiopulmonary)
Urinary elimination, altered

6. Skills and services identified

- ***Hospice nursing***

  a. *Comfort and symptom control*

  Observation and assessment of patient with long-standing congestive heart failure on multiple medications, admitted to hospice with severe edema, with poor activity tolerance, and on oxygen therapy 24 hours a day

  Observation and complete system assessment of patient with cardiac disease _____ (specify physician's orders)

  Presentation of hospice philosophy and services

  Explain patient rights and responsibilities

  Assess patient, family, and caregiver wishes and expectations regarding care

  Assess patient, family, and caregiver resources available for care

  Provision of volunteer support to patient and family

  Teach family or caregiver physical care of patient

  Assess pain and other symptoms, including site, duration, characteristics, and relief measures

  RN to monitor for presence and amount of lower leg edema

  Teach patient or caregiver record keeping for daily weights and other aspects of self-observational care skills

  Assess site, amount, and frequency of chest pain episodes

  Teach care of bedridden patient

  Measure vital signs and pain q visit

  Assess pain, and evaluate the pain management's effectiveness

  RN to observe for signs and symptoms of digoxin toxicity, including GI symptoms such as vomiting or nausea and neurological changes such as visual disturbances, headache, and cardiovascular manifestations

  RN to observe for signs and symptoms of infection

  Teach patient signs and symptoms of pacemaker problems or failure, including increased SOB, cough, pulse change, and increased edema

  RN to assess and monitor patient's pain, implement ordered pain control/relief measures, and assess patient's response to interventions—surgical or cardiac pain

  Assess for orthostatic hypotension

  Comprehensive patient/family education regarding signs, symptoms of CHF, daily records of weight, I & O, infusion pump care, etc.

  Assess cardiovascular, pulmonary, and respiratory status

  Assess for SOB and dyspnea, and promote rest and pacing of activities

  Comfort measures of backrub and hand or other therapeutic massage

  Oxygen on at _____ liters per _____ (specify physician orders)

  Teach caregivers symptom control and relief measures

  Pain assessment and management q visit

  Identify and monitor pain, symptoms, and relief measures

  Teach caregiver or family care of weak, terminally ill patient

RN to assess patient's pain or other symptoms q visit to identify need for change, addition, or other plan or dose adjustment

Observation and assessment, communication with physician related to signs and symptoms of continuing decompensation and increased symptoms, pain, discomfort, shortness of breath, and measures to alleviate and control

Teach caregiver/patient use of pain assessment tool/scale and reporting mechanism(s)

Effective management of pain and prevention of secondary symptoms

RN to provide and teach effective oral care and comfort measures

Intervention of symptoms directed toward comfort and palliation

Teach patient/family about realistic expectations of disease process

Teach care of dying and signs/symptoms of impending death

Presence and support

Other interventions, based on patient/family needs

b. *Safety and mobility considerations*

Patient provided with home safety information and instruction related to _____ and documented in the clinical record

Teach patient and family regarding energy conservation techniques

RN to teach care and safety regarding oxygen safety at home

Teach patient and family about planning and pacing activities

Teach family regarding safety of patient in home

Other interventions, based on patient/family needs

c. *Emotional/spiritual considerations*

Psychosocial assessment of patient and family regarding disease and prognosis

Assess mental status and sleep disturbance changes

Psychosocial aspects of pain control (e.g., depression) assessed and acknowledged with team support/intervention

RN to provide emotional support to patient and family

Inform patient/family/caregiver of available volunteer support

Ongoing acknowledgment of spirituality and related concerns of patient/family

Other interventions, based on patient/family needs

d. *Skin care*

RN to provide skilled observation and assessment of surgical sites, post–cardiac surgery care

Observation and assessment of skin

RN to assess wound site, change dressing (specify dressing orders and frequency per physician orders, and teach caregiver about wound and infection control care)

RN to culture wound site and send to lab for C & S

Pressure ulcer care as indicated

Assess skin integrity

Evaluate patient's need for equipment and supplies to decrease pressure, including alternating pressure mattress, gel foam seat cushion, and heel and elbow protectors

Observation and evaluation of wound and surrounding skin

Teach family to perform dressing between RN visits, specifically
_____

Teach patient, family, or caregiver about proper body alignment and positioning in bed to prevent skin tears from shearing skin

Observation and skilled assessment of areas for possible breakdown, including heels, hips, elbows, ankles, and other pressure-prone areas

Teach caregiver regarding skin care needs, including the need for frequent position changes, appropriate pressure pads and mattresses, and the prevention of breakdown

Other interventions, based on patient/family needs

e. *Elimination considerations*

Assess bowel regimen, and implement program as needed

Check for and remove impaction as needed (per physician orders)

Condom catheter or indwelling catheter as indicated

Assess amount and frequency of urinary output

RN to teach catheter care to caregiver

RN to teach caregiver daily care of catheter

RN to evaluate the patient's bowel patterns and need for stool softeners, laxatives, and dietary adjustments, and to develop bowel management plan

Other interventions, based on patient/family needs

f. *Hydration/nutrition*

Instruct patient about specified diet _____ (specify physician orders)

Teaching and training regarding diet and exercise

Assess nutrition and hydration statuses, and provide nutritional information/education

Diet counseling for patient with anorexia

Teach feeding-tube care to family

Obtain weights as ordered to assist in comfort and medication regulation

Nutrition/hydration supported by offering patient's choice of favorite or desired foods or liquids

Nutrition/hydration maintained by offering patient high-protein diet and foods of choice as tolerated

Teach patient and family to expect decreased nutritional and fluid intake as disease progresses

Other interventions, based on patient/family needs

g. *Therapeutic/medication regimens*

RN to instruct patient and caregiver regarding multiple medication, including schedule, functions, routes, knowledge, compliance, and possible side effects

RN to assess the patient's unique response to treatments or interventions, and to report changes, unfavorable responses, or reactions to the physician

Assess for nitroglycerin use, frequency, amount, and relief patterns

Patient education related to side effects and actions of multiple medications

Medication management related to complex regimen including beta
   blockers, anticoagulants, antihypertensives, etc. Consider drug/drug,
   drug/food interactions
Teach new pain and symptom control medication regimen
Medication assessment and management
Teach new medication regimen and side effects
Teach patient and caregiver use of PCA pump
RN to instruct in pain control measures and medications
Implement nonpharmacological interventions such as progressive muscle
   relaxation, imagery, positive visualization, music, massage and touch,
   and humor therapy of patient's choice
Other interventions, based on patient/family needs

h. *Other considerations*
   Assess disease progression of process
   RN to assess the patient's response to treatments and interventions and
      to report to the physician changes, unfavorable responses, or reac-
      tions
   Other interventions, based on patient/family needs

- *Home health aide or certified nursing assistant*
   Effective and safe personal care
   Safe ADL assistance and support
   Respite care and active listening skills
   Observation and reporting
   Meal preparation
   Homemaker services
   Comfort care
   Other duties

- *Hospice social worker*
   Psychosocial assessment of patient and family/caregiver, including adjust-
      ment to illness and its implications
   Identification of optimal coping strategies
   Financial assessment and counseling regarding food acquisition, ability to
      prepare, and costs of needed medications
   Intervention/support related to terminal illness and loss
   Emotional/spiritual support
   Depression/fear assessed and addressed
   Facilitate communication among patient, family, and hospice team
   Referral/linkage to community services and resources as indicated
   Grief counseling and intervention/support related to illness/loss
   Patient/caregiver counseling and support
   Identification of caregiver role strain necessitating respite/relief measures/
      support
   For patients who live alone with no support system (e.g., able, available,
      willing caregiver[s]): obtain linkage with necessary community re-
      sources to enable patient to remain in the home
   Identification of illness-related psychiatric condition

- *Volunteer(s)*
   Support, friendship, companionship, and presence
   Comfort and dignity maintained/provided for patient and family

Errands and transportation

Other services, based on interdisciplinary team recommendations and patient/caregiver needs

- **Spiritual counselor**

  Spiritual assessment and care

  Counseling, intervention, and support related to that dimension of life related to life's meaning (consistent with patient's beliefs)

  Support, listening, and presence

  Participation in sacred or spiritual rituals or practices

  Other supportive care, based on patient/family needs and belief systems

- **Dietitian/nutritional counseling**

  Assessment of patient with decreased intake, weight gain/loss, anorexia, and nausea

  Supportive counseling with patient/family indicating that patient will have a decreased appetite and usually at some point may not eat/drink

  Assessment and recommendations for swallowing difficulties

  Teaching and support of family members and caregivers

  Support and care with food and nourishment as desired by patient

  Evaluation/management of nutritional deficits and needs

  Encourage nutritional supplements and snacks to increase protein and caloric intake

  Food and dietary recommendations incorporating patient choice and wishes

- **Occupational therapist**

  Evaluation of ADL and functional mobility

  Assessment of need for adaptive equipment and assistive devices

  Safety assessment of patient's environment and ADL

  Assessment for energy conservation training

  Energy conservation techniques

- **Physical therapist**

  Evaluation

  Safety assessment of patient's environment

  Safe transfer training or bed mobility exercises

  Pain assessment/reduction factors

  Strengthening exercises/program

  Assessment of gait safety and home safety measures

  Instruct/supervise caregiver and volunteers on home exercise program for conditioning and strength

  Assistive, adaptive devices and evaluation of equipment and teaching

- **Bereavement counselor**

  Assessment of the needs of the bereaved family and friends

  Support and intervention, based on assessment and ongoing findings

  Presence and counseling

  Supportive visits and follow-up, other interventions (e.g., mailings, calls)

  Other services related to bereavement work and support

- **Pharmacist**

  Evaluation of hospice patient on multiple cardiac medications for possible food/drug, drug/drug interactions

  Medication monitoring regarding therapeutic levels and dosages

Pain consult and input into interdisciplinary plan of care related to pain control, palliation, and symptom management

Assessment of medication regimen and plan for safety and compliance

Other interventions, based on the unique needs of the patient/family

- *Music, massage, art, or other therapies or services*

  Evaluation and intervention based on patient's and caregiver's unique wishes and needs that support care, comfort, and death in the setting of the patient's choice

  Assessment plan to engage patient and support comfort, quality, enjoyment, and dignity

  Pet therapy (including patient's pet, if available) and therapeutic intervention

  Other interventions, based on the unique needs of the patient/family

7. **Outcomes for care**

- *Hospice nursing*

  Death with dignity and symptoms controlled in setting of patient/family choice

  Optimal comfort, support, and dignity provided throughout illness

  Death with maximum comfort through effective symptom control with specialized hospice support

  Patient/caregiver able to list adverse cardiac drug reactions/problems with infusion pump/site and whom to call for follow-up and resolution

  Patient reports decrease in SOB, chest pain by _____ (specify date)

  Caregiver effective in care management and knows whom to call for questions/concerns

  Skin integrity maintained as evidenced by problem-free skin

  Pain controlled and comfort needs met throughout POC

  IV access site remains patent without signs/symptoms of infection, and flushing/dressing care is provided per protocol

  Patient verbalizes understanding of and adheres to medication regimens

  Patient/caregiver verbalizes side effects and actions of anticoagulant therapy

  Regulated bowel program, as evidenced by regular bowel movements

  Patient will report being comfortable _____% of the day (*comfortable* defined as pain free)

  Compliance with and adherence to interdisciplinary care plan as demonstrated by observation and reporting by caregiver/patient

  Patient and caregiver verbalize satisfaction with care

  Educational tools/plans incorporated in daily care, and patient and caregiver verbalize understanding of safe, needed care

  Patient will decide on care, interventions, and evaluation

  Caregiver effective in care management and knows whom to call for questions/concerns

  Patient will express satisfaction with hospice support received and will experience increased comfort

  Patient will be made comfortable at home through death in accordance with the patient's wishes

Effective pain control and symptom control verbalized by patient

Patient verbalizes understanding of and adheres to care and medication regimens

Patient and caregiver supported through patient's death

Comfort maintained through course of care

The patient and family receive hospice support and care, and family members and friends are able to spend quality time with the patient

Caregiver able and verbalizes comfort with role and understands when to call hospice team members

Patient supported through and receives the maximum benefit from palliative chemotherapy and radiation with minimal complications

Patient and caregiver list adverse reactions, potential complications, signs/symptoms of infection (e.g., sputum change, chest congestion)

Comfort maintained through death with dignity

Pain effectively managed, and patient verbalizes comfort

Patient has stable respiratory status with patent airway (e.g., no dyspnea, infection free)

Optimal gas exchange and comfort as measured through oximetry and lab tests

Patient is protected from injury, has stable respiratory status, and is compliant with medication, safety, and care regimens

Comfort and individualized intervention of patient with immobility/bedbound status (e.g., skin, urinary, musculature, vascular)

Spiritual and psychosocial needs met (specify) as defined by patient and caregiver throughout course of care

Patient states pain is _____ on 0-10 scale by next visit

Patient and caregiver demonstrate appropriate backup or "rescue" therapies for breakthrough pain or other symptoms (e.g., dyspnea)

Pain and symptoms managed/controlled in setting of patient/family choice (e.g., patient/family report ability to eat, sleep, speak clearly with pacing)

Patient's/family's privacy, independence, and choices supported with respect and maintained through death

Enhancement and support of quality of life

Effective symptom relief and control (e.g., a peaceful and comfortable death at home, some enjoyment of life)

Maximizing the patient's quality of life (e.g., alert and pain free or as patient wishes)

Pharmacological and nonpharmacological interventions such as localized heat application, positioning, relaxation methods, and music

Patient cared for and family supported through death with physical, psychosocial, spiritual, and other concerns/needs acknowledged/addressed

Patient- and family-centered hospice care provided based on the patient's/family's unique situation and needs

Infection control and palliation

Grief/bereavement expression and support provided

Patient is pain free by next visit

Caregiver demonstrates ability to manage pain, where applicable

Patient maintains comfort and dignity throughout illness

Planned and effective bowel program, as evidenced by bowel movements and patient/family report of comfort

- *Home health aide or certified nursing assistant*
  Effective hygiene, personal care, and comfort
  ADL assistance
  Comfort and presence
  Observation and reporting
  Safe environment maintained

- *Hospice social worker*
  Problem identified and addressed, with patient/caregiver linked with
      appropriate support services and plan of care successfully imple-
      mented
  Patient and caregiver cope adaptively with illness and death
  Adaptive adjustment to changed body and body image
  Psychosocial support and counseling offered to patient/caregivers experi-
      encing loss and grief
  Caregiver system assessed and development of stable caregiver plan facili-
      tated
  Resources identified, community linkage as appropriate for patient/family

- *Volunteer(s)*
  Comfort, companionship, and friendship extended to patient/family
  Patient and caregiver support as defined by needs of patient/family
  Support and respite provided as defined by the patient/caregiver

- *Spiritual counselor*
  Spiritual support assessed, offered, and provided as defined by needs of
      patient/caregiver
  Participation in sacred or spiritual rituals or practices (consistent with pa-
      tient's beliefs)
  Provision of spiritual support and care as based on the assessed and
      ongoing needs of the patient and family
  Support, listening, and presence
  Spiritual support offered and patient/family needs met
  Patient/family express a relief of symptoms of spiritual suffering
  Intervention and support provided related to that dimension of life related
      to life's meaning (consistent with patient's beliefs)

- *Dietitian/nutritional counseling*
  Family and caregiver integrating recommendations into nutrition teaching
      (where appropriate)
  Patient and caregiver know whom and where to call for nutrition- and
      hydration-related questions/concerns
  Nutrition/hydration per patient/caregiver choices
  Caregiver demonstrates use of recommendations into daily meal planning
  Patient/family verbalize comprehension of changing nutritional needs

- *Occupational therapist*
  Patient and caregiver demonstrate maximum independence with ADL,
      adaptive techniques, and assistive devices
  Patient and caregiver demonstrate maximum safety in ADL and functional
      mobility
  Patient and caregiver demonstrate effective use of energy conservation

Verbalization/demonstration of improved functional activity level and enhanced quality of life

Patient and caregiver demonstrate effective use of diaphragmatic breathing to reduce shortness of breath and relaxation techniques to help in pain/symptom management

- *Physical therapist*

  Prevention of complications

  Home exercise and upper extremity program taught to caregiver

  Optimal strength, mobility, function maintained/achieved

  Compliance with home exercise program by _____ (specify date)

- *Bereavement counselor*

  Support services related to grief provided to patient and family

  Well-being and resolution process of grief initiated and followed through bereavement services

- *Pharmacist*

  Multiple drug regimen reviewed for food/drug and drug/drug interactions in patient on dobutamine infusions for end stage cardiac disease and other multiple medications

  Stability and safety in complex medication regimen with maximum benefit to patient

  Effective pain and symptom control and symptom management as reported by patient/caregiver

  Lab reports reviewed for therapeutic dosages and effective patient response

- *Music, massage, art, or other therapies or services*

  Therapeutic massage/touch effective for patient as self-reported or observed by caregivers/family

  Improved muscle tone, relaxation, and/or sleep

  Patient comfortable and relaxed (e.g., sleeping) after massage

  Music therapy intervention based on assessment to decrease pain perception and provide emotional expression and support

  Maintenance of comfort and physical, psychosocial, and spiritual health

  Holistic health maintained and comfort achieved through _____ (specify modality)

  Patient has pet's presence as desired—in all care sites, when possible

8. **Patient, family, and caregiver educational needs**

   Educational needs are the care regimens that contribute to safe and effective care at home between the hospice team's visits. These include the following:

   The basic tenets of hospice and the availability of support 24 hours a day, 7 days a week

   Home safety assessment and counseling

   The patient's medication regimen

   Safe and proper body mechanics to promote patient comfort and prevent caregiver safety problems

   Other teaching specific to the patient's and family's unique needs

Support groups available to patient's family, such as the hospice program's "Caregiver Support Group" meetings for family members and friends of the patient

Anticipated disease progression

Effective use of oxygen, including use, ordered liter flow, and safety

Other teaching specific to the patient and family/caregiver needs

9. **Specific tips for quality and reimbursement**

Document any variances to expected outcomes. There are many models of hospice programs. Those that are home health agency-based must work within the framework of the Medicare home care program. For example, sometimes a hospice patient reaches a stable period in the illness and has no further skilled needs or the patient is no longer homebound per Medicare home health care criteria. When this occurs, one option is to discharge the patient from Medicare home health agency reimbursement and maintain the patient on grant funds or other available resources. If the patient's status deteriorates and again meets the Medicare criteria, a new start of care is initiated on the HCFA form 485. Usually hospices continue volunteer support, nursing, and other services indicated during these periods of no reimbursement.

The Medicare hospice benefit does not require that the patient be homebound or have identified skilled needs. Though it is a needed and viable program, the Medicare hospice benefit may not be indicated for all Medicare eligible beneficiaries. For further information on this benefit, please refer to HCFA Hospice Manual 21.

Should the patient's status deteriorate and increased personal care be needed, obtain a telephone order for the increased service, noting frequency and estimating the duration.

Obtain a telephone order for all medication and treatment changes of the medical regimen and document these in the clinical record.

Unless the patient is in a hospice insurance program, some insurers will not pay for a skilled nurse visit that is made at death if the patient is dead when the nurse arrives at the home. From a Medicare home care perspective, the visit at the time of death may be covered when the orders and clinical record document assessment of the patient's status or signs of death/life or state law allows pronouncement of death by a nurse.

Document patient deterioration

Document dehydration, dehydrating

Document patient change or instability

Document pain, other symptoms not controlled

Document status after acute episode of _____ (specify)

Document positive urine, sputum, etc. culture; patient started on _____ (specify ordered antibiotic therapy)

Document patient impacted; impaction removed manually

Document RN in frequent communication with physician regarding _____ (specify)

Document febrile at _____, pulse change at _____, irr., irr.

Document change noted in _____

Document bony prominences red, opening

Document RN contacted physician regarding _____ (specify)

Document marked SOB

Document alteration in mental status

Document medications being adjusted, regulated, or monitored

Document unable to perform own ADLs, personal care

Document all interdisciplinary team meetings and communications in the POC and in the progress notes of the clinical record

All hospice team members should have input into the POC and document their interventions and goals

Remember that the clinical documentation is key to measuring compliance for quality and reimbursement purposes. Care coordination, timely verbal and initial physician orders, and assessment and addressing of spiritual and psychosocial needs should be ongoing and documented in the patient's clinical record

The documentation should support that all hospice care supports comfort and dignity while meeting patient/family needs

The documentation should include ongoing assessment and management of pain and other symptoms and the anticipation and prevention of secondary symptoms such as constipation

It is important to note that all team members, including nurses and social workers, should assess, identify, and "hear" spiritual needs that the patient and family want to be addressed. These spiritual issues are key to the provision of high-quality hospice care and cannot be addressed effectively and promptly by the spiritual counselor only

Document clearly symptoms, clinical changes, and assessment findings related to pain and patient care

Document weight loss, increased shortness of breath, dyspnea, infection, sepsis, new or changed medications, etc.

Document any skin changes (e.g., inflamed, painful, weeping skin site[s])

Remember that the "litmus test" of care coordination rests on the quality of the clinical documentation by all team members. Review one of your patient's clinical records and ask yourself the following: "If I was unable to give a verbal report/update on this patient/family's course of care, would a peer be able to pick up and provide the same level of care and know (from the documentation) the current orders, medications, and other details that contribute to effective hospice care?"

This patient population usually has many clinical changes that should be documented. These include weight loss and multiple and changed medication regimens with varying routes. Side effects of the drug regimen should be observed, noted, documented, and reported

Your assessments, observations, and clinical findings assist in painting a picture to support coverage and documentation requirements for hospice care

Document any hospitalizations and changed clinical findings

Document patient changes, symptoms, and psychosocial issues impacting the patient and family and plan of care

Document changes to the plan of care such as medications, services, frequency, communications, and concurrence of other team members

Document coordination of services or consultation of the other members of the IDT

Document communications and care coordination with other care providers, such as skilled nursing facility or nursing home staff, inpatient team members, and hired caregivers

Document any hospitalizations and changed clinical findings

In the clinical documentation, paint the picture of your end stage cardiac patient. The patient may be on multiple cardiac medications, have had multiple cardiac events or surgeries, have chronic edema, need oxygen at all times, be very short of breath, and have poor or no activity tolerance or energy. This is the kind of specificity in the clinical documentation that clearly shows why the hospice team was called in at this point along the patient's illness continuum and supports coverage and documentation requirements of an insurance provider, such as Medicare

For this and other noncancer diagnoses, document clearly the symptoms and clinical and assessment findings that support the end stage of the chronic illness process

Document patient changes, symptoms, psychosocial issues impacting the care, and information gathered at the patient/family visits and during team meetings

The documentation should reflect ongoing effects of the terminal condition, the patient's/family's difficulty with care or coping, and the continued desire for hospice care

Document angina episodes and relief interventions

Note easy fatigability or any episodes of palpitations

Document dyspnea, with or without activity

Document orthopnea, lower extremity or other edema

Document decreased tolerance to activity or other changes

10. **Resources for hospice care and practice**

Should the patient need to travel with oxygen, there are two resources that may assist. *Traveling with Oxygen* is a booklet published by the American Association of Respiratory Care (AARC). This booklet is available from the AARC at 11030 Ables Lane, Dallas, Texas, 77529 by calling (214) 243-2272.

Another publication is *Air Travel with Oxygen* by Gail Livingstone, a Lung Association volunteer. As a person who uses oxygen, she shares her experiences. The booklet is available from the American Lung Association, 1740 Broadway, New York, New York, 10019-4374, (212) 315-8700.

A helpful resource is the National Hospice Organization's (NHO) second edition of *Medical Guidelines for Determining Prognoses in Selected Non-Cancer Diseases*. Call NHO at 1-703-243-5900 for more information.

CEREBRAL VASCULAR ACCIDENT (CVA) CARE

1. **General considerations**
   Because of the high prevalence of hypertension, cerebral vascular accident (CVA), or stroke, continues to be a leading cause of illness and death.
   Please refer to "Bedbound Care," "Cardiac Care," or "Pain Care" should these sections pertain to your patient.

2. **Needs for visit**
   Physician order for hospice care, specific to the hospice program's admission criteria and policies
   Standard precautions supplies
   Vital signs equipment for baseline assessment
   Other supplies or equipment, based on physician orders

3. **Safety considerations**
   Infection control/standard precautions
   Night-light
   Extra caution on slippery surfaces
   Removal of scatter rugs
   Tub rail, grab bars for bathroom safety
   Supportive and nonskid shoes
   Handrail on stairs
   Fall precautions/protocol
   Protective skin measures
   Identification and report of any skin problems
   Protection of affected extremities from injury
   Bathroom safety supports, including shower bench, tub rails
   Wheelchair precautions/assisted ambulation and transfers
   Safety for home medical equipment (e.g., bed, cane)
   The phone number and name of person to call with a care problem
   Smoke detector and fire evacuation plan
   Others, based on the patient's unique condition and environment

4. **Potential diagnoses and codes**

AMI	410.92
Angina	413.9
Aphasia	784.3
Atrial fibrillation	427.31
Carotid artery occlusion	433.1
Catheter, indwelling	57.94
Cerebrovascular disease	437.9
CHF	428.0
COPD	496
Cor pulmonale	416.9
CVA	436
CVA with dysphasia	436 and 784.5

Diabetes mellitus, with complications, NIDDM	250.90
Diabetes mellitus, with complications, IDDM	250.91
Dysphagia	787.2
Dysphagia and CVA	782.2 and 436.0
Emphysema	492.8
Endarterectomy (surgical)	38.10
Esophageal stricture	530.3
Fluid and electrolyte imbalance	276.9
Foley catheter	57.94
Gastrostomy	43.19
Gastrostomy, tube insertion	43.11
Heart disease, chronic ischemic	414.9
Hemiplegia or hemiparesis	342.9
Hypertension	401.9
Hypertension, accelerated	401.0
Hypertensive nephrosclerosis	403.90
Incontinence of feces	787.6
Incontinence of urine	788.30
Left heart failure	428.1
Nasogastric tube feeding	96.6
Nasogastric tube insertion	96.07
Obesity	278.00
Paralysis agitans (Parkinson's disease)	332.0
Pneumonia	486
Pneumonia aspiration	507.0
Pressure (decubitus) ulcer	707.0
Protein-caloric malnutrition	263.9
Quadriplegia	436 and 344.00
Seizure disorder	780.3
TIA	435.9
Urinary retention	788.20
Urinary tract infection	599.0

5. **Associated nursing diagnoses**
   Activity intolerance
   Airway clearance, ineffective
   Anxiety
   Aspiration, risk for
   Body image disturbance
   Body temperature, altered, risk for
   Bowel incontinence
   Breathing pattern, ineffective
   Cardiac output, decreased
   Caregiver role strain
   Caregiver role strain, risk for
   Communication, impaired verbal
   Constipation
   Coping, family: potential for growth
   Coping, ineffective family: compromised

Coping, ineffective family: disabling
Coping, ineffective individual
Diarrhea
Denial, ineffective
Disuse syndrome, risk for
Diversional activity deficit
Family processes, altered
Fatigue
Fear
Fluid volume deficit, risk for
Fluid volume excess
Gas exchange, impaired
Home maintenance management, impaired
Hopelessness
Incontinence, total
Infection, risk for
Injury, risk for
Knowledge deficit (care regimen)
Management of therapeutic regimen (individuals), ineffective
Mobility, impaired physical
Nutrition, altered: less than body requirements
Oral mucous membrane, altered
Pain
Pain, chronic
Powerlessness
Role performance, altered
Self-care deficit, bathing/hygiene
Self-care deficit, dressing/grooming
Self-care deficit, feeding
Self-care deficit, toileting
Sensory/perceptual alterations (specify) (visual, auditory, kinesthetic, gustatory, tactile, olfactory)
Sexual dysfunction
Sexuality patterns, altered
Skin integrity, impaired
Skin integrity, impaired, risk for
Sleep pattern disturbance
Social interaction, impaired
Spiritual distress (distress of the human spirit)
Spiritual well-being, potential for enhanced
Swallowing, impaired
Thought processes, altered
Tissue integrity, impaired
Tissue perfusion, altered (specify type) renal, cerebral, cardiopulmonary, gastrointestinal, peripheral)
Unilateral neglect
Urinary elimination, altered
Urinary retention

6. **Skills and services identified**

- *Hospice nursing*

  a. *Comfort and symptom control*

    Skilled assessment and observation of all systems of patient with S/P CVA and terminal prognosis

    Observation and assessment of patient with _____ on multiple medications, admitted to hospice with increasing debility, right-sided weakness, and seizures in hospital

    Presentation of hospice philosophy and services

    Explain patient rights and responsibilities

    Assess patient, family, and caregiver wishes and expectations regarding care

    Assess patient, family, and caregiver resources available for care

    Provision of volunteer support to patient and family

    Teach family or caregiver physical care of patient

    RN to provide and teach effective oral care and comfort measures

    Assess pain and other symptoms, including site, duration, characteristics, and relief measures

    Assess pain, and evaluate pain management's effectiveness

    Teach care of bedridden patient

    Measure vital signs, including pain, q visit

    Assess cardiovascular, pulmonary, and respiratory status

    Teach new pain or symptom control medication regimen

    Teach caregivers symptom control and relief measures

    Oxygen on at _____liter per _____ (Specify physician orders)

    Identify and monitor pain, symptoms, and relief measures

    Teach caregiver or family care of weak, terminally ill patient

    RN to instruct in pain control measures and medications

    Teach family or caregiver care of the immobilized or bedridden patient

    Assess neurological status

    Assess respiratory, cardiovascular statuses and other systems

    Observe and monitor for neurological deficits

    Teach patient/family use of standardized form/tool to use between hospice team members' visits (and for care coordination between team members)

    Teach patient/family principles of effective pain management

    Observation and assessment, communication with physicians related to signs and symptoms of continuing decompensation and increased symptoms, pain, discomfort, shortness of breath, and measures to alleviate and control

    Effective management of pain and prevention of secondary symptoms

    Interventions of symptoms directed toward comfort and palliation

    Pain assessment and management q visit, including source of pain (e.g., cancer pain, infection, pathological fracture, other medical problems such as cardiac or arthritis pain)

    RN to teach patient and caregiver about disease process and management

    Teach patient and family about realistic expectations of disease process

Teach care of dying and signs/symptoms of impending death

Presence and support

Other interventions, based on patient/family needs

b. *Safety and mobility considerations*

Provide caregiver with home safety information and instruction related to _____ and documented in the clinical record

Teach family or caregiver about oxygen therapy, utilization, and associated safety information

Teach family regarding safety of patient in home

Teach family regarding energy conservation techniques

Other interventions, based on patient/family needs

c. *Emotional/spiritual considerations*

Psychosocial assessment of patient and family regarding disease and prognosis

RN to provide emotional support to patient and family

Assess mental status and sleep disturbance changes

RN to provide support and intervention for depression

Psychosocial aspects of pain control (e.g., depression, others) assessed and acknowledged with team support/intervention

Assess for and manage plans for psychosocial and/or spiritual pain (e.g., all pain, anxiety, interpersonal difficulties, other distress)

Teach patient/family about depression and signs/symptoms of exacerbation, needing more intervention

Ongoing acknowledgment of spirituality and related concerns of patient/family

Inform patient/family/caregiver of available volunteer support

Other interventions, based on patient/family needs

d. *Skin care*

Pressure ulcer care as indicated

Assess skin integrity

Observation and evaluation of wound and surrounding skin

Evaluate patient's need for equipment, including supplies to decrease pressure, alternating pressure mattress, gel foam seat cushion, and heel and elbow protectors

Teach family to perform dressing between RN visits, specifically

_____

Teach patient and family or caregiver about proper body alignment and positioning in bed to prevent skin tears from shearing skin

Observe and apply skilled assessment of areas for possible breakdown, including heels, hips, elbows, ankles, and other pressure-prone areas

Teach caregiver about patient's skin care needs, including the need for frequent position changes, appropriate pressure pads and mattresses, and the prevention of breakdown

Other interventions, based on patient/family needs

e. *Elimination considerations*

Assess bowel regimen, and implement program as needed

Check for and remove impaction as needed

Condom catheter or indwelling catheter as indicated

Assess amount and frequency of urinary output

Teach catheter care to caregiver

RN to teach caregiver daily care of catheter

RN to evaluate the patient's bowel patterns and need for stool softeners, laxatives, and dietary adjustments, and to develop bowel management plan

Check for and remove fecal impactions prn, per physician orders

Implement bowel and bladder training regimen

RN to change catheter (specify type, size) q _____ (specify ordered frequency)

Observation and complete systems assessment of patient with an indwelling catheter

RN to change catheter every 4 weeks and 3 prn visits for catheter problems, including patient complaints, signs and symptoms of infection, and other factors necessitating evaluation and possible catheter change

Teaching and ongoing assessment related to early prevention and identification of constipation and its correction/resolution

Initiate bowel management program per physician

Implement bowel assessment management program

Teach patient, family, and aide the importance of observing and noting bowel movements between scheduled nursing visits

Obtain patient history related to norms for bowel movements to date (e.g., "all my life I go only every other day")

Consider stool softeners and offer laxative of choice, Fleet's enemas prn, and other methods per patient wishes and physician orders

Other interventions, based on patient/family needs

f. *Hydration/nutrition*

Instruct patient about specified diet _____ (specify physician orders)

Assess nutrition and hydration statuses

Diet counseling for patient with anorexia

Teach family or caregiver about feeding tubes of pumps

Nutrition/hydration supported by offering patient's choice of favorite or desired foods or liquids

Nutrition/hydration maintained by offering patient high-protein diet and foods of choice as tolerated

Assessment and plan related to anorexia/cachexia, tube feedings, difficulty/painful swallowing, and/or transitional feedings (e.g., TPN to oral)

Teach patient and family to expect decreased nutritional and fluid intake as disease progresses

Other interventions, based on patient/family needs

g. *Therapeutic/medication regimens*

Medication assessment and management q visit

Teach new medications and effects

Assess for electrolyte imbalance

Teach patient and caregiver use of PCA pump

Nonpharmacological interventions such as progressive muscle relaxation, imagery, positive visualization, music, massage and touch, and humor therapy of patient's choice implemented

Teach new medication regimen

Assessment of effectiveness of new therapeutic med regimen

RN to assess the patient's response to therapeutic treatments and interventions and to report to the physician any changes or unfavorable responses

Encourage family/caregivers to give the patient medications on the schedule and around the clock

Medications changed using equianalgesic conversion tables/physician orders (e.g., from oral morphine to an equianalgesic dose of transdermal fentanyl)

Other interventions, based on patient/family needs

h. *Other considerations*

Observation and assessment of hospice patient with CVA and mental status changes, signs/complaints of depression

Observation of patient for neuropsychiatric complications of illness, including confusion, depression, and anxiety

Assess progression of disease process

RN to assess the patient's response to treatments and interventions and to report to the physician changes, unfavorable responses, or reactions

Other interventions, based on patient/family needs

- *Home health aide or certified nursing assistant*
  Effective and safe personal care
  Safe ADL assistance and support
  Observation and reporting
  Respite care and active listening skills
  Meal preparation
  Homemaker services
  Comfort care
  Other duties

- *Hospice social worker*
  Psychosocial assessment of patient and family/caregiver, including adjustment to long-term illness and its implications
  Identification of optimal coping strategies/caregiver role strain
  Financial assessment and counseling regarding food acquisition, ability to prepare, and costs of needed medications
  Intervention/support related to terminal illness and loss
  Emotional/spiritual support
  Depression/fear assessed and addressed
  Facilitate communication among patient, family, and hospice team
  Referral/linkage to community services and resources as indicated
  Grief counseling and intervention/support related to illness/loss
  Patient/caregiver counseling and support
  Patient lives alone with no support system (e.g., able, available, willing caregiver[s]): obtain necessary resources to allow patient to remain in home
  Identification of illness-related psychiatric condition necessitating care
  Facilitation of will/funeral arrangements

- *Volunteer(s)*
  Support, friendship, companionship, and presence
  Comfort and dignity maintained/provided for patient and family
  Errands and transportation
  Other services, based on interdisciplinary team recommendations and
      patient/caregiver needs

- *Spiritual counselor*
  Spiritual assessment and care
  Counseling, intervention, and support related to that dimension of life
      related to life's meaning (consistent with patient's beliefs)
  Support, listening, and presence
  Participation in sacred or spiritual rituals or practices
  Other supportive care, based on patient/family needs and belief systems

- *Dietitian/nutritional counseling*
  Assessment of patient with decreased intake, weight loss, anorexia, and
      pressure ulcer
  Supportive counseling with patient/family indicating that patient will have
      a decreased appetite and usually at some point may not eat/drink
  Assessment and recommendations for swallowing difficulties
  Teaching and support of family members and caregivers
  Support and care with soft food and nourishment as desired by patient
  Evaluation/management of nutritional deficits and needs
  Encourage nutritional supplements and snacks to increase protein and
      caloric intake
  Food and dietary recommendations incorporate patient choice and wishes
  Evaluation for tube feeding/TPN if condition warrants and per plan of care

- *Occupational therapist*
  Evaluation of ADL and functional mobility
  Assess for need for adaptive equipment and assistive devices
  Safety assessment of patient's environment and ADLs
  Assessment for energy conservation training
  Assessment of upper extremity function, retraining motor skills, and/or
      splinting for contracture(s)

- *Physical therapist*
  Evaluation
  Safety assessment of patient's environment
  Safe transfer training or bed mobility exercises
  Pain assessment/reduction factors
  Strengthening exercises/program
  Assessment of gait safety and home safety measures
  Instruct/supervise caregiver and volunteers on home exercise program for
      conditioning and strength
  Assistive, adaptive devices and evaluation of equipment and teaching

- *Speech-language pathologist*
  Evaluation for speech/swallowing problems
  Food texture recommendations
  Alternate functional communication

- *Bereavement counselor*
  Assessment of the needs of the bereaved family and friends
  Support and intervention, based on assessment and ongoing findings
  Presence and counseling
  Supportive visits and follow-up, other interventions (e.g., mailings, calls)
  Other services related to bereavement work and support

- *Pharmacist*
  Evaluation of hospice patient with constipation on cathartics, stool soften-
    ers, and other medications for possible food/drug, drug/drug interactions
  Medication monitoring regarding therapeutic levels and dosages
  Pain consult and input into interdisciplinary plan of care related to pain
    control, palliation, and symptom management
  Assessment of medication regimen and plan for safety and compliance

- *Music, massage, art, or other therapies or services*
  Evaluation and intervention based on patient's and caregiver's unique
    wishes and needs that support care, comfort, and death in the setting of
    the patient's choice
  Pet therapy (including patient's pet, if available) and therapeutic interven-
    tion
  Assessment plan to engage patient and support comfort, quality, enjoyment,
    and dignity

7. **Outcomes for care**

- *Hospice nursing*
  Supportive care and scopolamine patches per physician order
  Mental distress, depression, and fear of dying addressed throughout care by
    hospice team
  Patient and family able to care for and support patient
  Patient and caregiver can verbalize symptoms, changes, or accelerations
    that necessitate call to physician
  Patient and family demonstrate compliance to medication and other thera-
    peutic interventions
  Patient demonstrates stabilization and increased or enhanced coping skills
    related to functioning and depression
  Pain and symptoms managed/controlled in setting of patient/family choice
    (e.g., patient/family report ability to eat, sleep, speak with pacing)
  Planned and effective bowel program, as evidenced by regular bowel
    movements and patient/family report of comfort
  Death with dignity, and pain/symptoms controlled in setting of patient/
    family choice
  Optimal comfort, support, and dignity provided throughout illness
  Death with maximum comfort through effective symptom control with spe-
    cialized hospice support
  Patient and caregiver able to list adverse drug reactions/problems with
    medication regimen and whom to call for follow-up and resolution
  Patient's/family's privacy, independence, and choices supported with
    respect and maintained through death
  Enhancement and support of quality of life

Effective symptom relief and control (e.g., a peaceful and comfortable death at home, depression controlled, some enjoyment of life)

Maximizing the patient's quality of life (e.g., alert and pain free or as patient wishes)

Pharmacological and nonpharmacological interventions such as localized heat application, biofeedback, massage, positioning, relaxation methods, and music

Patient states pain is at _____ on 0-10 scale by next visit

Patient and caregiver verbalize satisfaction with care

Educational tools/plans incorporated in daily care, and patient/caregiver verbalizes understanding of safe, needed care

Patient will decide on care, interventions, and evaluation

Caregiver effective in care management and knows whom to call for questions/concerns

Patient will express satisfaction with hospice support received and will experience increased comfort

Patient will be made comfortable at home through death in accordance with the patient's wishes

Effective pain control and symptom control verbalized by patient

Patient verbalizes understanding of and adheres to care and medication regimens

Patient and caregiver supported through patient's death

Comfort maintained through course of care

Patient and family receive hospice support and care, and family members and friends are able to spend quality time with the patient

Caregiver is able and verbalizes comfort with role and lists when to call hospice team members

Patient supported through and receives the maximum benefit from palliative chemotherapy and radiation with minimal complications

Patient and caregiver list adverse reactions, potential complications, signs/symptoms of infection (e.g., sputum change, chest congestion)

Comfort maintained through death with dignity

Pain effectively managed, and patient verbalizes comfort

Patient is protected from injury, has stable respiratory status, and is compliant with medication, safety, and care regimens

Comfort and individualized intervention of patient with immobility/bedbound status (e.g., skin, urinary, musculature, vascular)

Spiritual and psychosocial needs met (specify) as defined by patient and caregiver throughout course of care

Adherence to POC as demonstrated and verbalized by caregiver and demonstrated by patient findings by _____ (specify date)

Wound healed by _____ with stabilization of site and no infection

Patient/caregiver demonstrates compliance with instructions related to medications, extremity elevation, and wound care

Lab values (e.g., CBC) will be within normal limits for patient by _____ (date)

Patient and family will report optimal function S/P CVA by _____

Weight lost/maintained/gained _____ lbs. by _____ (date)

Patient reports decrease in SOB, chest pain by _____

Patient's catheter will remain infection free and patent

Caregiver is effective in care management and knows whom to call for questions/concerns

Pain controlled and comfort needs met throughout POC

IV access site remains patent without signs/symptoms of infection, and flushing/dressing care is provided per protocol

Patient verbalizes understanding of and adheres to medication regimens

Regulated bowel program, as evidenced by regular bowel movements

Patient will report being comfortable _____% of the day (*comfortable* defined as pain free)

Patient cared for and family supported through death with physical, psychosocial, spiritual, and other concerns/needs acknowledged/addressed

Patient- and family-centered hospice care provided based on the patient's/family's unique situation and needs

Infection control and palliation

Grief/bereavement expression and support provided

Caregiver demonstrates ability to manage pain, where applicable

Patient maintains comfort and dignity throughout illness

- *Home health aide or certified nursing assistant*
  Effective hygiene, personal care, and comfort
  ADL assistance
  Safe environment maintained

- *Hospice social worker*
  Problem identified and addressed, with patient and caregiver linked with appropriate support services and plan of care successfully implemented
  Patient and caregiver cope adaptively with illness and death
  Adaptive adjustment to changed body and body image
  Psychosocial support and counseling offered to patient/caregivers experiencing loss and grief

- *Volunteer(s)*
  Comfort, companionship, and friendship extended to patient/family
  Support and respite provided as defined by the needs of the patient/caregiver
  Patient and family supported by team with care, comfort, and companionship

- *Spiritual counseling*
  Support, listening, and presence
  Spiritual support offered and provided as defined by needs of patient/caregiver
  Participation in sacred or spiritual rituals or practices
  Provision of spiritual support and care based on the assessed and ongoing needs of the patient and family
  Spiritual support offered, and patient and family needs met
  Patient and family express relief of symptoms of spiritual suffering

- *Dietitian/nutritional counseling*

  Family and caregiver integrate recommendations into nutrition teaching (where appropriate)

  Patient and caregiver know whom to call for nutrition- and hydration-related questions/concerns

  Nutrition/hydration per patient's choices

  Caregiver integrates recommendations into daily meal planning

- *Occupational therapist*

  Patient and caregiver demonstrate maximum independence with ADLs, adaptive techniques, and assistive devices

  Patient and caregiver demonstrate maximum safety in ADL and functional mobility

  Patient and caregiver demonstrate effective use of energy conservation

  Verbalization/demonstration of improved functional activity level and enhanced quality of life

  Patient and caregiver demonstrate effective use of diaphragmatic breathing to reduce shortness of breath and relaxation techniques to help in pain/symptom management

  Patient and caregiver demonstrate correct use of exercise and splints for maximum upper extremity function and joint position

- *Physical therapist*

  Prevention of complications

  Home exercise and upper extremity program taught to caregiver

  Optimal strength, mobility, and function maintained/achieved

  Compliance with home exercise program by _____ (specify date)

  Safety in mobility and transfers

- *Speech-language pathologist*

  Communication method implemented, and patient able to be understood as self-reported or reported by family/caregivers

  Safe swallowing and functional communication

  Recommended lists of food/textures for safety and patient choice

- *Bereavement counselor*

  Grief support services provided to patient and family

  Well-being and resolution process of grief initiated and followed through bereavement services

- *Music, massage, art, or other therapies or services*

  Therapeutic massage/touch effective for patient as self-reported or observed by caregivers/family

  Improved muscle tone, relaxation, and/or sleep

  Patient comfortable and relaxed (e.g., sleeping) after massage

  Music therapy intervention based on assessment to decrease pain perception and provide emotional expression and support

  Patient has pet's presence as desired—in all care sites, when possible

  Maintenance of comfort and physical, psychosocial, and spiritual health

  Holistic health maintained and comfort achieved through _____ (specify modality)

8. **Patient, family, and caregiver educational needs**

Educational needs are the care regimens that contribute to safe and effective care at home between the hospice team's visits. These include the following:

The basic tenets of hospice and the availability of support 24 hours a day, 7 days a week

Home safety assessment and counseling

The patient's medication regimen

Safe and proper body mechanics to promote patient comfort and prevent caregiver safety problems

Other teaching specific to the patient's and family's unique needs

Support groups available to patient's family, such as the hospice program's "Caregiver Support Group" meetings for family members and friends of the patient

The importance of and all aspects of effective skin care regimens to prevent breakdown, including the need for frequent position changes, proper body alignment, pressure pads or mattresses, and other measures for prevention.

Anticipated disease progression

Other information based on the patient's unique medical and other needs

9. **Specific tips for quality and reimbursement**

Document any variances to expected outcomes. Often the diagnosis of CVA indicates multiple identifiable nursing needs. There are many models of hospice programs. Those that are home health agency–based must work within the framework of the Medicare home care program. For example, sometimes a hospice patient reaches a stable period in the illness and has no further skilled needs or the patient is no longer homebound per Medicare home health care criteria. When this occurs, one option is to discharge the patient from Medicare home health agency reimbursement and maintain the patient on grant funds or other available resources. If the patient's status deteriorates and again meets the Medicare criteria, a new start of care is initiated on the HCFA form 485. Usually hospices continue volunteer support, nursing, and other services indicated during these periods of no reimbursement.

The Medicare hospice benefit does not require that the patient be homebound or have identified skilled needs. Though it is a needed and viable program, the Medicare hospice benefit may not be indicated for all Medicare eligible beneficiaries. For further information on this benefit, please refer to HCFA Hospice Manual 21.

Should the patient's status deteriorate and increased personal care be needed, obtain a telephone order for the increased service, noting frequency and estimating the duration.

Obtain a telephone order for all medication and treatment changes of the medical regimen, and document these in the clinical record. Document coordination of services and consultation with other members of the IDG.

Unless the patient is in a hospice insurance program, some insurers will not pay for a skilled nurse visit that is made at death if the patient is dead when the nurse arrives at the home. From a Medicare home care perspective, the visit at the time of death may be covered when the orders and clinical record document assessment of the patient's status or signs of death/life or state law allows pronouncement of death by a nurse.

Document patient deterioration

Document dehydration, dehydrating

Document patient change or instability

Document pain, other symptoms not controlled

Document status after acute episode of _____ (specify)

Document positive urine, sputum, etc. culture; patient started on _____ (specify ordered antibiotic therapy)

Document patient impacted; impaction removed manually

Document RN in frequent communication with physician regarding _____ (specify)

Document febrile at _____, pulse change at _____, irr., irr.

Document change noted in _____

Document bony prominences red, opening

Document RN contacted physician regarding _____ (specify)

Document marked SOB

Document alteration in mental status

Document medications being adjusted, regulated, or monitored

Document unable to perform own ADLs, personal care

Document all interdisciplinary team meetings and communications in the POC and in the progress notes of the clinical record

All hospice team members involved should have input into the POC and document their interventions and goals

Document in the clinical notes the clear progression and symptomatology and interventions that demonstrate the interventions and overall management of the patient with the stroke and attendant needs for hospice support

Document when/if the patient has respiratory changes, shortness of breath, exacerbation of conditions, dysphagia, changes in pain, and other symptoms and that they are identified and resolved

Remember that the clinical documentation is key to measuring compliance for quality and reimbursement purposes. Care coordination, timely verbal and initial physician orders, and assessment and addressing of spiritual and psychosocial needs should be ongoing and documented in the patient's clinical record

The documentation should support that all hospice care supports comfort and dignity while meeting patient/family needs

The documentation should include ongoing assessment and management of pain and other symptoms and the anticipation and prevention of secondary symptoms such as constipation

It is important to note that all team members, including nurses and social workers, should assess, identify, and "hear" spiritual needs that the patient/family want to be addressed. These spiritual issues are key to the provision of quality hospice care and cannot be addressed effectively and promptly by the spiritual counselor only

Document clearly symptoms, clinical changes, and assessment findings related to pain and patient care

Document patient changes, symptoms, and clinical information identified from visits and team conferences that support hospice care and a limited life expectancy

Clearly support in the documentation the rationale that supports/explains the progression of the illness from the chronic to terminal stages

Document patient changes, symptoms, psychosocial issues impacting the care, and information gathered at patient/family visits and during team meetings

The documentation should reflect ongoing effects of the terminal condition, the patient's/family's difficulty with care or coping, and the continued desire for hospice care

Document mentation, behavioral, and/or cognitive changes

Document dysphagia, weight loss, increased shortness of breath, dyspnea, infection, sepsis, new or changed medications, etc.

Document any skin changes (e.g., inflamed, painful, weeping skin site[s])

Document when the patient is actively dying, deteriorating, and progressing toward death

Remember that the "litmus test" of care coordination rests on the quality of the clinical documentation by all team members. Review one of your patient's clinical records and ask yourself the following: "If I was unable to give a verbal report/update on this patient, would a peer be able to pick up and provide the same level of care and know (from the documentation) the current orders, medications, and other details that contribute to effective hospice care?"

This patient population usually has many clinical changes that should be documented

Your assessments, observations, and clinical findings assist in painting a picture to support coverage and documentation requirements for hospice care

Document any hospitalizations and changed clinical findings

10. **Resources for hospice care and practice**
A helpful resource is the National Hospice Organization's (NHO) second edition of *Medical Guidelines for Determining Prognoses in Selected Non-Cancer Diseases.* Call NHO at 1-703-243-5900 for more information.

For more information, contact the American Heart Association at 1-214-373-6300 or 1-800-AHAUSA1 to connect with your local affiliate. The National Stroke Association also has information and can be reached at 1-800-STROKES.

CONSTIPATION CARE

1. **General considerations**

   Constipation is one of the most common secondary symptoms that cause distress for hospice patients and is also a source of concern for their family members. Dame Cicely Saunders, considered by many to be the founder of the modern hospice movement, is reported to have given a lecture in which every fourth slide read, "Nothing matters more than the bowels." Consequently, effective bowel management is a contributor to quality hospice care. Every patient should be evaluated on admission and monitored every visit for this problem, and the entire team should be aware of this problematic area because prevention is the best cure. Many hospices use a flow chart method to identify/prevent constipation problems in the course of care. Constipation can lead to other pain problems, including hemorrhoidal pain and bleeding, anorexia, nausea, diarrhea, and impactions. See Table 2-1 for a bowel regimen to prevent narcotic-induced constipation.

2. **Needs for visit**

   Physician order for hospice care, specific to the hospice program's admission criteria and policies

   Standard precautions supplies

   Vital signs equipment for baseline assessment

   Other supplies or equipment, based on physician orders

3. **Safety considerations**

   Infection control/standard precautions

   Night-light

   Extra caution on slippery surfaces

   Removal of scatter rugs

   Tub rail, grab bars for bathroom safety

   Supportive and nonskid shoes

   Handrail on stairs

   Fall precautions

   Protective skin measures

   Identification and report of any skin problems

   Smoke detector and fire evacuation plan

   Assistance with ambulation

   Others, based on the patient's unique condition and environment

4. **Potential diagnoses and codes**

Bowel impaction	560.30
Cancer, colon	153.9
Cancer, rectosigmoid	154.0
Constipation	564.0
Dehydration	276.5
Ileus	560.1
Impaction	560.30

TABLE 2-1

BOWEL REGIMEN TO PREVENT
NARCOTIC-INDUCED CONSTIPATION

Medication	Suggested Beginning Dose	Usual Range of Dosage
1. Begin with *one* of the combined stool softener and mild peristaltic stimulants:		
Dioctyl sodium sulfosuccinate, 100 mg plus casanthranol 30 mg (Peri-Colace)	1 capsule tid	1 capsule qd to 2 capsules tid
or		
Docusate sodium, 50 mg, plus senna 187 mg (Senokot-S)	1 tablet tid	1 tablet qd to 4 tablets tid
or		
Docusate calcium, 60 mg, plus danthron, 50 mg (Doxidan)	1 capsule bid	1 capsule qd to 2 capsules tid
2. If no bowel movement occurs in any 48 hr period, add *one* to *two* of the following:		
Senna 187 mg (Senokot)	2-3 tablets hs	2 tablets hs to 4 tablets tid
Bisacodyl (Dulcolax)	10-15 mg PO hs	5 mg PO hs to 15 mg PO tid
Milk of Magnesia	30-60 ml hs	30-60 ml qd or bid
Lactulose (Chronulac: 10 g/15 ml)	30-45 ml hs	15-60 ml qd or bid
Perdiem (avoid if fluid intake is reduced)	2 teaspoons hs	1 teaspoon to 2 tablespoons qd
3. If no bowel movement occurs within 72 hr, perform rectal examination to rule out impaction. If not impacted, go to #4. If impacted, go to #5.		
4. If not impacted, try *one* of the following:		
Bisacodyl (Dulcolax) suppository	10 mg	
Magnesium Citrate	8 oz PO	
Senna extract (X-prep liquid)	2½ oz PO	
Mineral Oil	30-60 ml PO	
Milk of Magnesia 25 ml *and* Cascara 5 ml suspension		
Fleet Enema		
5. If impacted:		
Manually disempact if stool is soft enough.		
If not, soften with glycerin suppository or oil retention enema, then disempact manually.		
Follow up with enema (tap water, soapsuds) until clear.		
Increase daily bowel regimen		

Adapted from Levy MH: Pain management in advanced cancer, *Semin Oncol* 12:404, 1985.

5. **Associated nursing diagnoses**
   Activity intolerance
   Body image disturbance
   Bowel incontinence
   Caregiver role strain
   Caregiver role strain, risk for
   Constipation
   Constipation, colonic
   Constipation, perceived
   Diarrhea
   Fatigue
   Fear
   Fluid volume deficit, risk for
   Grieving, anticipatory
   Hyperthermia
   Incontinence, total
   Injury, risk for
   Knowledge deficit (bowel management program)
   Management of therapeutic regimen (individual), ineffective
   Mobility, impaired physical
   Nutrition, altered: less than body requirements
   Pain
   Pain, chronic
   Self-care deficit, toileting
   Sexuality patterns, altered
   Skin integrity impaired, risk for
   Sleep pattern disturbance
   Social interaction, impaired
   Spiritual distress (distress of the human spirit)
   Spiritual well-being, potential for enhanced
   Swallowing, impaired
   Urinary elimination, altered
   Urinary retention

6. **Skills and services identified**

   - *Hospice nursing*

     a. *Comfort and symptom control*
        Skilled observation and assessment of the patient with impaction/
           constipation
        Observation and assessment of patient with _____ on mul-
           tiple medications, admitted to hospice with _____ (e.g.,
           restrictive lung disease)
        Presentation of hospice philosophy and services
        Explain patient rights and responsibilities
        Assess patient, family, and caregiver wishes and expectations regarding
           care
        Assess patient, family, and caregiver resources available for care
        Provision of volunteer support to patient and family
        Teach family or caregiver physical care of patient

Assess pain and other symptoms, including site, duration, characteristics, and relief measures

RN to provide and teach effective oral care and comfort measures

Pain assessment and management q visit

Teach caregiver/patient use of pain assessment tool/scale and reporting mechanism(s)

Effective management of pain and prevention of secondary symptoms

Interventions of symptoms directed toward comfort and palliation

Observation and assessment, communication with physician related to signs and symptoms of continuing decompensation and increased symptoms, pain, discomfort, shortness of breath, and measures to alleviate and control

Teach patient and family about realistic expectations for the disease process

Teach care of dying and signs/symptoms of impending death

Presence and support

Other interventions, based on patient/family needs

b. *Safety and mobility considerations*

Provide patient with home safety information and instruction related to _____ and documented in the clinical record

Rehabilitation management related to safe bed mobility and transfers

Teach family about safety of patient in home

Teach patient and family about energy conservation techniques

Teach caregiver to observe for increased secretions and teach safe suctioning, when needed

Other interventions, based on patient/family needs

c. *Emotional/spiritual considerations*

Psychosocial assessment of patient and family regarding disease and prognosis

Psychosocial aspects of pain control (e.g., depression) assessed and acknowledged with team support/intervention

Inform patient/family/caregiver of available volunteer support

Ongoing acknowledgment of spirituality and related concerns of patient/family

Other interventions, based on patient/family needs

d. *Skin care*

Pressure ulcer care as indicated

Assess skin integrity

Observation and evaluation of wound and surrounding skin

Evaluate patient's need for equipment, including supplies to decrease pressure, alternating pressure mattress, gel foam seat cushion, and heel and elbow protectors

Teach family to perform dressing between RN visits, specifically _____

Teach patient and family or caregiver about proper body alignment and positioning in bed to prevent skin tears from shearing skin

Observe and apply skilled assessment of areas for possible breakdown, including heels, hips, elbows, ankles, and other pressure-prone areas

Teach caregiver about skin care needs, including the need for frequent position changes, appropriate pressure pads and mattresses, and the prevention of breakdown

Other interventions, based on patient/family needs

e. *Elimination considerations*

Assess bowel regimen and implement program as needed

Evaluation and examination for, and manual removal of, fecal impaction (per orders)

Teach new bowel training regimen

Administer enema per order

Teach suppository administration

Assess bowel sounds, all four quadrants

Digital rectal exam per physician orders

Implement bowel and bladder training regimen

Teach patient/family and aide the importance of observing and noting bowel movements between scheduled nursing visits

Obtain patient history related to norms for bowel movements to date (e.g., "all my life I go only every other day")

Consider stool softeners and offer laxative of choice, Fleet's enemas prn, and other methods per patient wishes and physician orders

Other interventions, based on patient/family needs

f. *Hydration/nutrition*

Assess nutrition/hydration status

Teach about need for increased fiber, fruit, and fluid diet, as appropriate

Other interventions, based on patient/family needs

g. *Other considerations*

Assess progression of disease process

RN to assess the patient's response to treatments and interventions and to report to the physician changes, unfavorable responses, or reactions

Other interventions, based on patient/family needs

- **Home health aide or certified nursing assistant**

Effective and safe personal care

Safe ADL assistance and support

Respect for privacy while supporting patient safety

Observation and reporting

Respite care and active listening skills

Meal preparation

Homemaker services

Assistance with toileting activities and support of patient habits

Comfort care

Other duties

- **Hospice social worker**

Psychosocial assessment of patient and family/caregiver, including adjustment to long-term illness and its implications

Identification of optimal coping strategies

Financial assessment and counseling regarding food acquisition, ability to prepare, and costs of needed medications

Intervention/support related to terminal illness and loss

Emotional/spiritual support

Identification of caregiver role strain necessitating respite/relief measures/support

Depression/fear assessed and addressed

Facilitate communication among patient, family, and hospice team

Referral/linkage to community services and resources as indicated

Grief counseling and intervention/support related to illness/loss

Patient/caregiver counseling and support

For patient who lives alone with no support system (e.g., able, available, willing caregiver[s]): obtain linkage with necessary community resources to allow patient to remain at home

Identification of illness-related psychiatric condition necessitating care

- *Volunteer(s)*

Support, friendship, companionship, presence, and respite care

Comfort and dignity maintained/provided for patient and family

Errands and transportation

Other services, based on interdisciplinary team recommendations and patient/caregiver needs

- *Spiritual counselor*

Spiritual assessment and care

Counseling, intervention, and support related to that dimension of life related to life's meaning (consistent with patient's beliefs)

Support, listening, and presence

Participation in sacred or spiritual rituals or practices

Other supportive care, based on patient's/family's needs and belief systems

- *Dietitian/nutritional counseling*

Assessment of patient with decreased intake, weight loss, anorexia, and increased shortness of breath (e.g., "don't feel like eating")

Supportive counseling with patient/family indicating that patient will have a decreased appetite and usually at some point may not eat/drink

Assessment and recommendations for swallowing difficulties

Teaching and support of family members and caregivers

Increased fluid intake as tolerated, especially fruit juices (e.g., prune, apple)

Support and care with food and nourishment as desired by patient

Evaluation/management of nutritional deficits and needs

Encourage nutritional supplements and snacks to increase protein and caloric intake

Suggest foods high in fiber (e.g., bran, whole grains, and fruits, especially pineapple, prunes, raisins, vegetables, nuts, and legumes). Avoid increased fiber if patient is dehydrated, or severe constipation or obstruction/ileus is anticipated

- *Bereavement counselor*

Assessment of the needs of the bereaved family and friends

Support and intervention, based on assessment and ongoing findings

Presence and counseling

Supportive visits and follow-up, other interventions (e.g., mailings, calls)
Other services related to bereavement work and support

- *Pharmacist*
  Evaluation of hospice patient with constipation on cathartics, stool softeners, and other medications for possible food/drug, drug/drug interactions
  Medication monitoring regarding therapeutic levels and dosages
  Pain consult and input into interdisciplinary plan of care related to pain control, palliation, and symptom management
  Assessment of medication regimen and plan for safety and compliance

- *Music, massage, art, or other therapies or services*
  Evaluation and intervention based on patient's and caregiver's unique wishes and needs that support care, comfort, and death in the setting of the patient's choice
  Assessment plan to engage patient and support comfort, quality, enjoyment, and dignity
  Pet therapy (including patient's pet, if available) and therapeutic intervention

7. **Outcomes for care**

- *Hospice nursing*
  Planned and effective bowel program, as evidenced by regular bowel movements and patient/family report of comfort
  Death with dignity, and symptoms controlled in setting of patient/family choice
  Optimal comfort, support, and dignity provided throughout illness
  Death with maximum comfort through effective symptom control with specialized hospice support
  Patient and caregiver able to list adverse drug reactions/problems with medication regimen and whom to call for follow-up and resolution
  Pain and symptoms managed/controlled in setting of patient/family choice (e.g., patient/family report ability to eat, sleep, speak clearer with pacing)
  Patient's/family's privacy, independence, and choices supported with respect and maintained through death
  Enhancement and support of quality of life
  Effective symptom relief and control (e.g., a peaceful and comfortable death at home, some enjoyment of life)
  Maximizing the patient's quality of life (e.g., alert and pain free or as patient wishes)
  Pharmacological and nonpharmacological interventions, such as localized heat application, positioning, relaxation methods, and music
  Patient cared for and family supported through death, with physical, psychosocial, spiritual, and other concerns/needs acknowledged/addressed
  Patient- and family-centered hospice care provided based on the patient's/family's unique situation and needs
  Infection control and palliation
  Grief/bereavement expression and support provided
  Patient is pain free by next _____ visit

Caregiver demonstrates ability to manage pain, where applicable

Patient maintains comfort and dignity throughout illness

- *Home health aide or certified nursing assistant*

  Effective hygiene, personal care, and comfort

  ADL assistance

  Safe environment maintained

- *Hospice social worker*

  Problem identified and addressed, with patient/caregiver and linked with appropriate support services and plan of care successfully implemented

  Patient and caregiver cope adaptively with illness and death

  Adaptive adjustment to changed body and body image

  Psychosocial support and counseling offered to patient/caregivers experiencing loss and grief

  Resources identified, community linkage as appropriate for patient and family

- *Volunteer(s)*

  Comfort, companionship, and friendship extended to patient/family

  Support and respite provided as defined by the needs of the patient/caregiver

  Patient and family supported by team with care, comfort, and companionship

- *Spiritual counseling*

  Spiritual support, listening, and presence offered and provided as defined by needs of patient/caregiver

  Provision of spiritual support and care as based on the assessed and ongoing needs of the patient and family

  Spiritual support offered, and patient and family needs met

  Patient and family express relief of symptoms of spiritual suffering

- *Dietitian/nutritional counseling*

  Family and caregiver integrate dietary recommendations into nutrition teaching (where appropriate)

  Patient and caregiver know whom to call for nutrition- and hydration-related questions/concerns

  Nutrition/hydration per patient's choices

  Caregiver integrates dietary recommendations into daily meal planning

- *Bereavement counselor*

  Grief support services provided to patient and family

  Well-being and resolution process of grief initiated and followed through bereavement services

- *Pharmacist*

  Multiple drug regimen reviewed for food/drug and drug/drug interactions in patient on multiple meds

  Stability and safety in complex medication regimen with maximum benefit to patient

  Effective pain and symptom control and symptom management as reported by patient/caregiver (e.g., constipation)

  Lab reports reviewed for therapeutic dosages and effective patient response

- *Music, massage, art, or other therapies or services*
    Therapeutic massage/touch effective for patient as self-reported or observed
        by caregivers/family
    Improved muscle tone, relaxation, and/or sleep
    Patient comfortable and relaxed (e.g., sleeping) after massage
    Music therapy intervention based on assessment to decrease pain percep-
        tion and provide emotional expression and support
    Maintenance of comfort and physical, psychosocial, and spiritual health
    Holistic health maintained and comfort achieved through _____
        (specify modality)
    Patient has pet's presence as desired—in all care sites, when possible

8. **Patient, family, and caregiver educational needs**
    Educational needs are the care regimens that contribute to safe and effective
    care at home between the hospice team's visits. These include the following:
    The basic tenets of hospice and the availability of support 24 hours a day, 7
        days a week
    Home safety assessment and counseling
    The patient's medication regimen
    Safe and proper body mechanics to promote patient comfort and prevent
        caregiver safety problems
    Other teaching specific to the patient's and family's unique needs
    Support groups available to patient's family, such as the hospice program's
        "Caregiver Support Group" meetings for family members and friends of
        the patient
    The bowel training regimen and schedule
    The need to call the hospice program should the patient experience discom-
        fort (and need to be disimpacted)
    The importance of prevention, where possible
    Anticipated disease progression
    Any other information, based on the patient's unique medical condition and
        needs

9. **Specific tips for reimbursement and quality**
    Document any variances to expected outcomes. There are many models of
    hospice programs. Those that are home health agency–based must work
    within the framework of the Medicare home care program. For example,
    sometimes a hospice patient reaches a stable period in the illness and has no
    further skilled needs or the patient is no longer homebound per Medicare
    home health care criteria. When this occurs, one option is to discharge the
    patient from Medicare home health agency reimbursement and maintain the
    patient on grant funds or other available resources. If the patient's status de-
    teriorates and again meets the Medicare criteria, a new start of care is initi-
    ated on the HCFA form 485. Usually hospices continue volunteer support,
    nursing, and other services indicated during these periods of no reimburse-
    ment.
        The Medicare hospice benefit does not require that the patient be home-
    bound or have identified skilled needs. Though it is a needed and viable
    program, the Medicare hospice benefit may not be indicated for all Medicare
    eligible beneficiaries. For further information on this benefit, please refer to
    HCFA Hospice Manual 21.

Should the patient's status deteriorate and increased personal care be needed, obtain a telephone order for the increased service, noting frequency and estimating the duration.

Obtain a telephone order for all medication and treatment changes of the medical regimen and document these in the clinical record.

Unless the patient is in a hospice insurance program, some insurers will not pay for a skilled nurse visit that is made at death if the patient is dead when the nurse arrives at the home. From a Medicare home care perspective, the visit at the time of death may be covered when the orders and clinical record document assessment of the patient's status or signs of death/life or state law allows pronouncement of death by a nurse.

Document the last bowel movement (if known) before RN visit

Document distention noted, as indicated

Document actual removal of fecal material

Document family and caregiver teaching regarding bowel training program

Document family and caregiver teaching regarding new diet regimen

Be aware that these patients are considered intermittent and, as such, can remain home care patients while receiving infrequent RN visits for occasional disimpactions

Document patient deterioration

Document dehydration, dehydrating

Document patient change or instability

Document pain, other symptoms not controlled

Document status after acute episode of _____ (specify)

Document positive urine, sputum, etc. culture; patient started on _____ (specify ordered antibiotic therapy)

Document patient impacted; impaction removed manually

Document RN in frequent communication with physician regarding _____ (specify)

Document febrile at _____, pulse change at _____, irr., irr.

Document change noted in _____

Document bony prominences red, opening

Document RN contacted physician regarding _____ (specify)

Document marked SOB

Document alteration in mental status

Document medications being adjusted, regulated, or monitored

Document unable to perform own ADLs, personal care

Document all interdisciplinary team meetings and communications in the POC and in the progress notes of the clinical record

All hospice team members should have input into the POC and document their interventions and goals

Remember that the clinical documentation is key to measuring compliance for quality and reimbursement purposes. Care coordination, timely verbal and initial physician orders, and assessment and addressing of spiritual and psychosocial needs should be ongoing and documented in the patient's clinical record

The documentation should support that all hospice care supports comfort and dignity while meeting patient/family needs

The documentation should include ongoing assessment and management of pain and other symptoms and the anticipation and prevention of secondary symptoms such as constipation

It is important to note that all team members, including nurses and social workers, should assess, identify, and "hear" spiritual needs that the patient/family want to be addressed. These spiritual issues are key to the provision of quality hospice care and cannot be addressed effectively and promptly by the spiritual counselor only

Document clearly symptoms, clinical changes, and assessment findings related to pain and patient care

Document weight loss, increased shortness of breath, dyspnea, infection, sepsis, new or changed medications, etc.

Document any skin changes (e.g., inflamed, painful, weeping skin site[s])

Remember that the "litmus test" of care coordination rests on the quality of the clinical documentation by all team members. Review one of your patient's clinical records and ask yourself the following: "If I was unable to give a verbal report/update on this child/family's course of care, would a peer be able to pick up and provide the same level of care and know (from the documentation) the current orders, medications, and other details that contribute to effective hospice care?"

This patient population usually has many clinical changes that should be documented. These include weight loss, multiple and changed medication regimens with varying routes. Side effects to the drug regimen should be observed, noted, documented, and reported

Your assessments, observations, and clinical findings assist in painting a picture to support coverage and documentation requirements for hospice care

Document any hospitalizations and changed clinical findings

Document patient changes, symptoms, and psychosocial issues impacting the patient and family and plan of care (e.g., patient was DNR, and now DNR status has changed with patient/family input and decision)

Document coordination of services and consultation with other members of the IDG

Document coordination with other team members at SNF, nursing home, etc.

10. **Resources for hospice care and practice**

The National Digestive Diseases Information Clearinghouse has a flyer on constipation. For more information, call 1-301-644-3810.

DEPRESSION AND PSYCHIATRIC CARE

1. **General considerations**

   Though usually not a primary reason for admission to hospice, the hospice patient's and family's depression and psychiatric problems can present challenges to the hospice team. See also "Cancer Care," "Pain Care," or other sections that may pertain to your hospice patient.

2. **Needs for visit**

   Physician order for hospice care, specific to the hospice program's admission criteria and policies

   Standard precautions supplies

   Vital signs equipment for baseline assessment

   Other supplies or equipment, based on physician orders

3. **Safety considerations**

   Infection control/standard precautions

   Depression/confusion precautions

   Disposal of sharps and related supplies

   Supervised medication administration

   Night-light

   The phone number and name of the person to call with a care problem

   Extra caution on slippery surfaces

   Removal of scatter rugs

   Tub rail, grab bars for bathroom safety

   Supportive and nonskid shoes

   Handrail on stairs

   Fall precautions

   Protective skin measures

   Identification and report of any skin problems

   Smoke detector and fire evacuation plan

   Assistance with ambulation

   Others, based on the patient's unique condition and environment

4. **Potential diagnoses and codes**

AIDS dementia	042 and 294.1
Agoraphobia	300.22
Alcoholism	303.90
Alzheimer's	331.0
Anemia	285.9
Anorexia nervosa	307.1
Anxiety state	300.00
Bipolar disorder	296.50
Bulimia	307.51
Constipation	564.0
Creutzfeldt-Jakob disease and dementia	046.1 and 294.1
CVA	436
Dementia	294.8

Depression, reactive	300.4
Depressive disorder	311
Depressive psychosis	296.20
Drug addiction	304.90
Electroshock therapy	94.27
Hypochondriasis	300.7
Korsakoff's dementia	294.0
Malaise and fatigue	780.7
Mania	296.00
Nonpsychotic brain syndrome	310.9
Obesity	278.00
Obsessive-compulsive disorder	300.3
Organic brain syndrome	310.9
Panic disorder	300.01
Panic disorder with agoraphobia	300.21
Personality disorder	301.9
Polyaddiction	304.80
Post traumatic stress disorder	309.81
Presenile dementia	290.13
Psychosis	296.20
Schizophrenia, simple	295.90
Schizophrenia, undifferentiated	295.8
Senile dementia	290.0
Traumatic stress disorder	308.3
Unipolar affective disorder	296.00

5. **Associated nursing diagnoses**
   Anxiety
   Body image disturbance
   Caregiver role strain
   Caregiver role strain, risk for
   Communication, impaired verbal
   Constipation
   Coping, ineffective family: disabling
   Coping, ineffective individual
   Decisional conflict (specify)
   Family processes, altered
   Fatigue
   Fear
   Fluid volume deficit, risk for
   Grieving, anticipatory
   Grieving, dysfunctional
   Hopelessness
   Injury, risk for
   Knowledge deficit (self-care management)
   Management of therapeutic regimen (individuals), ineffective
   Mobility, impaired physical
   Noncompliance
   Nutrition, altered: less than body requirements
   Nutrition, altered: more than body requirements

Pain
Pain, chronic
Parenting, altered
Parenting, altered, potential
Post-trauma response
Powerlessness
Rape-trauma syndrome
Rape-trauma syndrome: compound reaction
Self-care deficit (specify)
Self-esteem disturbance
Self-esteem, chronic low
Self-esteem, situational low
Sensory/perceptual alterations (specify) (visual, auditory, kinesthetic, gustatory, tactile, olfactory)
Sexual dysfunction
Sexuality patterns, altered
Sleep pattern disturbance
Social interaction, impaired
Spiritual distress (distress of the human spirit)
Spiritual well-being, potential for enhanced
Thought processes, altered
Trauma, risk for
Violence, risk for, self-directed or directed at others

6. **Skills and services identified**

   • *Hospice nursing*

       a. *Comfort and symptom control*
           Skilled assessment of the patient with _____ (specify the psychiatric disorder) admitted for hospice care
           Observation and assessment of patient with _____ (specify) on multiple medications, admitted to hospice with increasing shortness of breath and pain
           Psychotherapeutic interventions, including _____ (specify)
           Evaluation and psychotherapy
           Assessment and observation of cognitive/affective behaviors
           RN to initiate psychotherapy after acute hospitalization
           Skilled observation and assessment of all systems
           Teach family or caregiver care of patient
           Assess pain and other symptoms, including site, duration, characteristics, and relief measures
           Assess pain, and evaluate pain management's effectiveness
           RN to instruct in pain control measures and medications
           Presentation of hospice philosophy and services
           Explain patient rights and responsibilities
           Assess patient, family, and caregiver wishes and expectations regarding care
           Assess patient, family, and caregiver resources available for care
           Provision of volunteer support to patient and family
           RN to provide and teach effective oral care and comfort measures

RN to assess patient's pain or other symptoms q visit to identify need
for change, addition, or other dose adjustment(s)

Teach caregiver or family care of weak, terminally ill patient

Comfort measures of backrub, hand, and other therapeutic massage

Teach patient and caregiver about disease and management

Observe for sleeping, eating, and other changes in patterns

RN to observe and assess patient's hygiene, personal care, independence
with disease

RN to evaluate behavior medication plan, including support, teaching,
and evaluation of compliance

Teach patient/family about depression and signs/symptoms of exacerbation that require more intervention

Teach patient/family use of standardized form/tool to use between
hospice team members' visits (and for care coordination between
team members)

Teach patient/family principles of effective pain management

Effective management of pain and prevention of secondary symptoms

Interventions of symptoms directed toward comfort and palliation

Observation and assessment, communication with physician related to
signs and symptoms of continuing decompensation and increased
symptoms, pain, discomfort, shortness of breath, and measures to
alleviate and control

Teach caregiver/patient use of pain assessment tool/scale and reporting
mechanism(s)

Pain assessment and management q visit, including source of pain (e.g.,
cancer pain, infection, pathological fracture, other medical problems,
such as cardiac or arthritis pain)

Teach patient and family about realistic expectations of disease
process

Teach care of dying and signs/symptoms of impending death

Presence and support

Other interventions, based on patient/family needs

b. *Safety and mobility considerations*

Provide caregiver with home safety information and instruction related
to _____ and documented in the clinical record

Home safety evaluation and plan to help ensure safety

Other interventions, based on patient/family needs

c. *Emotional/spiritual considerations*

Psychosocial assessment of patient and family regarding disease and
prognosis

RN to provide emotional support to patient with severe grief reaction

RN to provide emotional support to patient and family

Inform patient/family/caregiver of available volunteer support

Assess mental status and sleep disturbance changes

RN to monitor patient's mental status for signs and symptoms of depression or _____ (specify)

Active, nonjudgmental listening to patient expression of a desire to "end
it all" and referral to other team members for counseling, intervention

Reality orientation and counseling

Crisis intervention and counseling

Observation and assessment of hospice patient mental status changes/ complaints of situational/other depressions

Observation of patient for neuropsychiatric complications of illness, including confusion, depression, and anxiety

RN to provide support and intervention for depression

Active listening to patients/families related to their loss, grief, and anticipation of death

Assess for and manage plans for psychosocial and/or spiritual pain (e.g., all pain, anxiety, interpersonal and other distress)

Ongoing acknowledgment of spirituality and related concerns of patient/ family

Psychosocial aspects of pain control (e.g., depression) addressed and acknowledged with team support/intervention

Other interventions, based on patient/family needs

d. *Skin care*

Observation of skin and patient's overall physical status

Teach patient and family or caregiver about proper body alignment and positioning in bed to prevent skin tears from shearing skin

Observe and apply skilled assessment of areas for possible breakdown, including heels, hips, elbows, ankles, and other pressure-prone areas

Teach caregiver about skin care needs, including the need for frequent position changes, appropriate pressure pads and mattresses, and the prevention of breakdown

Assess skin integrity

Observation and evaluation of wound and surrounding skin

Evaluate patient's need for equipment, including supplies to decrease pressure, alternating pressure mattress, gel foam seat cushion, and heel and elbow protectors

Teach family to perform dressing between RN visits, specifically

Other interventions, based on patient/family needs

e. *Elimination considerations*

RN to evaluate the patient's bowel patterns and need for stool softeners, laxatives, and dietary adjustments, and to develop bowel management plan

Initiate bowel management program per hospice physician

Teaching and ongoing assessment regarding early prevention and identification of constipation and its correction/resolution

Implement bowel assessment and management program

Teach patient/family and aide the importance of observing and noting bowel movements between scheduled nursing visits

Obtain patient history related to norms for bowel movements to date (e.g., "all my life I go only every other day")

Consider stool softeners and offer laxative of choice, Fleet's enemas prn, and other methods per patient wishes and physician orders

Other interventions, based on patient/family needs

f. *Hydration/nutrition*

Instruct patient about specified diet _____ (specify physician orders)

Nutrition/hydration supported by offering patient's choice of favorite or desired foods or liquids

Monitor hydration and nutrition intake

Assessment and plan related to anorexia/cachexia, tube feedings, difficult/painful swallowing, and/or transitional feedings (e.g., TPN to oral)

Teach patient and family to expect decreased nutritional and fluid intake as disease progresses

Other interventions, based on patient/family needs

g. *Therapeutic/medication regimens*

RN to teach regarding antidepressive medication and side effects

RN to monitor medication regimen and compliance with _____ therapy (specify)

Medication assessment and management q visit

Nonpharmacological interventions such as progressive muscle relaxation, imagery, positive visualization, music, massage and touch, and humor therapy of patient's choice implemented

RN to monitor/assess effectiveness of new antipsychotic drug(s) for severe agitation, psychotic behavior, and suicidal thoughts or planning

RN to monitor effectiveness of new tranquilizer regimen for severe anxiety

RN to administer injection of psychotropic medication _____ q _____ (specify orders)

RN to weigh patient (specify ordered frequency)

Medication teaching and management

Weekly venipunctures for _____ (specify)

Teach about and observe side effects of palliative chemotherapy, including constipation, anemia, and fatigue

Evaluation of medication response

Assess the patient's response to therapeutic treatments and interventions, and report any changes or unfavorable responses to the physician (i.e., extrapyramidal symptoms)

Assessment of effectiveness of new therapeutic medication regimen

Evaluate with interdisciplinary team and physician the hospice patient's need for antidepressants

Observation and assessment of patient on tricyclic antidepressants to assist in pain relief of neuropathic origin

Evaluation/observation of patient's mood and appetite as recently started on corticosteroids

Teaching of patient/family, including information on medications and the management program (e.g., strength, type, actions, times, and compliance tips)

Encourage family/caregivers to give the patient medications on the schedule and around the clock

Medications changed using equianalgesic conversion tables/physician orders (e.g., from oral morphine to an equianalgesic dose of transdermal fentanyl)

Other interventions, based on patient/family needs

h. *Other considerations*

Assess progression of disease process

RN to assess the patient's response to treatments and interventions and to report changes, unfavorable responses, or reactions to the physician

Other interventions, based on patient/family needs

- ***Home health aide or certified nursing assistant***

Effective and safe personal care

Safe ADL assistance and support

Respite care and active listening skills

Observation and reporting

Meal preparation

Homemaker services

Comfort care

Other duties

- ***Hospice social worker***

Psychosocial assessment of patient and family/caregiver, including adjustment to long-term illness and its implications

Identification of optimal coping strategies

Financial assessment and counseling regarding food acquisition, ability to prepare, and costs of needed medications

Intervention/support related to terminal illness and loss

Emotional/spiritual support

Depression/fear assessed and addressed

Facilitate communication among patient, family, and hospice team

Referral/linkage to community services and resources as indicated

Grief counseling and intervention/support related to illness/loss

Patient/caregiver counseling and support

Identification of caregiver role strain necessitating respite/relief measures/support

For patient who lives alone with no support system (e.g., able, available, willing caregiver[s]): obtain necessary resources to enable patient to remain in the home.

Identification of illness-related psychiatric condition necessitating care

Suicidal ideation assessment and evaluation, follow-up

Other interventions, based on the patient's/family's unique needs

- ***Volunteer(s)***

Support, friendship, companionship, and presence

Comfort and dignity maintained/provided for patient and family

Errands and transportation

Other services, based on interdisciplinary team recommendations and patient/caregiver needs

- *Spiritual counselor*
  Spiritual assessment and care
  Counseling, intervention, and support related to that dimension of life
    related to life's meaning (consistent with patient's beliefs)
  Support, listening, and presence
  Participation in sacred or spiritual rituals or practices
  Other supportive care, based on patient's/family's needs and belief systems

- *Dietitian/nutritional counseling*
  Assessment of patient with decreased intake, weight loss, anorexia, and
    increased shortness of breath (e.g., "don't feel like eating")
  Supportive counseling with patient/family indicating that patient will have
    a decreased appetite and usually at some point may not eat/drink
  Assessment and recommendations for swallowing difficulties
  Teaching and support of family members and caregivers
  Support and care with food and nourishment as desired by patient
  Evaluation/management of nutritional deficits and needs
  Encourage nutritional supplements and snacks to increase protein and
    caloric intake
  Food and dietary recommendations incorporate patient choice and wishes

- *Occupational therapist*
  Evaluation of ADLs, functional mobility, need for adaptive techniques and
    assistive devices
  Safety assessment of patient's environment and ADLs
  Assessment for energy conservation training
  Instruct/supervise caregivers and volunteers in the home exercise program
    for safety/conditioning/strength

- *Bereavement counselor*
  Assessment of the needs of the bereaved family and friends
  Support and intervention, based on assessment and ongoing findings
  Presence and counseling
  Supportive visits and follow-up, other interventions (e.g., mailings, calls)
  Other services related to bereavement work and support

- *Pharmacist*
  Evaluation of hospice patient with depression and constipation on cathar-
    tics, stool softeners, and other medications for possible food/drug, drug/
    drug interactions
  Medication monitoring regarding therapeutic levels and dosages
  Medication consult and input into interdisciplinary plan of care related to
    pain control, palliation, and symptom management
  Assessment of medication regimen and plan for safety and compliance

- *Music, massage, art, or other therapies or services*
  Evaluation and intervention based on patient's and caregiver's unique
    wishes and needs that support care, comfort, and death in the setting of
    the patient's choice
  Assessment plan to engage patient and support comfort, quality, enjoyment,
    and dignity

Pet therapy (including patient's pet, if available) and therapeutic intervention

7. **Outcomes for care**

   • *Hospice nursing*

   Pharmacological and nonpharmacological interventions, such as localized heat application, positioning, relaxation methods, and music

   Mental distress, depression, and fear of dying addressed throughout care by hospice team

   Patient and family able to care for and support patient

   Patient and caregiver can verbalize symptoms, changes, or accelerations that necessitate call to physician

   Patient and family demonstrate compliance with medication regimen and other therapeutic interventions

   Patient demonstrates stabilization and increased or enhanced coping skills related to functioning and depression

   Pain and symptoms managed/controlled in setting of patient/family choice (e.g., patient and family report ability to eat, sleep, speak with pacing)

   Planned and effective bowel program, as evidenced by regular bowel movements and patient/family report of comfort

   Death with dignity, and pain/symptoms controlled in setting of patient/family choice

   Optimal comfort, support, and dignity provided throughout illness

   Death with maximum comfort through effective symptom control with specialized hospice support

   Patient verbalizes feelings in a safe environment

   Patient and caregiver demonstrate compliance with instructions related to medications, positive coping skills and other behaviors, and decision making

   Lab values (i.e., lithium) will be within normal limits for patient by _____ (date)

   Symptoms stabilized as evidenced by _____ (define) by _____ (date)

   Caregiver effective in care management and knows whom to call for questions/concerns

   Patient verbalizes understanding of and adheres to medication regimens

   Anxiety decreased as noted by behaviors and self-report by patient/caregiver

   Patient self-reports decreased episodes of panic and is able to leave home without spouse by _____ (specify)

   Compliance with and adherence to interdisciplinary care plan as demonstrated by observation and reporting by caregiver/patient

   Other goals/outcomes based on the patient's unique needs and problems

   Educational tools/plans incorporated in daily care, and patient/caregiver verbalizes understanding of safe, needed care

   Adherence to POC as demonstrated and verbalized by caregiver and demonstrated by patient findings by _____ (specify date)

   Patient states pain is _____ on 0-10 scale by next visit

Patient/caregiver demonstrates appropriate backup or "rescue" therapies for breakthrough pain or other symptoms (e.g., dyspnea)

Patient will decide on care, interventions, and evaluation

Patient will express satisfaction with hospice support received and will experience increased comfort

Patient will be made comfortable at home through death in accordance with the patient's wishes

Effective pain control and symptom control verbalized by patient

Patient and caregiver supported through patient's death

Comfort maintained through course of care

The patient and family receive hospice support and care, and family members and friends are able to spend quality time with the patient

Caregiver able and verbalizes comfort with role and lists when to call hospice team members

Patient supported through and receives the maximum benefit from palliative chemotherapy and radiation with minimal complications

Patient/caregiver lists adverse reactions, potential complications, signs/symptoms of infection (e.g., sputum change, chest congestion)

Comfort maintained through death with dignity

Pain effectively managed, and patient verbalizes comfort

Patient/caregiver able to list adverse drug reactions/problems with medication regimen and whom to call for follow-up and resolution

Patient's/family's privacy, independence, and choices supported with respect and maintained through death

Enhancement and support of quality of life

Effective symptom relief and control (e.g., a peaceful and comfortable death at home, depression controlled, some enjoyment of life)

Maximizing the patient's quality of life (e.g., alert and pain-free or as patient wishes)

Pharmacological and nonpharmacological interventions, such as localized heat application, biofeedback, massage, positioning, relaxation methods, and music

Patient cared for and family supported through death with physical, psychosocial, spiritual, and other concerns/needs acknowledged/addressed

Patient- and family-centered hospice care provided based on the patient's/family's unique situation and needs

Infection control and palliation

Grief/bereavement expression and support provided

Patient is pain free by next _____ visit

Caregiver demonstrates ability to manage pain, where applicable

Patient maintains comfort and dignity throughout illness

- *Home health aide or certified nursing assistant*
  Effective hygiene, personal care, and comfort
  ADL assistance
  Safe environment maintained

- *Hospice social worker*
  Problem identified and addressed, with patient and caregiver linked with appropriate community support services and plan of care successfully implemented

Patient and caregiver cope adaptively with illness and death

Psychosocial support and counseling offered to patient/caregivers experiencing loss and grief

Counseling/support related to ideation of suicide

Caregiver system assessed, and development of stable caregiver plan facilitated

- *Volunteer(s)*

Comfort, companionship, and friendship extended to patient/family

Support and respite provided as defined by the needs of the patient/caregiver

Patient and family supported by team with care, comfort, and companionship

- *Spiritual counseling*

Intervention/support provided related to that dimension of life related to life's meaning

Spiritual support offered and provided as defined by needs of patient/caregiver

Participation in sacred or spiritual rituals or practices

Provision of spiritual support and care based on the assessed and ongoing needs of the patient and family

Spiritual support offered, and patient and family needs met

Patient and family express relief of symptoms of spiritual suffering

Support, listening, and presence

- *Dietitian/nutritional counseling*

Patient and family verbalize comprehension of changing nutritional needs

Family and caregiver integrate recommendations into nutrition teaching (where appropriate)

Patient and caregiver know whom to call for nutrition- and hydration-related questions/concerns

Nutrition/hydration per patient's choices

Caregiver integrates recommendations into daily meal planning

- *Occupational therapy*

Patient and caregiver demonstrate maximum independence with ADL

Patient and caregiver demonstrate maximum safety in ADL and functional mobility

Patient and caregiver demonstrate effective use of energy conservation to improve quality of life

- *Bereavement counselor*

Bereavement support provided

- *Pharmacist*

Regimen for bowel regimen successful as self-reported by patient and in update at team meeting

Multiple drug regimen reviewed for food/drug and drug/drug interactions in patient on multiple meds

Stability and safety in complex medication regimen, with maximum benefit to patient

Effective symptom control and symptom management as reported by
patient/caregiver

Lab reports reviewed for therapeutic dosages and effective patient response

* *Music, massage, art, or other therapies or services*

Therapeutic massage/touch effective for patient as self-reported or observed
by caregivers/family

Improved muscle tone, relaxation, and/or sleep

Patient comfortable and relaxed (e.g., sleeping) after massage

Music therapy intervention based on assessment to decrease pain perception and provide emotional expression and support

Maintenance of comfort and physical, psychosocial, and spiritual health

Holistic health maintained and comfort achieved through _____
(specify modality)

Patient has pet's presence as desired—in all care sites, when possible

8. **Patient, family, and caregiver educational needs**

Educational needs are the care regimens that contribute to safe and effective
care at home between the hospice team's visits. These include the following:

The basic tenets of hospice and the availability of support 24 hours a day, 7
days a week

Home safety assessment and counseling

The patient's medication regimen

Safe and proper body mechanics to promote patient comfort and prevent
caregiver safety problems

Other teaching specific to the patient's and family's unique needs

Support groups available to patient's family, such as the hospice program's
"Caregiver Support Group" meetings for family members and friends of
the patient

Anticipated disease progression

Safety concerns, medication compliance, and importance of keeping psycho-
therapeutic appointments at the mental health center

Importance of adequate hydration and nutrition

Signs and symptoms of recurring depression or other behaviors; side effects
related to drugs that necessitate seeking medical follow-up

Home safety concerns and issues

The importance of medical follow-up, including drug levels if indicated, and
family therapy

9. **Specific tips for quality and reimbursement**

Document any variances to expected outcomes. There are many models of
hospice programs. Those that are home health agency–based must work
within the framework of the Medicare home care program. For example,
sometimes a hospice patient reaches a stable period in the illness and has no
further skilled needs or the patient is no longer homebound per Medicare
home health care criteria. When this occurs, one option is to discharge the
patient from Medicare home health agency reimbursement and maintain the
patient on grant funds or other available resources. If the patient's status deteriorates and again meets the Medicare criteria, a new start of care is initiated on the HCFA form 485. Usually hospices continue volunteer support,

nursing, and other services indicated during these periods of no reimbursement.

The Medicare hospice benefit does not require that the patient be homebound or have identified skilled needs. Though it is a needed and viable program, the Medicare hospice benefit may not be indicated for all Medicare eligible beneficiaries. For further information on this benefit, please refer to HCFA Hospice Manual 21.

Should the patient's status deteriorate and increased personal care be needed, obtain a telephone order for the increased service, noting frequency and estimating the duration.

Obtain a telephone order for all medication and treatment changes of the medical regimen, and document these in the clinical record.

Unless the patient is in a hospice insurance program, some insurers will not pay for a skilled nurse visit that is made at death if the patient is dead when the nurse arrives at the home. From a Medicare home care perspective, the visit at the time of death may be covered when the orders and clinical record document assessment of the patient's status or signs of death/life or state law allows pronouncement of death by a nurse.

Document patient deterioration

Document dehydration, dehydrating

Document patient change or instability

Document pain, other symptoms not controlled

Document status after acute episode of _____ (specify)

Document positive urine, sputum, etc. culture; patient started on
_____ (specify ordered antibiotic therapy)

Document patient impacted; impaction removed manually

Document RN in frequent communication with physician regarding
_____ (specify)

Document febrile at _____, pulse change at _____, irr.,
irr.

Document change noted in _____

Document bony prominences red, opening

Document RN contacted physician regarding _____ (specify)

Document marked SOB

Document alteration in mental status

Document medications being adjusted, regulated, or monitored

Document unable to perform own ADLs, personal care

Document all interdisciplinary team meetings and communications in the
POC and in the progress notes of the clinical record

All disciplines involved should have input into the POC and document their
interventions and goals

Document in the clinical notes the clear progression and symptomatology and
interventions that demonstrate the interventions and overall management
of the patient with pain

Document when/if the patient has respiratory changes, shortness of breath,
exacerbation of conditions, dysphagia, changes in pain, and other symptoms and that they are identified and resolved

Remember that the clinical documentation is key to measuring compliance
for quality and reimbursement purposes. Care coordination, timely verbal
and initial physician orders, and assessment and addressing of spiritual

and psychosocial needs should be ongoing and documented in the patient's clinical record

The documentation should support that all hospice care supports comfort and dignity while meeting patient/family needs

The documentation should include ongoing assessment and management of pain and other symptoms and the anticipation and prevention of secondary symptoms such as constipation

It is important to note that all team members, including nurses and social workers, should assess, identify, and "hear" spiritual needs that the patient/family want to be addressed. These spiritual issues are key to the provision of quality hospice care and cannot be addressed effectively and promptly by the spiritual counselor only.

Document clearly symptoms, clinical changes, and assessment findings related to pain and patient care

Document patient changes, symptoms, and clinical information identified from visits and team conferences that support hospice care and a limited life expectancy

Document coordination of services or consultation of the other members of the IDT

Document changes to the plan of care, such as medications, services, frequency, communication, and concurrence of other team members

Clearly support in the documentation the rationale that supports/explains the progression of the illness from the chronic to terminal stages

Document mentation, behavioral, and/or cognitive changes

Document dysphagia, weight loss, increased shortness of breath, dyspnea, infection, sepsis, new or changed medications, etc.

Document any skin changes (e.g., inflamed, painful, weeping skin site[s])

Document when the patient is actively dying, deteriorating, or progressing toward death

Remember that the "litmus test" of care coordination rests on the quality of the clinical documentation by all team members. Review one of your patient's clinical records and ask yourself the following: "If I was unable to give a verbal report/update on this patient, would a peer be able to pick up and provide the same level of care and know (from the documentation) the current orders, medications, and other details that contribute to effective hospice care?"

This patient population usually has many clinical changes that should be documented. These include weight loss and multiple and changed medication regimens with varying routes. Side effects to the drug regimen should be observed, noted, documented, and reported

Your assessments, observations, and clinical findings assist in painting a picture to support coverage and documentation requirements for hospice care

Document any hospitalizations and changed clinical findings

Document patient changes, symptoms, psychosocial issues impacting the care, and information gathered at the patient/family visits and during team meetings

The documentation should reflect ongoing effects of the terminal condition, the patient's/family's difficulty with care or coping, and the continued desire for hospice care

Document communications and care coordination with other care providers, such as skilled nursing facility or nursing home staff, inpatient team members, and hired caregivers

10. **Resources for hospice care and practice**

The Agency for Health Care Policy and Research offers *Depression Is a Treatable Illness: Patient Guide* (AHCPR Pub. No. 93-0053). Call 1-800-358-9295.

The American Psychiatric Association (1-800-682-6220) offers free pamphlets entitled *Psychiatric Medications; Mental Illness: An Overview; Depression; Manic-Depressive/Bipolar Disorder; Anxiety Disorders; Obsessive-Compulsive Disorder; Mental Health of the Elderly; Phobias; Schizophrenia;* and many more.

DIABETES MELLITUS AND OTHER VASCULAR CONDITIONS

1. **General considerations**

   Diabetes mellitus and comorbid conditions such as peripheral vascular disease, cellulitis, and amputation care present challenges to the hospice team. All of these patient problems usually indicate a long-term chronic disease process for the new hospice patient and family. See also "Cancer Care," "Pain Care," and other sections that may pertain to your hospice patient.

2. **Needs for visit**

   Physician order for hospice care, specific to the hospice program's admission criteria and policies

   Standard precautions/supplies

   Vital signs equipment for baseline assessment

   Other supplies or equipment, based on physician orders

3. **Safety considerations**

   Infection control/standard precautions

   Night-light

   Extra caution on slippery surfaces

   Removal of scatter rugs

   Tub rail, grab bars for bathroom safety

   Supportive and nonskid shoes

   Handrail on stairs

   Fall precautions

   Protective skin measures

   Identification and report of any skin problems

   Smoke detector and fire evacuation plan

   Assistance with ambulation

   Foot care and protection

   Avoidance of heating pads, electric blankets, extremes of hot/cold

   Disposal of sharps and related supplies

   Safety related to decreased sensation in extremities and protection from heat and cold

   Disposal of soiled dressings and related supplies

   Anticoagulant precautions

   Supervised medication administration

   Multiple medications (e.g., side effects, needles, safe storage)

   Safety for home medical equipment

   Supportive and well-fitting shoes and socks

   Emergency symptoms and actions to take

   The phone number and name of person to call with a care problem

   Others, based on the patient's unique condition and environment

4. **Potential diagnoses and codes**

AKA right or left	V49.76
AMI	410.92

Amputee, bilateral	736.89
Amputation, infected right or left BKA, AKA	997.62
Amputation, transmetatarsal (right or left) (surgical)	84.12
Angina	413.9
Arterial graft, S/P	39.58
Arterial insufficiency	447.1
Arterial occlusive disease	447.1
Atherosclerosis	440.9
Bilateral amputee	V49.70 (after care)
BKA, right or left (surgical)	84.15
Bullous pemphigoid	694.5
Cellulitis of the arm	682.3
Cellulitis of the trunk	682.2
Cellulitis RLE, LLE	682.6
Cellulitis and abscess (legs)	682.6
Cellulitis of the trunk	682.2
CHF	428.0
Chronic ischemic heart disease	414.9
Chronic renal failure	585
Circulatory disease	459.9
COPD	496
Coronary artery disease	414.00
CVA	436
Decubitus ulcer (pressure ulcer)	707.0
Diabetes glaucoma	250.50 and 365.44
Diabetes mellitus, with complications (NIDDM)	250.90
Diabetes mellitus, with complications (IDDM)	250.91
Diabetic neuropathy	250.60 and 357.2
Diabetic retinopathy (insulin dependent)	250.51 and 362.01
Diabetic retinopathy (non–insulin dependent)	250.50 and 362.01
Electrolyte/fluid imbalance	276.9
Excoriation of skin	919.8
Femoral-popliteal bypass (surgical)	39.29
Foot abscess	682.7
Gangrene, right or left foot	250.70 and 785.4
Gangrene toe	785.4
Hyperglycemia	790.6
Hypertension and diabetes	250.80 and 401.9
Hypoglycemia	250.80
Ketoacidosis, insulin dependent	250.11
Ketoacidosis, non–insulin dependent	250.10
Left heart failure	428.1
Obesity	278.00
Pain in limb	729.5
Peripheral vascular disease	250.70 and 443.9
Pressure (decubitus) ulcer	707.0
Staph infection	041.10
Stasis ulcer	454.2
Thrombophlebitis	451.9

Toe amputation (surgical)	84.11
Ulcer, right or left	707.1
Urinary tract infection	599.0
Vascular insufficiency	459.81
Vasculitis	250.70 and 447.6

5. **Associated nursing diagnoses**
   Activity intolerance
   Activity intolerance, risk for
   Adjustment, impaired
   Anxiety
   Aspiration, risk for
   Body image disturbance
   Body temperature, altered, risk for
   Bowel incontinence
   Breathing pattern, ineffective
   Cardiac output, decreased
   Caregiver role strain
   Caregiver role strain, risk for
   Communication, impaired verbal
   Constipation
   Coping, ineffective family: compromised
   Coping, ineffective family: disabling
   Coping, ineffective individual
   Denial, ineffective
   Diarrhea
   Disuse syndrome, risk for
   Family processes, altered
   Fatigue
   Fear
   Fluid volume deficit, risk for
   Fluid volume excess
   Gas exchange, impaired
   Grieving, anticipatory
   Growth and development, altered
   Home maintenance management, impaired
   Hyperthermia
   Hypothermia
   Incontinence, total
   Infection, risk for
   Injury, risk for
   Knowledge deficit (disease and self-care management)
   Mobility, impaired physical
   Noncompliance (specify)
   Nutrition, altered: less than body requirements
   Oral mucous membrane, altered
   Pain
   Pain, chronic
   Parenting, altered
   Peripheral neurovascular dysfunction, risk for

Protection, altered
Role performance, altered
Self-care deficit, bathing/hygiene
Self-care deficit, dressing/grooming
Self-care deficit, feeding
Self-care deficit, toileting
Sensory/perceptual alterations (specify) (visual, auditory, kinesthetic, gustatory, tactile, olfactory)
Sexual dysfunction
Sexuality patterns, altered
Skin integrity, impaired
Skin integrity, impaired, risk for
Sleep pattern disturbance
Social interaction, impaired
Spiritual distress (distress of the human spirit)
Spiritual well-being, potential for enhanced
Swallowing, impaired
Thought processes, altered
Tissue integrity, impaired
Tissue perfusion, altered (specify type) (renal, cerebral, cardiopulmonary, gastrointestinal, peripheral)
Trauma, potential for
Unilateral neglect
Urinary elimination, altered
Urinary retention

6. **Skills and services identified**

   • *Hospice nursing*

      a. *Comfort and symptom control*
         Complete initial systems assessment of the patient with
         _____ (specify) admitted to hospice for _____
         (specify problem necessitating care)
         Skilled observation and all systems assessment of patient with diabetes mellitus
         Presentation of hospice philosophy and services
         Explain patient rights and responsibilities
         Assess patient, family, and caregiver wishes and expectations regarding care
         Assess patient, family, and caregiver resources available for care
         Provision of volunteer support to patient and family
         Teach family or caregiver physical care of patient
         Assess pain and other symptoms, including site, duration, characteristics, and relief measures
         Assess pain and evaluate the pain management's effectiveness
         Teach care of bedridden patient
         Measure vital signs and pain, q visit
         Assess cardiovascular, pulmonary, and respiratory status
         Teach patient/family principles of effective pain management

Teach caregivers symptom control and relief measures

Identify and monitor pain, symptoms, and relief measures

Teach patient and family about use of home glucose monitoring

Teach insulin administration and other DM care regimens including foot care, skin care, and emergency measures for signs and symptoms of hyper/hypoglycemia

RN to assess patient's pain or other symptoms q visit to identify need for change, addition, or other plan or dose adjustment

Assess peripheral circulation

Check pedal pulses for equality, rate, and strength

Assess amount, site(s) of edema

Pain management and relief interventions

Teach patient correct application of compression stockings

Assess pain, site, frequency, and duration

Teach effective personal hygiene and proper hand-washing techniques

Teach signs and symptoms of (further) infection

Teach signs/symptoms of hyperglycemia and hypoglycemia and emergency measures to patient and family

Assess for long-term ability of patient and family to comply with regimen

Teaching and training, observation and assessment related to diabetes care and management

Ongoing monitoring and assessment of blood glucose readings and patient's management of compliance with new DM regimen

Instruct patient in equipment and use of blood glucose monitoring program

Assess for signs of decreased circulation and report to physician

Teach patient's family care regimen

Teach patient/family use of standardized form/tool to use between hospice team members' visits (and for care coordination between team members)

RN to teach patient and family on all aspects of care of the patient with diabetes, including foot care, signs/care of hypo- or hyperglycemia, and the importance of medical follow-up

Observation and assessment, communication with physician related to signs and symptoms of continuing decompensation and increased symptoms, pain, discomfort, shortness of breath, and measures to alleviate and control

Pain assessment and management q visit

Pain assessment and management q visit, including source of pain (e.g., neuropathy, phantom pain, claudification, infection, and other problems, such as cardiac or arthritis pain)

Effective management of pain and prevention of secondary symptoms

RN to provide and teach effective oral care and comfort measures

Teach patient/family about realistic expectations of disease process

Teach care of dying and signs/symptoms of impending death

Presence and support

Other interventions, based on patient/family needs

b. *Safety and mobility considerations*

Patient provided with home safety information and instruction related to _____ and documented in the clinical record

Teach patient or family member safe home blood glucose monitoring process

Teach patient all aspects of safe care with new SQ insulin infusion pump at home

Teach family about safety of patient in home

Teach family about energy conservation techniques

Assess safety related to amputation and balance/mobility

Other interventions, based on patient/family needs

c. *Emotional/spiritual considerations*

Psychosocial assessment of patient and family regarding disease and prognosis

RN to provide emotional support to patient and family

Assess patient's and caregiver's coping skills

Interventions of symptoms directed toward comfort and palliation

Observation and assessment of mental status changes/complaints of depression in new hospice patient with pain and wound

Observation of patient for neuropsychiatric complications of illness, including confusion, depression, and anxiety

RN to provide support and intervention for depression

Teach patient/family about depression and signs/symptoms of exacerbation that require more intervention

Inform patient/family/caregiver of available volunteer support

Assess for and manage plans for psychosocial and/or spiritual pain (e.g., all pain, anxiety, interpersonal and other distress)

Psychosocial aspects of pain control (e.g., depression) assessed and acknowledged with team support/intervention

Ongoing acknowledgment of spirituality and related concerns of patient/family

Other interventions, based on patient/family needs

d. *Skin care*

Pressure ulcer care as indicated

Assess skin integrity

Evaluate patient's need for equipment, including supplies to decrease pressure, alternating pressure mattress, gel foam seat cushion, and heel and elbow protectors

Observation and evaluation of wound and surrounding skin

Teach patient, family, or caregiver about proper body alignment and positioning in bed to prevent skin tears from shearing skin

Observation and skilled assessment of areas for possible breakdown, including heels, hips, elbows, and ankles

Teach family to perform dressing between RN visits, specifically _____

Teach caregiver about skin care needs, including the need for frequent position changes, appropriate pressure pads and mattresses, and the prevention of breakdown

Medicate patient with pain medication before dressing change

Dressing change _____ site (specify physician orders)

Gently wash and dry site

Evaluate temperature, redness of site, and amount of swelling

Culture open wound as ordered, and send for culture and sensitivity test

Instruct patient or caregiver on dressing change procedure

Apply occlusive (or other ordered) dressing to wound

Assess and objectively document wound progress

Obtain specific wound dressing orders, including sterile or nonsterile procedure(s)

Specify dressing regimen and frequency of wound changes every visit

Observation, assessment, and supportive care related to vascular problems, including diabetes and cellulitis with weeping skin sites

Comprehensive management of diabetes and wound care regimens

Other interventions, based on patient/family needs

e. *Elimination considerations*

Assess bowel regimen, and implement program as needed

Check for and remove impaction as needed

Condom catheter or indwelling catheter as indicated

Assess amount and frequency of urinary output

RN to teach caregiver daily catheter care

RN to evaluate the patient's bowel patterns and need for stool softeners, laxatives, and dietary adjustments, and to develop bowel management plan

Teach patient or family urine check procedures, as ordered

Teaching and ongoing assessment related to early prevention and identification of constipation and its correction/resolution

Initiate bowel management program per hospice physician

Implement bowel assessment and management program

Teach patient/family and aide the importance of observing and noting bowel movements between scheduled nursing visits

Obtain patient history related to norms for bowel movements to date (e.g., "all my life I go only every other day")

Consider stool softeners and offer laxative of choice, Fleet's enemas prn, and other methods per patient wishes and physician orders

Other interventions, based on patient/family needs

f. *Hydration/nutrition*

Detailed nutritional assessment related to diabetes, weight, constipation, and immobility

Assess nutrition and hydration statuses

Diet counseling for patient with anorexia

Teach feeding-tube care to family

Nutrition/hydration supported by offering patient's choice of favorite or desired foods or liquids

Nutrition/hydration maintained by offering patient high-protein diet and foods of choice as tolerated

Teach patient and family to expect decreased nutritional and fluid intake as disease progresses

Other interventions, based on patient/family needs

g. *Therapeutic/medication regimens*

Comprehensive management of medications, including antibiotics and those for pain and diabetes

Teaching of patient/family, including medications and the management program (e.g., strength, type, actions, times, and compliance tips)

Encourage family/caregivers to give patient medications on the schedule and around the clock

Monitor patient for side effects of drugs and drug/food and drug/drug interactions

Teach new pain and symptom control medication regimen

RN to assess the patient's unique response to treatments or interventions, and to report changes, unfavorable responses, or reactions to the physician

Medication assessment and management

Teach patient and caregiver use of PCA pump

Assess for electrolyte imbalance

Nonpharmacological interventions such as progressive muscle relaxation, imagery, positive visualization, music, massage and touch, and humor therapy of patient's choice implemented

Teach new antibiotic regimen of _____ (specify)

Teaching and training related to IV antibiotic therapy (e.g., infusion hook-up and discontinuance, signs and symptoms of infiltration, reaction)

Teach new medication regimen

Teach patient or family to mix insulin(s)

Venipuncture for FBS as indicated

Teach about new insulin and medication regimen

Teach action of ordered insulin(s)

Teach use of single-site rotations for injections or other ordered rotation method

Medications changed using equianalgesic conversion tables/physician orders (e.g., from oral morphine to an equianalgesic dose of transdermal fentanyl)

Other interventions, based on patient/family needs

h. *Other considerations*

Administer or teach foot care regimen

Assess need for podiatrist to provide needed foot care

Assess progression of disease process

RN to assess the patient's response to treatments and interventions and to report to the physician changes, unfavorable responses, or reactions

Other interventions, based on patient/family needs

- ***Home health aide or certified nursing assistant***

Effective and safe personal care

Safe ADL assistance and support

Respite care and active listening skills

Observation and reporting

Meal preparation

Homemaker services
Comfort care
Other duties

- *Hospice social worker*
Psychosocial assessment of patient and family/caregiver, including adjust-
ment to long-term illness and its implications
Identification of optimal coping strategies
Identification of caregiver role strain necessitating respite/relief measures/
support
Financial assessment and counseling regarding food acquisition, ability to
prepare, and costs of needed medications
Intervention/support related to terminal illness and loss
Emotional/spiritual support
Depression/fear assessed and addressed
Facilitate communication among patient, family, and hospice team
Referral/linkage to community services and resources as indicated
Grief counseling and intervention/support related to illness/loss
Patient/caregiver counseling and support
For patient who lives alone with no support system (e.g., able, available,
willing caregiver[s]): obtain resources that enable patient to remain in
the home
Identification of illness-related psychiatric condition necessitating care

- *Volunteer(s)*
Support, friendship, companionship, and presence
Comfort and dignity maintained/provided for patient and family
Errands and transportation
Other services, based on interdisciplinary team recommendations and
patient/caregiver needs

- *Spiritual counselor*
Spiritual assessment and care
Counseling, intervention, and support related to that dimension of life
related to life's meaning (consistent with patient's beliefs)
Support, listening, and presence
Participation in sacred or spiritual rituals or practices
Other supportive care, based on patient/family needs and belief systems

- *Dietitian/nutritional counseling*
Assessment of patient with decreased intake, weight loss, anorexia, and
increased shortness of breath (e.g., "don't feel like eating")
Supportive counseling with patient/family indicating that patient will have
a decreased appetite and usually at some point may not eat/drink
Assessment and recommendations for swallowing difficulties
Teaching and support of family members and caregivers
Support and care with food and nourishment as desired by patient
Evaluation/management of nutritional deficits and needs
Encourage nutritional supplements and snacks to increase protein and
caloric intake
Food and dietary recommendations incorporate patient choice and wishes

- *Occupational therapist*
  Evaluation of ADL and functional mobility
  Assess for need for adaptive equipment and assistive devices
  Safety assessment of patient's environment and ADLs
  Assessment for energy conservation training
  Assessment of upper extremity function, retraining motor skills

- *Physical therapist*
  Evaluation
  Safety assessment of patient's environment
  Safe transfer training or bed mobility exercises
  Pain assessment/reduction factors
  Strengthening exercises/program
  Assessment of gait safety and home safety measures
  Instruct/supervise caregiver and volunteers on home exercise program for
      conditioning and strength
  Assistive, adaptive devices and evaluation of equipment and teaching

- *Speech-language pathologist*
  Evaluation for speech/swallowing problems
  Food texture recommendations
  Alternate functional communication

- *Bereavement counselor*
  Assessment of the needs of the bereaved family and friends
  Support and intervention, based on assessment and ongoing findings
  Presence and counseling
  Supportive visits and follow-up, other interventions (e.g., mailings, calls)
  Other services related to bereavement work and support

- *Pharmacist*
  Evaluation of hospice patient with constipation on cathartics, stool soften-
      ers, and other medications for possible food/drug, drug/drug interac-
      tions
  Medication monitoring regarding therapeutic levels and dosages
  Pain consult and input into interdisciplinary plan of care related to pain
      control, palliation, and symptom management
  Assessment of medication regimen and plan for safety and compliance

- *Music, massage, art, or other therapies or services*
  Evaluation and intervention based on patient's and caregiver's unique
      wishes and needs that support care, comfort, and death in the setting of
      the patient's choice
  Assessment plan to engage patient and support comfort, quality, enjoyment,
      and dignity
  Pet therapy (including patient's pet, if available) and therapeutic interven-
      tion

7. **Outcomes for care**

- *Hospice nursing*
  Death with dignity, and symptoms controlled in setting of patient/family
      choice

Mental distress, depression, and fear of dying addressed throughout care by hospice team

Patient and family able to care for and support patient

Patient and caregiver can verbalize symptoms, changes, or accelerations that necessitate call to physician

Patient and family demonstrate compliance with medication regimen and other therapeutic interventions

Patient demonstrates stabilization and increased or enhanced coping skills related to functioning and depression

Pain and symptoms managed/controlled in setting of patient/family choice (e.g., patient/family report ability to eat, sleep, speak with pacing)

Planned and effective bowel program, as evidenced by regular bowel movements and patient/family report of comfort

Optimal comfort, support, and dignity provided throughout illness

Death with maximum comfort through effective symptom control with specialized hospice support

Patient and caregiver able to list adverse drug reactions/problems with medication regimen and whom to call for follow-up and resolution

Patient's and family's privacy, independence, and choices supported with respect and maintained through death

Enhancement and support of quality of life

Effective symptom relief and control (e.g., a peaceful and comfortable death at home, depression controlled, some enjoyment of life)

Maximizing the patient's quality of life (e.g., alert and pain free or as patient wishes)

Pharmacological and nonpharmacological interventions such as localized heat application, biofeedback, massage, positioning, relaxation methods, and music

Patient cared for and family supported through death with physical, psychosocial, spiritual, and other concerns/needs acknowledged/addressed

Patient- and family-centered hospice care provided based on the patient/family's unique situation and needs

Patient states pain is _____ on 0-10 scale by next visit

Patient and caregiver demonstrate appropriate backup or "rescue" therapies for breakthrough pain or other symptoms (e.g., dyspnea)

Patient and family verbalize satisfaction with care

Compliance with wound care and associated regimen by _____ (specify date)

Pain control/comfort achieved as verbalized by patient

Teaching program related to the prevention of infection and injuries demonstrated by caregivers

Wound healed and site infection free (e.g., no redness, swelling)

Patient/caregiver will demonstrate _____% (specify) compliance with instructions related to care

Patient and caregiver demonstrate and practice effective hand washing and other infection control measures (specify, e.g., disposal of dressings)

Adherence to POC by patient and caregivers and ability to demonstrate safe and supportive care

Symptoms stabilized as evidenced by _____ (define) by _____ (date)

Caregiver effective in care management and knows whom to call for questions/concerns

Patient verbalizes understanding of and adheres to medication regimens

Patient compliant with self-care regarding DM and aspects of regimen by _____ (date)

Blood sugar in normal patient range, and patient verbalizes understanding of factors that contribute to prevention of complications

Patient/caregiver will demonstrate _____% behavioral compliance with instructions related to medications, leg elevation, diet, and care

Adherence to POC by patient and caregivers and ability to demonstrate safe and supportive care

Optimal circulation for patient

Educational tools/plans incorporated in daily care, and patient/caregiver verbalizes understanding of safe, needed care

Patient will decide on care, interventions, and evaluation

Caregiver effective in care management and knows whom to call for questions/concerns

Patient will express satisfaction with hospice support received and will experience increased comfort

Patient will be made comfortable at home through death in accordance with the patient's wishes

Effective pain control and symptom control verbalized by patient

Patient verbalizes understanding of and adheres to care and medication regimens

Patient and caregiver supported through patient's death

Comfort maintained through course of care

Patient and family receive hospice support and care, and family members and friends are able to spend quality time with the patient

Caregiver able and verbalizes comfort with role and understands when to call hospice team members

Patient supported through and receives the maximum benefit from palliative chemotherapy and radiation with minimal complications

Patient/caregiver lists adverse reactions, potential complications, signs/symptoms of infection (e.g., sputum change, chest congestion)

Comfort maintained through death with dignity

Pain effectively managed, and patient verbalizes comfort

Patient is protected from injury, has stable respiratory status, and is compliant with medication, safety, and care regimens

Comfort and individualized intervention of patient with immobility/bedbound status (e.g., skin, urinary, musculature, vascular)

Spiritual and psychosocial needs met (specify) as defined by patient and caregiver throughout course of care

Infection control and palliation of wound site

Grief/bereavement expression and support provided

Caregiver demonstrates ability to manage pain, where applicable

Patient maintains comfort and dignity throughout illness

Other goals/outcomes, based on the patient's unique needs and problems

- *Home health aide or certified nursing assistant*
  Effective hygiene, personal care, and comfort
  ADL assistance
  Safe environment maintained

- *Hospice social worker*
  Problem identified and addressed, with patient/caregiver linked with appropriate support services and plan of care successfully implemented
  Patient and caregiver cope adaptively with illness and death
  Adaptive adjustment to changed body and body image
  Psychosocial support and counseling offered to patient/caregivers experiencing loss and grief
  Resources identified, community linkage as appropriate for patient/family
  Caregiver system assessed, and development of stable caregiver plan facilitated

- *Volunteer(s)*
  Comfort, companionship, and friendship extended to patient/family
  Support and respite provided as defined by the needs of the patient/caregiver
  Patient and family supported by team with care, comfort, and companionship

- *Spiritual counseling*
  Spiritual support offered and provided as defined by needs of patient/caregiver
  Provision of spiritual support and care based on the assessed and ongoing needs of the patient and family
  Spiritual support offered, and patient and family needs met
  Patient and family express relief of symptoms of spiritual suffering
  Support, listening, and presence
  Intervention and support provided related to that dimension of life related to life's meaning (consistent with patient's beliefs)
  Participation in sacred or spiritual rituals or practices

- *Dietitian/nutritional counseling*
  Family and caregiver integrate recommendations into nutrition teaching (where appropriate)
  Patient and caregiver know whom to call for nutrition- and hydration-related questions/concerns
  Nutrition/hydration per patient's choices
  Caregiver integrates recommendations into daily meal planning
  Patient and family verbalize comprehension of changing nutritional needs

- *Occupational therapist*
  Patient and caregiver demonstrate maximum independence with ADLs, adaptive techniques, and assistive devices
  Patient and caregiver demonstrate maximum safety in ADLs and functional mobility
  Patient and caregiver demonstrate effective use of energy conservation

Verbalization/demonstration of improved functional activity level and enhanced quality of life

Patient and caregiver demonstrate effective use of diaphragmatic breathing to reduce shortness of breath and relaxation techniques to help in pain/symptom management

Patient and caregiver demonstrate correct use of exercise and splints

- *Physical therapist*

Prevention of complications

Home exercise and upper extremity program taught to caregiver

Optimal strength, mobility, function maintained/achieved

Compliance with home exercise program by _____ (specify date)

- *Speech-language pathologist*

Communication method implemented, and patient able to be understood as self-reported or reported by family/caregivers

Safe swallowing and functional communication

Recommended lists of foods/textures for safety and patient choice

- *Bereavement counselor*

Support services related to grief provided to patient and family

Well-being and resolution process of grief initiated and followed through bereavement services

- *Pharmacist*

Regimen for bowel/other regimen successful as self-reported by patient and in update at team meeting

Multiple drug regimen reviewed for food/drug and drug/drug interactions in patient on multiple meds

Stability and safety in complex medication regimen, with maximum benefit to patient

Effective pain and symptom control and symptom management as reported by patient/caregiver

- *Music, massage, art, or other therapies or services*

Therapeutic massage/touch effective for patient as self-reported or observed by caregivers/family

Improved muscle tone, relaxation, and/or sleep

Patient comfortable and relaxed (e.g., sleeping) after massage

Pet therapy (including patient's pet, if available) and therapeutic intervention

Music therapy intervention based on assessment to decrease pain perception and provide emotional expression and support

Maintenance of comfort and physical, psychosocial, and spiritual health

Holistic health maintained and comfort achieved through _____ (specify modality)

8. **Patient, family, and caregiver educational needs**

Educational needs are the care regimens that contribute to safe and effective care at home between the hospice team's visits. These include the following:

The basic tenets of hospice and the availability of support 24 hours a day, 7 days a week

Home safety assessment and counseling

The patient's medication regimen

Safe and proper body mechanics to promote patient comfort and prevent
   caregiver safety problems

Anticipated disease progression

Other teaching specific to the patient's and family's unique needs

Support groups available to patient's family, such as the hospice program's
   "Caregiver Support Group" meetings for family members and friends of
   the patient

9. **Specific tips for quality and reimbursement**

   Document any variances to expected outcomes. There are many models of hospice programs. Those that are home health agency–based must work within
   the framework of the Medicare home care program. For example, sometimes a
   hospice patient reaches a stable period in the illness and has no further skilled
   needs or the patient is no longer homebound per Medicare home health care
   criteria. When this occurs, one option is to discharge the patient from Medicare
   home health agency reimbursement and maintain the patient on grant funds or
   other available resources. If the patient's status deteriorates and again meets the
   Medicare criteria, a new start of care is initiated on the HCFA form 485. Usually hospices continue volunteer support, nursing, and other services indicated
   during these periods of no reimbursement.

   The Medicare hospice benefit does not require that the patient be homebound or have identified skilled needs. Though it is a needed and viable
   program, the Medicare hospice benefit may not be indicated for all Medicare
   eligible beneficiaries. For further information on this benefit, please refer to
   HCFA Hospice Manual 21.

   Should the patient's status deteriorate and increased personal care be
   needed, obtain a telephone order for the increased service, noting frequency
   and estimating the duration.

   Obtain a telephone order for all medication and treatment changes of the
   medical regimen, and document these in the clinical record.

   Unless the patient is in a hospice insurance program, some insurers will
   not pay for a skilled nurse visit that is made at death if the patient is dead
   when the nurse arrives at the home. From a Medicare home care perspective,
   the visit at the time of death may be covered when the orders and clinical
   record document assessment of the patient's status or signs of death/life or
   state law allows pronouncement of death by a nurse.

   Document patient deterioration

   Document dehydration, dehydrating

   Document patient change or instability

   Document pain, other symptoms not controlled

   Document status after acute episode of _____ (specify)

   Document positive urine, sputum, etc. culture; patient started on
      _____ (specify ordered antibiotic therapy)

   Document patient impacted; impaction removed manually

   Document RN in frequent communication with physician regarding
      _____ (specify)

   Document febrile at _____, pulse change at _____, irr.,
      irr.

Document change noted in _____

Document bony prominences red, opening

Document RN contacted physician regarding _____ (specify)

Document marked SOB

Document alteration in mental status

Document medications being adjusted, regulated, or monitored

Document unable to perform own ADLs, personal care

Document all interdisciplinary team meetings and communications in the POC and in the progress notes of the clinical record

All hospice team members involved should have input into the POC and document their interventions and goals

Document the wound, indicate stage, drainage, color, amount, and the specific care provided

Communicate any POC changes in your documentation

Document progress in wound healing or deterioration in wound status and measure in progress notes at least 1 time a week, noting other pertinent diagnoses that impede progress

Decrease visit frequency as appropriate

If wound culture is obtained, document the results

Document if patient or family member unable to do dressing (retinopathy, severity of wound, etc.)

Document any other learning barriers

Document the specific teaching accomplished and the behavioral outcomes of that teaching

Document patient's level of independence in care

Document the care coordination between disciplines and interdisciplinary care planning

Wound care is an area in which some managed-care companies and other payors are attempting to decrease the allowed numbers of visits. It is the professional nurse's responsibility to remember that it is not just the dressing change that occurs. When a nurse makes the home visit, an assessment of the wound healing or deterioration and teaching occur. These skills usually require the skills of a nurse. All these components contribute to safer, effective wound care

In addition, for home care, remember that daily insulin injections (and only in those cases where the patient is unable or unwilling) is the exception to daily. Please review the HHA Manual 11 or information from your manager obtained from the home health intermediary for further information

Remember that the clinical documentation is key to measuring compliance for quality and reimbursement purposes. Care coordination, timely verbal and initial physician orders, and assessment and addressing of spiritual and psychosocial needs should be ongoing and documented in the patient's clinical record

The documentation should support that all hospice care supports comfort and dignity while meeting patient/family needs

The documentation should include ongoing assessment and management of pain and other symptoms and the anticipation and prevention of secondary symptoms such as constipation

It is important to note that all team members, including nurses and social
workers, should assess, identify, and "hear" spiritual needs that the
patient/family want to be addressed. These spiritual issues are key to the
provision of quality hospice care and cannot be addressed effectively and
promptly by the spiritual counselor only

Document clearly symptoms, clinical changes, and assessment findings
related to pain and patient care

Document weight loss, increased shortness of breath, dyspnea, infection,
sepsis, new or changed medications, etc.

Document any skin changes (e.g., inflamed, painful, weeping skin site[s])

Remember that the "litmus test" of care coordination rests on the quality
of the clinical documentation by all team members. Review one of your
patient's clinical records and ask yourself the following: "If I was
unable to give a verbal report/update on this child/family's course
of care, would a peer be able to pick up and provide the same level of
care and know (from the documentation) the current orders,
medications, and other details that contribute to effective hospice
care?"

This patient population usually has many clinical changes that should be
documented. These include weight loss and multiple and changed medication regimens with varying routes. Side effects to the drug regimen should
be observed, noted, documented, and reported

Your assessments, observations, and clinical findings assist in painting a
picture to support coverage and documentation requirements for hospice
care

Document any hospitalizations and changed clinical findings.

Document patient changes, symptoms, and psychosocial issues impacting the
patient, family, and plan of care

Document changes to the plan of care such as medications, services, frequency, communication, and concurrence of other team members

Document coordination of services or consultation of the other members of
the IDT

Document communications and care coordination with other care providers,
such as skilled nursing facility or nursing home staff, inpatient team
members, and hired caregivers

10. **Resources for hospice care and practice**

The American Diabetes Association (ADA) has resources available for patients and their families. It can be reached at 1-800-342-2383. It offers literature, meal planning, videos, weight planning and management services, and
patient advocates. It also has a monthly magazine entitled *Forecast* for all
ADA members.

The Department of Health & Human Services National Diabetes Information Clearinghouse can be reached at 1-301-654-3327 for a listing of professional and patient education publications.

The Agency for Health Care Policy and Research offers *Preventing Pressure Ulcers: Patient Guide* (AHCPR Pub. No. 92-0048) and *Treating Pressure Sores: Consumer Guide* (AHCPR Pub. No. 95-0654) and can be reached
at 1-800-358-9295.

In Motion is the magazine of the Amputee Coalition of America. It can be reached at 1-423-524-8772.

Another helpful resource is the NHO's second edition of *Medical Guidelines for Determining Prognoses in Selected Non-Cancer Diseases.* Call NHO at 1-703-243-5900 for more information.

HEAD AND NECK CANCER CARE

1. **General considerations**

   Patients and their families often seek or are referred to hospice care after a long battle with cancer and surgeries and resulting tracheostomies and laryngectomies. This patient population may be on alternative feeding mechanisms and have feeding tubes or be on total parenteral nutrition (TPN). Hospice can positively impact the symptoms and side effects of the surgeries and disease processes for patients and families. Body image adjustments with depression, pain, dyspnea, bleeding, and food intolerance with nutritional depletion may be seen in this patient population. See also "Cancer Care," "Constipation Care," "Brain Tumor Care," and "Pain Care" should these sections pertain to your hospice patients and families.

2. **Needs for visit**

   Physician order for hospice care, specific to the hospice program's admission criteria and policies

   Standard precautions supplies

   Vital signs equipment for baseline assessment

   Other supplies or equipment, based on physician orders

3. **Safety considerations**

   Infection control/standard precautions

   Avoid respiratory irritants (e.g., powder), and keep site covered during activities (e.g., shaving) that may lead to inhalation

   Importance of shielding the stoma site

   Avoid swimming or any contact with water near stoma site

   A working phone

   Supportive and well-fitting nonslip shoes

   Night-light

   Tub rail, grab bars, shower seat for bathroom safety

   Fall precautions/protocol

   Protective skin measures and skin site care

   Medication safety (e.g., side effects, storage)

   Safety related to home medical equipment

   Emergency symptoms that necessitate immediate reporting/assistance and actions to take

   The phone number and name of person to call with a care problem

   Identification and report of any skin problems

   Smoke detector and fire evacuation plan

   Others, based on the patient's unique condition and environment

4. **Potential diagnoses and codes**

Airway obstruction, chronic	496
Attention to tracheostomy	V55.0
Brain cancer	191.9
Bronchitis, acute	466.0
Cancer of the esophagus	150.9

Cancer of the head or neck	195.0
Cancer of the larynx	161.9
Cancer of the pharynx	149.0
Cancer of the tongue	141.9
Cancer of the trachea	162.0
Candidiasis, esophageal	112.84
Candidiasis, oral	112.0
Dysphagia	787.2
Esophagus, cancer of the	150.9
Gastrostomy tube insertion (surgical)	43.11
Gastrostomy (other) (surgical)	43.19
Head and neck cancer	195.0
Laryngeal cancer	161.9
Laryngectomy (surgical)	30.4
Metastases, general	199.1
Nasogastric tube feeding (surgical)	96.6
Nasogastric tube insertion	96.07
Nasopharyngeal cancer	147.9
Oropharyngeal cancer	146.9
Pharynx, cancer of the	149.0
Pneumonia	486
Pneumonia, aspiration	50.70
Respirator, dependence on	V46.1
Respiratory failure	518.81
Respiratory insufficiency (acute)	518.82
Seizure disorder	780.3
Tongue, cancer of the	141.9
Trachea, cancer of the	162.0
Tracheitis, acute	464.10
Tracheostomy, attention to	V55.0
Tracheostomy closure (surgical)	31.72
Tracheostomy permanent (surgical)	31.29

5. **Associated nursing diagnoses**
   Activity intolerance
   Airway clearance, ineffective
   Anxiety
   Aspiration, potential for
   Body image disturbance
   Body temperature, altered, risk for
   Caregiver role strain
   Caregiver role strain, risk for
   Communication, impaired verbal
   Family processes, altered
   Fatigue
   Fear
   Fluid volume deficit, risk for
   Gas exchange, impaired
   Grieving, anticipatory
   Home maintenance management, impaired

Hyperthermia
Infection, risk for
Injury, risk for
Knowledge deficit (self-care management)
Management of therapeutic regimen (individual), ineffective
Mobility, impaired physical
Nutrition, altered: less than body requirements
Oral mucous membrane, altered
Pain
Pain, chronic
Self-care deficit, feeding
Sexuality patterns, altered
Skin integrity, impaired
Skin integrity, impaired, risk for
Sleep pattern disturbance
Social interaction, impaired
Spiritual distress (distress of the human spirit)
Spiritual well-being, potential for enhanced
Swallowing, impaired
Tissue integrity, impaired

6. **Skills and services identified**

- *Hospice nursing*

  a. *Comfort and symptom control*
     Skilled observation and complete system assessment of the patient with
        head and neck cancer/tracheostomy admitted to hospice
     Skilled observation and assessment of the patient with a laryngectomy
        resulting from _____ (specify)
     Presentation of hospice philosophy and services
     Explain patient rights and responsibilities
     Assess patient, family, and caregiver wishes and expectations regarding
        care
     Assess patient, family, and caregiver resources available for care
     Provision of volunteer support to patient and family
     Teach family or caregiver physical care of patient
     Assess pain and other symptoms, including site, duration, characteris-
        tics, and relief measures
     RN to provide and teach effective oral care and comfort measures
     Comfort measures of backrub and hand or other therapeutic massage
     Assess pulmonary status in patient with new tracheostomy
     Pain assessment and management
     Suction per physician orders
     Teach patient and caregiver infection control measures (e.g., cleaning
        cannula)
     Implement and teach respiratory therapy program
     Teach care of tracheostomy
     Provide care of tracheostomy
     Teach signs and symptoms of URI and infection at site
     Assess pulmonary status

Assessment of respiratory status, including the amount and character of secretions

Assess vital signs

Teach patient, family, and caregiver suction procedure(s) with return demonstration

Measure weight

RN to instruct in pain control measures and medication

RN to assess patient's pain or other symptoms q visit to identify need for change, addition, or other plan or dose adjustment

Provide and teach daily tracheostomy management, including tube changes and stoma site care

Teach patient, family, and caregiver regimen for inner cannula care

Assessment of breath sounds and rate and rhythm of respirations

Teach signs and symptoms of respiratory infections

Review back-up ventilator support system and compressor system back-up

Effective management of pain and prevention of secondary symptoms

Interventions of symptoms directed toward comfort and palliation

Observation and assessment, communication with physician related to signs and symptoms of oncological emergencies (e.g., spinal cord compression, superior vena cava syndrome, hypercalcemia) and measures and symptom treatment

Teach caregiver/patient use of pain assessment tool/scale and reporting mechanism(s)

Observation and assessment of patient with nausea and vomiting who is receiving palliative radiation and chemotherapy

Assessment and relief/comfort measures related to dry mouth due to radiation therapy (e.g., mouth wetting product or medications to stimulate salivary glands, if appropriate per physician)

Comfort measures of "fake saliva, spit" through frequent use of squirt bottle and mouth rinses and chewing of sugarless gum or candy

Avoidance of antihistamines and other drying products that exacerbate the mouth dryness, if possible

Teach caregiver or family care of weak, terminally ill patient

Teach patient/family about realistic expectations of disease process

Teach care of dying, signs/symptoms of impending death

Presence and support

Other interventions, based on patient/family needs

b. *Safety and mobility considerations*

Provide caregiver with home safety information and instruction related to _____ and documented in the clinical record

Teach patient, family, and caregiver oxygen utilization and safety concerns

Teach patient, family, and caregiver environmental safety concerns

Teach patient, family, or caregiver environmental safety concerns regarding airway aspiration

Teach family regarding safety of patient in home

Teach family regarding energy conservation techniques

Other interventions, based on patient/family needs

c. *Emotional/spiritual considerations*

Psychosocial assessment of patient and family regarding disease and prognosis

RN to provide emotional support to patient and family

Emotional support of patient/family during radiation and chemotherapy in regards to loss, grief, and isolation

Provide support to patient during chemotherapy/radiation for cancer treatment

Psychosocial aspects of pain control (e.g., depression) assessed and acknowledged with team support/intervention

Ongoing acknowledgment of spirituality and related concerns of patient/ family

Inform patient/family/caregiver of available volunteer support

Assessment and care/support related to depression, changed body image concerns, fever, mouth sores/ulcers, complaints of extreme tiredness, and dry/cracking skin in patient receiving palliative chemotherapy

Other interventions, based on patient/family needs

d. *Skin care*

RN to teach patient care of irradiated skin sites

Observation and evaluation of wound and surrounding skin

Evaluate patient's need for equipment, including supplies to decrease pressure, alternating pressure mattress, gel foam seat cushion, and heel and elbow protectors

Teach family to perform dressing between RN visits, specifically

_____

Teach patient, family, or caregiver about proper body alignment and positioning in bed to prevent skin tears from shearing skin

Observe and apply skilled assessment of areas for possible breakdown including heels, hips, elbows, ankles, and other pressure-prone areas

Teach caregiver about skin care needs, including the need for frequent position changes, appropriate pressure pads and mattresses, and the prevention of breakdown

Teach patient, family, and caregiver site care

Other interventions, based on patient/family needs

e. *Elimination considerations*

Assess bowel regimen, and implement program as needed

Observation and complete systems assessment of the patient with an indwelling catheter

RN to change catheter every 4 weeks and make 3 prn visits for catheter problems, including patient complaints, signs and symptoms of infection, and other factors necessitating evaluation and possible catheter change

RN to teach caregiver daily care of catheter

RN to evaluate the patient's bowel patterns and need for stool softeners, laxatives, dietary adjustments, and develop bowel management plan

Other interventions, based on patient/family needs

f. *Hydration/nutrition*

Instruct patient/caregiver about specific diet _____ (specify physician orders)

Assess nutrition/hydration statuses

Nutrition/hydration supported by offering patient's choice of favorite or desired foods or liquids

Nutrition/hydration maintained by offering patient high-protein diet and foods of choice as tolerated

Encourage optimal nutrition through high-calorie, high-protein snacks

Assessment and plan related to anorexia/cachexia, tube feedings, difficulty swallowing, and/or transitional feedings (e.g., TPN to oral)

Assessments and interventions/plan related to patient/family complaints of dry mouth, with painful chewing, difficulty speaking, and denture fit concerns after radiation and surgery

Teach patient and family to expect decreased nutritional and fluid intake as disease progresses

Other interventions, based on patient/family needs

g. *Therapeutic/medication regimens*

Teach and observe regarding side effects of palliative chemotherapy, including constipation, anemia, and fatigue

RN to assess the patient's unique response to treatments or interventions, and to report changes or unfavorable responses or reactions to the physician

Medication information and instruction regarding drug/drug and drug/food interactions

Nonpharmacological interventions such as progressive muscle relaxation, imagery, positive visualization, music, massage and touch, and humor therapy of patient's choice implemented

Medication teaching and management

Teach patient and caregiver use of PCA pump

Other interventions, based on patient/family needs

h. *Other considerations*

Assess progression of disease process

RN to assess the patient's response to treatments and interventions and to report to physician changes, unfavorable responses, or reactions

Other interventions, based on patient/family needs

• *Home health aide or certified nursing assistant*

Effective and safe personal care

Safe ADL assistance and support

Respite care and active listening skills

Observation and reporting

Meal preparation

Homemaker services

Comfort care

Other duties

• *Hospice social worker*

Psychosocial assessment of patient and family/caregiver, including adjustment to illness and its implications

Identification of optimal coping strategies

Financial assessment and counseling regarding food acquisition, ability to prepare, and costs of needed medications

Intervention/support related to terminal illness and loss

Emotional/spiritual support

Depression/fear assessed and addressed

Facilitate communication among patient, family, and hospice team

Referral/linkage to community services and resources as indicated

Grief counseling and intervention/support related to illness/loss

Patient/caregiver counseling and support

For patients who live alone with no support system (e.g., able, available, willing caregiver[s]): obtain resources to enable patient to remain in home setting

Identification of caregiver role strain necessitating respite/relief measures/support

Identification of illness-related psychiatric condition necessitating care

- *Volunteer(s)*

  Support, friendship, companionship, and presence

  Advocacy and respite

  Comfort and dignity maintained/provided for patient and family

  Errands and transportation

  Other services, based on interdisciplinary team recommendations and patient/caregiver needs

- *Spiritual counselor*

  Spiritual assessment and care

  Counseling, intervention, and support related to that dimension of life related to life's meaning (consistent with patient's beliefs)

  Support, listening, and presence

  Participation in sacred or spiritual rituals or practices

  Other supportive care, based on patient's/family's needs and belief systems

- *Dietitian/nutritional counseling*

  Assessment of patient with decreased intake, weight loss, anorexia, and increased shortness of breath (e.g., "don't feel like eating")

  Supportive counseling with patient/family indicating that patient will have a decreased appetite and usually at some point may not eat/drink

  Assessment and recommendations for safety and swallowing difficulties

  Teaching and support of family members and caregivers

  Support and care with food and nourishment as desired by patient

  Evaluation/management of nutritional deficits and needs

  Encourage nutritional supplements and snacks to increase protein and caloric intake

  Food and textural dietary recommendations incorporate patient choice and wishes

  Tube-feeding considerations/counseling related to swallowing, other problems

- *Occupational therapist*

  Evaluation of ADLs and functional mobility

  Assess for need for adaptive equipment and assistive devices

  Safety assessment of patient's environment and ADLs

  Assessment for energy conservation training

  Assessment of upper extremity function, retraining motor skills

- *Physical therapist*
  Evaluation
  Safety assessment of patient's environment
  Safe transfer training or bed mobility exercises
  Pain assessment/reduction factors
  Strengthening exercises/program
  Assessment of gait safety and home safety measures
  Instruct/supervise caregiver and volunteers on home exercise program for
      conditioning and strength
  Assistive, adaptive devices evaluation of equipment and teaching

- *Speech-language pathologist*
  Evaluation for speech/swallowing problems
  Food texture recommendations
  Alternate functional communication/alaryngeal speech

- *Bereavement counselor*
  Assessment of the needs of the bereaved family and friends
  Support and intervention, based on assessment and ongoing findings
  Presence and counseling
  Supportive visits and follow-up, other interventions (e.g., mailings,
      calls)
  Other services related to bereavement work and support

- *Pharmacist*
  Evaluation of hospice patient with constipation on cathartics, stool soften-
      ers, and other meds for possible food/drug, drug/drug interactions
  Medication monitoring regarding therapeutic levels and dosages
  Pain consult and input into interdisciplinary plan of care related to pain
      control, palliation, and symptom management
  Assessment of medication regimen and plan for safety and compliance
  Assessment for need for liquid medications

- *Music, massage, art, or other therapies or services*
  Evaluation and intervention based on patient's and caregiver's unique
      wishes and needs that support care, comfort, and death in the setting of
      the patient's choice
  Assessment plan to engage patient and support comfort, quality, enjoyment,
      and dignity
  Pet therapy (including patient's pet, if available) and therapeutic interven-
      tion

7. **Outcomes for care**

- *Hospice nursing*
  Planned and effective bowel program, as evidenced by regular bowel
      movements and patient/family report of comfort
  Death with dignity, and symptoms controlled in setting of patient/family
      choice
  Optimal comfort, support, and dignity provided throughout illness
  Death with maximum comfort through effective symptom control with spe-
      cialized hospice support

Patient/caregiver able to list adverse drug reactions/problems with medication regimen and whom to call for follow-up and resolution

Pain and symptoms managed/controlled in setting of patient/family choice (e.g., patient/family report ability to eat, sleep, speak clearer with pacing)

Patient's/family's privacy, independence, and choices supported with respect and maintained through death

Enhancement and support of quality of life

Effective symptom relief and control (e.g., a peaceful and comfortable death at home, some enjoyment of life)

Maximizing the patient's quality of life (e.g., alert and pain free or as patient wishes)

Pharmacological and nonpharmacological interventions, such as localized heat application, positioning, relaxation methods, and music

Patient cared for and family supported through death, with physical, psychosocial, spiritual, and other concerns/needs acknowledged/ addressed

Patient- and family-centered hospice care provided based on the patient's/ family's unique situation and needs

Infection control and palliation

Grief/bereavement expression and support provided

Patient is pain free by next _____ visit

Caregiver demonstrates ability to manage pain, where applicable

Patient maintains comfort and dignity throughout illness

Patient and caregiver verbalize satisfaction with care

Educational tools/plans incorporated in daily care, and patient and caregiver verbalize understanding of safe, needed care

Patient will decide on care, interventions, and evaluation

Caregiver effective in care management and knows whom to call for questions/concerns

Patient will express satisfaction with hospice support received and will experience increased comfort

Patient will be made comfortable at home through death in accordance with the patient's wishes

Effective pain control and symptom control verbalized by patient

Patient verbalizes understanding of and adheres to care and medication regimens

Patient and caregiver supported through patient's death

Comfort maintained through course of care

The patient and family receive hospice support and care, and family members and friends are able to spend quality time with the patient

Caregiver able and verbalizes comfort with role and lists when to call hospice team members

Patient supported through and receives the maximum benefit from palliative chemotherapy and radiation with minimal complications

Patient and caregiver list adverse reactions, potential complications, signs/ symptoms of infection (e.g., sputum change, chest congestion)

Comfort maintained through death with dignity

Pain effectively managed, and patient verbalizes comfort

Patient has stable respiratory status with patent airway

Comfort and individualized intervention of patient with immobility/ bedbound status (e.g., skin, urinary, musculature, vascular)

Spiritual and psychosocial needs met (specify) as defined by patient and caregiver throughout course of care

Patient is protected from injury, has stable respiratory status, and is compliant with medication, safety, and care regimens

Patient self-care related to daily trach care

Early detection and intervention regarding problems of patients with immobility/bedbound status (e.g., skin, urinary, musculature, vascular)

Patient states pain is _____ on 0-10 scale by next visit

Patient and caregiver demonstrate appropriate back-up or "rescue" therapies for breakthrough pain or other symptoms (e.g., dyspnea)

- *Home health aide or certified nursing assistant*
  Effective hygiene, personal care, and comfort
  ADL assistance
  Safe environment maintained

- *Hospice social worker*
  Problem identified and addressed, with patient/caregiver linked with appropriate support services and plan of care successfully implemented
  Patient and caregiver cope adaptively with illness and death
  Adaptive adjustment to changed body and body image
  Psychosocial support and counseling offered to patient/caregivers experiencing loss and grief
  Caregiver system assessed, and development of stable caregiver plan facilitated

- *Volunteer(s)*
  Comfort, companionship, and friendship extended to patient/family
  Support and respite provided as defined by the needs of the patient/ caregiver
  Patient and family supported by team with care, comfort, and companionship

- *Spiritual counseling*
  Support, listening, and presence
  Spiritual support offered and provided as defined by needs of patient/ caregiver
  Provision of spiritual support and care as based on the assessed and ongoing needs of the patient and family
  Spiritual support offered, and patient and family needs met
  Patient and family express relief of symptoms of spiritual suffering

- *Dietitian/nutritional counseling*
  Patient and family verbalize comprehension of changing nutritional needs
  Family and caregiver integrate recommendations into nutrition teaching (where appropriate)
  Patient and caregiver know whom to call for nutrition- and hydration-related questions/concerns
  Nutrition/hydration per patient's choices
  Caregiver integrates dietary recommendations into daily meal planning

- *Occupational therapist*
  Patient and caregiver demonstrate maximum independence with ADLs, adaptive techniques, and assistive devices
  Patient and caregiver demonstrate maximum safety in ADL and functional mobility
  Patient and caregiver demonstrate effective use of energy conservation
  Verbalization/demonstration of improved functional activity level and enhanced quality of life
  Patient and caregiver demonstrate effective use of diaphragmatic breathing to reduce shortness of breath and relaxation techniques to help in pain/symptom management
  Patient and caregiver demonstrate correct use of exercises

- *Physical therapist*
  Prevention of complications
  Home exercise and upper extremity program taught to caregiver
  Optimal strength, mobility, function maintained/achieved
  Compliance with home exercise program by _____ (date)

- *Speech-language pathologist*
  Communication method implemented, and patient able to be understood as self-reported or reported by family/caregivers
  Safe swallowing and functional communication
  Recommended lists of foods/textures for safety and patient choice

- *Bereavement counselor*
  Grief support services provided to patient and family
  Well-being and resolution process of grief initiated and followed through bereavement services

- *Pharmacist*
  Regimen for bowel regimen successful as self-reported by patient and in update at team meeting
  Multiple drug regimen reviewed for food/drug and drug/drug interactions in patient on multiple meds
  Stability and safety in complex medication regimen with maximum benefit to patient
  Effective pain and symptom control and symptom management as reported by patient/caregiver
  Lab reports reviewed for therapeutic dosages and effective patient response

- *Music, massage, art, or other therapies or services*
  Therapeutic massage/touch effective for patient as self-reported or observed by caregivers/family
  Improved muscle tone, relaxation, and/or sleep
  Patient comfortable and relaxed (e.g., sleeping) after massage
  Patient has pet's presence as desired—in all care sites, when possible
  Music therapy intervention based on assessment to decrease pain perception and provide emotional expression and support
  Maintenance of comfort and physical, psychosocial, and spiritual health
  Holistic health maintained and comfort achieved through _____ (specify modality)

8. **Patient, family, and caregiver educational needs**

   Educational needs are the regimens that the caregiver will be managing with or for the patient. These include the following:

   The basic tenets of hospice and the availability of support 24 hours a day, 7 days a week

   Home safety assessment and counseling

   The patient's medication regimen

   Safe and proper body mechanics to promote patient comfort and prevent caregiver safety problems

   Other teaching specific to the patient's and family's unique needs

   Support groups available to patient's family, such as the hospice program's "Caregiver Support Group" meetings for family members and friends of the patient

   Importance of adequate hydration, optimal nutrition, and rest for healing and recovery

   Effective hand-washing techniques, prevention of infections, and avoidance of respiratory irritants such as cigarette smoke

   All aspects of stoma site care, including self-observational skills, cleansing routines, need for humidity, hygiene measures, and safety care related to stoma

   Anticipated disease progression

   Other information based on the patient's unique medical history and other identified needs

9. **Specific tips for quality and reimbursement**

   Unless the patient is in a hospice insurance program, some insurers will not pay for a skilled nurse visit that is made at death if the patient is dead when the nurse arrives at the home. From a Medicare home care perspective, the visit at the time of death may be covered when the orders and clinical record document assessment of the patient's status or signs of death/life or state law allows pronouncement of death by a nurse.

   Document patient deterioration

   Document dehydration, dehydrating

   Document patient change or instability

   Document pain, other symptoms not controlled

   Document status after acute episode of _____ (specify)

   Document positive urine, sputum, etc. culture; patient started on _____ (specify ordered antibiotic therapy)

   Document patient impacted; impaction removed manually

   Document RN in frequent communication with physician regarding _____ (specify)

   Document febrile at _____, pulse change at _____, irr., irr.

   Document change noted in _____

   Document bony prominences red, opening

   Document RN contacted physician regarding _____ (specify)

   Document marked SOB

   Document alteration in mental status

   Document medications being adjusted, regulated, or monitored

   Document unable to perform own ADLs, personal care

Document all interdisciplinary team meetings and communications in the POC and in the progress notes of the clinical record

All hospice team members involved should have input into the POC and document their interventions and goals

Document changes to the plan of care, such as medications, services, frequency, communication, and concurrence of other team members

Document coordination of services or consultation of the other members of the IDT

Document communications and care coordination with other care providers, such as skilled nursing facility or nursing home staff, inpatient team members, hired caregivers, and others

Document any variances to expected outcomes. There are many models of hospice programs. Those that are home health agency–based must work within the framework of the Medicare home care program. For example, sometimes a hospice patient reaches a stable period in the illness and has no further skilled needs or the patient is no longer homebound per Medicare home health care criteria. When this occurs, one option is to discharge the patient from Medicare home health agency reimbursement and maintain the patient on grant funds or other available resources. If the patient's status deteriorates and again meets the Medicare criteria, a new start of care is initiated on the HCFA form 485. Usually hospices continue volunteer support, nursing, and other services indicated during these periods of no reimbursement.

The Medicare hospice benefit does not require that the patient be homebound or have identified skilled needs. Though it is a needed and viable program, the Medicare hospice benefit may not be indicated for all Medicare eligible beneficiaries. For further information on this benefit, please refer to HCFA Hospice Manual 21.

Should the patient's status deteriorate and increased personal care be needed, obtain a telephone order for the increased service, noting frequency and estimating the duration.

Obtain a telephone order for all medication and treatment changes of the medical regimen, and document these in the clinical record.

Document in the clinical notes the clear progression and symptomatology and interventions that demonstrate caring for a patient with terminal cancer

Document when/if the patient has respiratory changes, shortness of breath, exacerbation of conditions, dysphagia, pain, and other symptoms and that they are identified and resolved

Remember that the clinical documentation is key to measuring compliance for quality and reimbursement purposes. Care coordination, timely verbal and initial physician orders, and assessment and addressing of spiritual and psychosocial needs should be clearly documented in the patient's clinical record.

The documentation should support that all hospice care supports comfort and dignity while meeting patient/family needs

The documentation should include the ongoing assessment and management of pain and other symptoms and the anticipation and prevention of secondary symptoms such as constipation

It is important to note that all team members, including nurses and social workers, should assess, identify, and "hear" spiritual needs that the patient/family want to be addressed. These spiritual issues are key to the provision of quality hospice care and cannot be addressed effectively and promptly by the spiritual counselor only

Document clearly symptoms, clinical changes, and assessment findings that support the end stage of the cancer process

Document patient changes, symptoms, and clinical information identified from visits and team conferences that support hospice care and a limited life expectancy

Clearly support in the documentation the rationale that supports/explains the progression of the illness from the chronic to terminal stages

Document mentation, behavioral, and/or cognitive changes

Document dysphagia, weight loss, increased shortness of breath, dyspnea, infection, sepsis, new or changed medications, etc.

Document any skin changes (e.g., inflamed, painful, weeping skin site[s])

Document when the patient is actively dying, deteriorating, or progressing toward death

Remember that the "litmus test" of care coordination rests within the quality of the clinical documentation by all team members. Review one of your patient's clinical records and ask yourself the following: "If I was unable to give a verbal report/update on this patient, would a peer be able to pick up and provide the same level of care and know (from the documentation) the current orders, medications, and other details that contribute to effective hospice care?"

10. **Resources for hospice care and practice**

Reference Guide for Clinicians: Management of Cancer Pain: Adults and *Consumer's Guide: Management of Cancer Pain* can be ordered by calling 1-800-358-9295. The patient guides are available in English and Spanish.

Get Relief From Cancer Pain is a pamphlet available from the National Cancer Institute's Cancer Information Service. Call 1-800-4-CANCER (1-800-422-6237).

Questions and Answers About Pain Control is a 76-page booklet available free from the National Cancer Institute's Cancer Information Service. Call 1-800-4-CANCER (1-800-422-6237).

The American Cancer Society has a resource entitled *Speech after Laryngectomy* that addresses the kinds of speech and artificial devices for patients. This resource can be obtained by calling 1-800-ACS-2345.

There is an oral cancer website at http://www.oralcancer.org and Oncolink at http://www.oncolink.upenn.edu. Oncolink is a service provided by the University of Pennsylvania Cancer Center that includes general information about cancer, head and neck cancers, and radiation oncology.

Support for People with Oral and Head and Neck Cancer (SPOHNC) (pronounced "spunk") is dedicated to meeting the needs of oral and head and neck cancer patients. They offer a "News from SPOHNC" newsletter and offer support and encouragement. They call be reached at (516) 759-5333 or at http://www.spohnc.org.

INFUSION CARE

1. **General considerations**

   The reasons for infusion therapy vary depending on the hospice's policies and the unique problems of the patient and family and may include medications for pain control and improvement of cardiac symptoms, transfusions to maintain function and quality of life, and parenteral hydration and palliative chemotherapy in some cases.

   Please refer to "AIDS Care," "Breast Cancer and Mastectomy Care," Cardiac Care (End Stage) and "Pain Care", should these sections also pertain to your patients and families.

2. **Needs for visit**

   Physician order for hospice care, specific to the hospice program's admission criteria and policies

   Standard precautions supplies

   Vital signs equipment for baseline assessment

   Specific initial and ongoing physician orders, including solution ordered, rate, site change, frequency

   Solution

   Tubing

   Catheter(s)

   Pump

   Tape

   Tourniquet

   2 × 2s

   Alcohol swabs

   Anaphylaxis kit

   Other equipment as directed per organizational protocol(s)

3. **Safety considerations**

   Infection control/standard precautions

   Night-light

   Chemical spill kit at the home

   Clean area for storage of infusion supplies

   Access to running water and electricity

   Multiple medications (e.g., side effects, safe storage)

   Safety for home medical equipment (pump)

   Emergency symptoms and actions to take

   The phone number and name of person to call with a care problem

   Smoke detector and fire evacuation plan

   Others, based on the patient's unique condition and environment

   Medical equipment safety and storage (e.g., infusion pump)

   A working phone, running water, and refrigerator

   Infusion protocol precautions

   Reactions or other symptoms that necessitate immediate reporting/assistance

4. Potential diagnoses and codes

AIDS (general)	042
Amputation	997.62
Appendix abscess	540.1
Bacteremia	790.7
Bone, aseptic necrosis	733.40
Bone marrow transplant	41.00
Bone metastases	198.5
Breast cancer	174.9
Cancer of the head/neck	195
Cardiomyopathy	425.4
Cellulitis, right or left lower leg	682.6
Cervix, cancer of	180.9
COPD	496
Colon cancer	153.9
Congestive heart failure	428.0
CVA	436
Cytomegalovirus (colitis)	078.5 and 558.9
Cytomegalovirus (esophagitis)	078.5 and 530.10
Cytomegalovirus (kidney)	078.5 and 593.9
Cytomegalovirus (retinitis)	078.5 and 363.20
Dehydration	276.5
Diabetes mellitus, with complications, adult	250.90
Diabetes mellitus, with complications, juv.	250.91
Dysphagia	787.2
Endocarditis	424.00
Esophagus, cancer of	150.9
Fluid and electrolyte imbalance	276.9
Foot abscess	682.7
Fracture, pathological	733.10
Gastric cancer, metastatic	197.8
Head or neck, cancer of the	195.0
Heart disease, end stage	429.9
Heart transplant (surgical)	37.5
Hickman catheter insertion	38.93
Hyperemesis gravidarum	643.03
Hypertension	401.9
Hypovolemia	276.5
Liver, end stage disease	571.8
Lung transplant (surgical)	33.50
Lyme disease	088.81
Metastases, general	199.1
Osteomyelitis	730.20
Osteomyelitis, ankle	730.27
Osteomyelitis, foot	730.27
Osteomyelitis, leg	730.26
Osteomyelitis (foot, ankle)	730.27
Osteomyelitis (lower leg, knee)	730.26
Osteomyelitis (pelvic region and thighs)	730.25

Osteomyelitis (site unspecified) acute	730.20
Ovarian cancer	183.0
Pancreatic cancer	157.9
Pelvic inflammatory disease (acute)	614.9
Pericarditis, acute	420.90
Pneumonia	486
Pneumonia, aspiration	507.0
Retinitis	363.20
Seizure disorder	780.3
Sinusitis	473.9
Spinal cord tumor	239.7
Staph infection	041.10
Syphilis	097.9
Urinary tract infection	453.9
Venous thrombosis	453.8
Viral meningitis	047.9
Wound infection	998.59

5. **Associated nursing diagnoses**
   Aspiration, risk for
   Body image disturbance
   Body temperature, altered, risk for
   Bowel incontinence
   Breathing pattern, ineffective
   Cardiac output, decreased
   Caregiver role strain
   Caregiver role strain, risk for
   Communication, impaired verbal
   Constipation
   Coping, ineffective family: compromised
   Coping, ineffective family: disabling
   Coping, ineffective individual
   Diarrhea
   Disuse syndrome, risk for
   Family processes, altered
   Fatigue
   Fear
   Fluid volume deficit, risk for
   Fluid volume excess
   Gas exchange, impaired
   Grieving, anticipatory
   Growth and development, altered
   Home maintenance management, impaired
   Hyperthermia
   Hypothermia
   Incontinence, total
   Infection, risk for
   Injury, risk for
   Knowledge deficit (specify)
   Mobility, impaired physical

Noncompliance (specify)
Nutrition, altered: less than body requirements
Oral mucous membrane, altered
Pain
Pain, chronic
Parenting, altered
Protection, altered
Role performance, altered
Self-care deficit, bathing/hygiene
Self-care deficit, dressing/grooming
Self-care deficit, feeding
Self-care deficit, toileting
Sensory/perceptual alterations (specify) (visual, auditory, kinesthetic, gustatory, tactile, olfactory)
Sexual dysfunction
Sexuality patterns, altered
Skin integrity, impaired
Skin integrity, impaired, risk for
Sleep pattern disturbance
Social interaction, impaired
Spiritual distress (distress of the human spirit)
Spiritual well-being, potential for enhanced
Swallowing, impaired
Thought processes, altered
Tissue integrity, impaired
Tissue perfusion, altered (specify type) (renal, cerebral, cardiopulmonary, gastrointestinal, peripheral)
Trauma, potential for
Urinary elimination, altered
Urinary retention

6. **Skills and services identified**

- *Hospice nursing*

   a. *Comfort and symptom control*
      Observation and complete systems assessment of the patient needing infusion therapy for _____ (specify)
      Presentation of hospice philosophy and services
      Explain patient rights and responsibilities
      Assess patient, family, and caregiver wishes and expectations regarding care
      Assess patient, family, and caregiver resources available for care
      Provision of volunteer support to patient and family
      Teach family or caregiver physical care of patient
      RN to provide and teach effective oral care and comfort measures
      Assess pain and other symptoms, including site, duration, characteristics, and relief measures
      Provide site care and implement therapy program
      Assess needle, supplies, and site for contamination
      Teach patient, family, and caregiver effective hand-washing techniques

Teach signs and symptoms of impeded or rapid flow of medication solution

Comfort measures of backrub and hand or other therapeutic massage

RN to change tubing and filter q_____ per hospice protocol

Teach family or caregiver to document date and time for all infusions started and completed

Teach patient, family, and caregiver about position of site with IV

Teach patient, family, and caregiver signs and symptoms of infection, phlebitis

Teach patient, family, and caregiver when to contact on-call RN or physician

Teach patient and family signs and symptoms of phlebitis, occlusion, displacement, infection, and other possible problems

RN to monitor patient for evidence of infection, metabolic problems, or other complications in patient on TPN

Teach self-observational and record-keeping skills to patient and caregiver for documenting response to _____ therapy

Pain assessment and ongoing management

PICC line flushed per organizational policy

Teaching and training related to the operation and troubleshooting of access device and pump (e.g., alarms, 800 numbers, whom to call)

Patient and caregiver provided with information and instruction about care and maintenance of the line, insertion site, and dressing changes

Teaching provided regarding the meticulous care that must be provided to prevent contamination and possible infection

Dressing change q heparin lock change, flush at end of therapy with _____ (specify); cap change q heparin lock change per organizational policy

Change battery q_____ (per protocol)

Perform sterile dressing change and site care q_____ (specify)

RN to restart peripheral IV q_____ (specify orders)

Assess pain, and evaluate the pain management's effectiveness

Teach care of bedridden patient

Measure vital signs, including pain, q visit

Assess cardiovascular, pulmonary, and respiratory status

Teach new pain- or symptom-control medication regimen

Teach caregivers symptom control and relief measures

Oxygen on at _____ liter per _____ (specify physician orders)

Identify and monitor pain, symptoms, and relief measures

RN to assess patient's pain or other symptoms q visit to identify need for change, addition, or other plan or dose adjustment

Observation and assessment, communication with physicians related to signs and symptoms of continuing decompensation and increased symptoms, pain, discomfort, shortness of breath, and measures to alleviate and control

Effective management of pain and prevention of secondary symptoms

Interventions of symptoms directed toward comfort and palliation

Teach caregiver/patient use of pain assessment tool/scale and reporting mechanism(s)

Teach patient and family about realistic expectations of disease process

Teach care of dying, and signs/symptoms of impending death

Presence and support

Other interventions, based on patient/family needs

b. *Safety and mobility considerations*

Provide caregiver with home safety information and instruction related to _____ and documented in the clinical record

Teach signs and symptoms of infiltration and home safety

RN to teach patient and caregiver in correct operation and care related to safe use of PCA pump for pain management

Teach family about safety of patient in home

Teach family about energy conservation techniques

Other interventions, based on patient/family needs

c. *Emotional/spiritual considerations*

Psychosocial assessment of patient and family regarding disease and prognosis

RN to provide emotional support to patient and family

Assess mental status and sleep disturbance changes

Assessment and care/support related to depression, changed body image concerns, fever, mouth sores/ulcers, complaints of extreme tiredness and dry/cracking skin in patient receiving palliative chemotherapy

Psychosocial aspects of pain control (e.g., depression) assessed and acknowledged with team support/intervention

Ongoing acknowledgment of spirituality and related concerns of patient/family

Other interventions, based on patient/family needs

d. *Skin care*

Pressure ulcer care as indicated

Assess skin integrity

RN to teach patient about care of irradiated skin sites

Provide site care per protocols

Observation and evaluation of wound and surrounding skin

Evaluate patient's need for equipment, including supplies to decrease pressure, alternating pressure mattress, gel foam seat cushion, and heel and elbow protectors

Teach family to perform dressing between RN visits, specifically

_____

Teach patient, family, or caregiver about proper body alignment and positioning in bed to prevent skin tears from shearing skin

Observe and apply skilled assessment of areas for possible breakdown, including heels, hips, elbows, ankles, and other pressure-prone areas

Teach caregiver about skin care needs, including the need for frequent position changes, appropriate pressure pads and mattresses, and the prevention of breakdown

Other interventions, based on patient/family needs

e. *Elimination considerations*

Assess bowel regimen, and implement program as needed

Assess urinary elimination changes related to hydration, change, status

Observation and assessment of patient with a peripherally inserted
central catheter (PICC) for long-term therapy

Check for and remove impaction as needed

Condom catheter or indwelling catheter as indicated

Assess amount and frequency of urinary output

RN to teach caregiver daily care of catheter

RN to evaluate the patient's bowel patterns and need for stool softeners,
laxatives, and dietary adjustments and to develop bowel management
plan

Implement bowel assessment and management program

Teach patient/family and aide the importance of observing and noting
bowel movements between scheduled nursing visits

Obtain patient history related to norms for bowel movements to date
(e.g., "all my life I go only every other day")

Consider stool softeners, and offer laxative of choice, Fleet's Enemas
prn, and other methods per patient wishes and physician orders

Other interventions, based on patient/family needs

f. *Hydration/nutrition*

Assess nutrition/hydration status

Diet counseling for patient with anorexia

Teach family or caregiver about feeding tubes or pumps

Nutrition/hydration supported by offering patient's choice of favorite or
desired foods or liquids

Nutrition/hydration maintained by offering patient high-protein diet and
foods of choice as tolerated

Assessment and plan related to anorexia/cachexia, tube feedings,
difficult/painful swallowing, and/or transitional feedings (e.g., TPN
to oral)

Assessment and interventions/plan related to patient/family complaints
of dry mouth, with painful chewing, difficulty speaking, and denture
fit concerns after radiation and surgery

Teach patient and family to expect decreased nutritional and fluid intake
as disease progresses

Other interventions, based on patient/family needs

g. *Therapeutic/medication regimens*

RN to assess the patient's response to therapeutic treatments and interventions and to report any changes or unfavorable responses to the
physician

Teach and observe regarding side effects of palliative chemotherapy,
including constipation, anemia, and fatigue

Venipuncture q_____ (specify ordered frequency) for monitoring platelet and other counts

Teach flush of heparin with NS solution techniques to ensure patency of
heparin lock and use of line for ordered medications

RN to instruct patient and caregiver regarding multiple medications, including schedule, route, functions, and possible side effects

RN to obtain blood for _____ (specify test and frequency)
from central venous catheter per protocol

Medication assessment and management

Teach new pain and symptom control medication regimen

Morphine pump (specify pump, doses, etc.) for increased comfort

Obtain venipuncture as ordered q_____ (ordered frequency)

Teach about new medications and effects

Assess for electrolyte imbalance

Teach patient and caregiver use of PCA pump

RN to instruct in pain control measures and medications

Nonpharmacological interventions, such as progressive muscle relaxation, imagery, positive visualization, music, massage and touch, and humor therapy of patient's choice implemented

Other interventions, based on patient/family needs

h. *Other considerations*

Assess progression of disease process

RN to assess the patient's response to treatments and interventions and to report to the physician changes, unfavorable responses, or reactions

Other interventions, based on patient/family needs

- *Home health aide or certified nursing assistant*

Effective and safe personal care

Safe ADL assistance and support

Respite care and active listening skills

Observation and reporting

Meal preparation

Homemaker services

Comfort care

Other duties

- *Hospice social worker*

Psychosocial assessment of patient and family/caregiver, including adjustment to long-term illness and its implications

Identification of optimal coping strategies

Identification of caregiver role strain necessitating respite/relief/support measures

Financial assessment and counseling regarding food acquisition, ability to prepare, and costs of needed medications

Intervention/support related to terminal illness and loss

Emotional/spiritual support

Depression/fear assessed and addressed

Facilitate communication among patient, family, and hospice team

Referral/linkage to community services and resources as indicated

Grief counseling and intervention/support related to illness/loss

Patient/caregiver counseling and support

For patients who live alone with no support system (e.g., able, available, willing caregiver[s]): obtain resources to enable patient to remain in home

Identification of illness-related psychiatric condition necessitating care

- *Volunteer(s)*

Support, friendship, companionship, and presence

Comfort and dignity maintained/provided for patient and family

Advocacy and respite

Errands and transportation

Other services, based on interdisciplinary team recommendations and
  patient/caregiver needs

- *Spiritual counselor*

  Spiritual assessment and care

  Counseling, intervention, and support related to that dimension of life
    related to life's meaning (consistent with patient's beliefs)

  Support, listening, and presence

  Participation in sacred or spiritual rituals or practices

  Other supportive care, based on patient's/family's needs and belief systems

- *Dietitian/nutritional counseling*

  Assessment of patient with decreased intake, weight loss, anorexia, and
    increased shortness of breath (e.g., "don't feel like eating")

  Supportive counseling with patient/family indicating that patient will have
    a decreased appetite and usually at some point may not eat/drink

  Assessment and recommendations for swallowing difficulties

  Teaching and support of family members and caregivers

  Support and care with food and nourishment as desired by patient

  Evaluation/management of nutritional deficits and needs

  Encourage nutritional supplements and snacks to increase protein and
    caloric intake

  Food and dietary recommendations incorporate patient choice and wishes

  Assist care team related to fluid needs and prevention of overhydration,
    overfeeding, and other problems

  Counseling related to infusion therapy

- *Occupational therapist*

  Evaluation of ADL and functional mobility

  Assessment of need for adaptive equipment and assistive devices

  Safety assessment of patient's environment and ADLs

  Assessment for energy conservation training

  Assessment of upper extremity function, retraining motor skills

- *Physical therapist*

  Evaluation

  Safety assessment of patient's environment

  Safe transfer training or bed mobility exercises

  Pain assessment/reduction factors

  Strengthening exercises/program

  Assessment of gait safety and home safety measures

  Instruct/supervise caregiver and volunteers on home exercise program for
    safety conditioning and strength

  Assistive, adaptive devices and evaluation of equipment and teaching

- *Speech-language pathologist*

  Evaluation for speech/swallowing problems

  Food texture recommendations

  Alternate functional communication

- *Bereavement counselor*

  Assessment of the needs of the bereaved family and friends

  Support and intervention, based on assessment and ongoing findings

Presence and counseling

Supportive visits, follow-up, and other interventions (e.g., mailings, calls)

Other services related to bereavement work and support

- *Pharmacist*

  Evaluation of hospice patient with constipation on cathartics, stool softeners, and other medications for possible food/drug, drug/drug interactions

  Medication monitoring regarding therapeutic levels and dosages

  Pain consult and input into interdisciplinary plan of care related to pain
  control, palliation, and symptom management

  Assessment of medication regimen and plan for safety and compliance

- **Music, massage, art, or other therapies or services**

  Evaluation and intervention based on patient's and caregiver's unique
  wishes and needs that support care, comfort, and death in the setting of
  the patient's choice

  Assessment plan to engage patient and support comfort, quality, enjoyment,
  and dignity

  Pet therapy (including patient's pet, if available) and therapeutic intervention

7. **Outcomes for care**

- *Hospice nursing*

  Patient cared for and family supported through death, with physical, psychosocial, spiritual, and other needs acknowledged/addressed

  Mental distress, depression, and fear of dying addressed throughout care by
  hospice team

  Patient and family able to care for and support patient

  Patient and caregiver can verbalize symptoms, changes, or accelerations
  that necessitate call to physician

  Patient and family demonstrate compliance with medication regimen and
  other therapeutic interventions

  Patient demonstrates stabilization and increased or enhanced coping skills
  related to functioning and depression

  Pain and symptoms managed/controlled in setting of patient/family choice
  (e.g., patient/family report ability to eat, sleep, speak with pacing)

  Planned and effective bowel program, as evidenced by regular bowel
  movements and patient/family report of comfort

  Death with dignity, and pain/symptoms controlled in setting of patient/
  family choice

  Optimal comfort, support, and dignity provided throughout illness

  Death with maximum comfort through effective symptom control with specialized hospice support

  Patient and caregiver able to list adverse drug reactions/problems with
  medication regimen and whom to call for follow-up and resolution

  Patient's/family's privacy, independence, and choices supported with
  respect and maintained through death

  Enhancement and support of quality of life

  Effective symptom relief and control (e.g., a peaceful and comfortable
  death at home, depression controlled, some enjoyment of life)

Maximizing the patient's quality of life (e.g., alert and pain free or as patient wishes)

Pharmacological and nonpharmacological interventions, such as localized heat application, biofeedback, massage, positioning, relaxation methods, and music

Patient- and family-centered hospice care provided based on the patient's/family's unique situation and needs

Patient verbalizes understanding of and adheres to medication regimens

Patient receives the maximum benefit from infusion therapy, with no evidence of complications (specify)

Patient and caregiver list adverse reactions, potential complications, signs/symptoms of infection

Infusion therapy catheter will remain patent and infection free through course of therapy

Patient and caregiver demonstrate understanding of care and associated regimens

Pain effectively managed (or other goal of infusion therapy, e.g., hydration achieved, infection controlled) as patient's pain is controlled and patient verbalizes comfort

Other goals/outcomes based on the patient's unique needs and problems

Effective and safe personal care

Activities of daily living completion

Patient and caregiver will cope adaptively with stress and illness

Caregiver or patient demonstrates safe and supportive care and coping skills related to the successful implementation of the POC

Linkage to community resources accomplished by _____ (specify date)

Patient and caregiver will verbalize/demonstrate activities related to plan for accessing community resources and ongoing support by _____ (specify date)

Nutrition optimal for patient on infusion therapy for _____

Patient reports understanding and compliance as evidenced in food diary reviewed with dietitian

Patient and caregiver know whom to call for nutrition-related questions/concerns

Medication regimen evaluated for drug/drug and drug/food interactions and problems

Lab reports reviewed for therapeutic dosages and safe, effective patient response

Stability and safety in complex multiple medication regimens

Patient is protected from injury, has stable respiratory status, and is compliant with medication, safety, and care regimens

Comfort and individualized intervention of patient with immobility/bedbound status (e.g., skin, urinary, musculature, vascular)

Spiritual and psychosocial needs met (specify) as defined by patient and caregiver throughout course of care

Patient states pain is _____ on 0-10 scale by next visit

Patient/caregiver demonstrates appropriate back-up or "rescue" therapies for breakthrough pain or other symptoms (e.g., dyspnea)

Patient and caregiver verbalize satisfaction with care

Educational tools/plans incorporated in daily care, and patient and caregiver verbalize understanding of safe, needed care

Patient will decide on care, interventions, and evaluation

Caregiver effective in care management and knows whom to call for questions/concerns

Patient will express satisfaction with hospice support received and will experience increased comfort

Patient will be made comfortable at home through death in accordance with the patient's wishes

Effective pain control and symptom control verbalized by patient

Patient verbalizes understanding of and adheres to care and medication regimens

Patient and caregiver supported through patient's death

Comfort maintained through course of care

Patient and family receive hospice support and care, and family members and friends are able to spend quality time with the patient

Caregiver able and verbalizes comfort with role and understands when to call hospice team members

Patient supported through and receives the maximum benefit from palliative chemotherapy and radiation with minimal complications

Patient and caregiver list adverse reactions, potential complications, signs/ symptoms of infection (e.g., sputum change, chest congestion)

Comfort maintained through death with dignity

Pain effectively managed and patient verbalizes comfort

Patient and family demonstrate compliance with self-observational and other care regimen skills taught

Patient's wound site shows evidence of healing as demonstrated by _____ (specify factors that identify improvement for this patient)

Patient and family verbalize troubleshooting for IV line care and when to call for assistance

IV line is patent, skin site is without problems (e.g., pain, infection), and patient receives course of IV therapy without problems

Infection control and palliation

Grief/bereavement expression and support provided

Patient is pain free by next _____ visit

Caregiver demonstrates ability to manage pain, where applicable

Patient maintains comfort and dignity throughout illness

- *Home health aide or certified nursing assistant*
Effective hygiene, personal care, and comfort
ADL assistance
Safe environment maintained

- *Hospice social worker*
Problem identified and addressed, with patient and caregiver linked with appropriate support services and plan of care successfully implemented
Patient and caregiver cope adaptively with illness and death
Psychosocial support and counseling offered to patient/caregivers experiencing loss and grief

Resources identified, community linkage as appropriate for patient/family
Identification of effective coping strategies
Caregiver system assessed, and development of stable caregiver plans facilitated

- *Volunteer(s)*
  Comfort, companionship, and friendship extended to patient/family
  Support provided as defined by the needs of the patient/caregiver
  Patient and family supported by team with care, comfort, and companionship

- *Spiritual counseling*
  Spiritual support offered and provided as defined by needs of patient/caregiver
  Provision of spiritual support and care based on the assessed and ongoing needs of the patient and family
  Support, listening, and presence
  Participation in sacred or spiritual rituals or practices
  Intervention and support related to that dimension of life related to life's meaning (consistent with patient's beliefs)
  Spiritual support offered, and patient and family needs met

- *Dietitian/nutritional counseling*
  Family and caregiver integrate recommendations into nutrition teaching (where appropriate)
  Patient and caregiver know whom to call for nutrition- and hydration-related questions/concerns
  Nutrition/hydration per patient's choices
  Caregiver integrates recommendations into daily meal planning
  Patient and family verbalize comprehension of changing nutritional needs
  Patient and caregiver know whom to call for nutrition- and hydration-related questions and concerns

- *Occupational therapist*
  Patient and caregiver demonstrate maximum independence with ADL, adaptive techniques, and assistive devices
  Patient and caregiver demonstrate maximum safety in ADL and functional mobility
  Patient and caregiver demonstrate effective use of energy conservation techniques
  Verbalization/demonstration of improved functional activity level and enhanced quality of life
  Patient and caregiver demonstrate effective use of diaphragmatic breathing to reduce shortness of breath and relaxation techniques to help in pain/symptom management
  Patient and caregiver demonstrate correct use of exercise and splints for maximum upper extremity function and joint position

- *Physical therapist*
  Prevention of complications
  Home exercise and upper extremity program taught to caregiver

Optimal strength, mobility, and function maintained/achieved

Compliance with home exercise program by _____ (specify
  date)

Safety in mobility and transfers

- *Speech-language pathologist*

  Communication method implemented, and patient able to be understood as
    self-reported or reported by family/caregivers

  Safe swallowing and functional communication

  Recommended lists of foods/textures for safety and patient choice

- *Bereavement counselor*

  Support services related to grief provided to patient and family

  Well-being and resolution process of grief initiated and followed through
    bereavement services

- *Pharmacist*

  Regimen for bowel regimen successful as self-reported by patient and in
    update at team meeting

  Multiple drug regimen reviewed for food/drug and drug/drug interactions in
    patient on multiple medications

  Stability and safety in complex medication regimen, with maximum benefit
    to patient

  Infusion medication(s) and blood level lab report reviewed for therapeutic
    dosage and safe, effective patient response and results reported to phy-
    sician

  Effective pain and symptom control and symptom management as reported
    by patient/caregiver

- *Music, massage, art, or other therapies or services*

  Therapeutic massage/touch effective for patient as self-reported or observed
    by caregivers/family

  Improved muscle tone, relaxation, and/or sleep

  Patient comfortable and relaxed (e.g., sleeping) after massage

  Music therapy intervention based on assessment to decrease pain percep-
    tion and provide emotional expression and support

  Maintenance of comfort and physical, psychosocial, and spiritual health

  Patient has pet's presence as desired—in all care sites, when possible

  Holistic health maintained and comfort achieved through _____
    (specify modality)

8. **Patient, family, and caregiver educational needs**

   Educational needs are the care regimens that contribute to safe and effective
   care at home between the hospice team's visits.

   These include the following:

   The basic tenets of hospice and the availability of support 24 hours a day, 7
     days a week

   Home safety assessment and counseling

   Anticipated disease progression

   Patient's medication regimen

Safe and proper body mechanics to promote patient comfort and prevent
  caregiver safety problems

Teach safe needle disposal, and provide container

Support groups available to patient's family, such as the hospice program's
  "Caregiver Support Group" meetings for family members and friends of
  the patient

Signs and symptoms that necessitate calling the physician

Teach patient and caregiver all aspects of care related to wound, including
  effective hand washing, disposal of soiled dressings, and other infection-
  control measures

The importance of nutrition in the healing process

Teach patient about all medications, including schedule, route, functions, and
  possible side effects

The patient's medications and their relationship to each other

Simple IV troubleshooting techniques and problem resolution

Care of the Groshong (or other catheter) and all aspects of care related to the
  safe delivery of the therapy, including teaching catheter function, potential
  problems, self-observational skills, safety, and site care

The importance of compliance to the regimen

The importance of medical follow-up

Effective hand-washing techniques and other infection-control measures

Safe disposal of needles and other sharps in the home

The symptoms that would necessitate calling emergency services

Other teaching specific to the patient and caregiver's needs based on the patient's unique medical condition

9. **Specific tips for quality and reimbursement**

   Document any variances to expected outcomes. Many models of hospice
   programs exist. Those that are home health agency–based must work within
   the framework of the Medicare home care program. For example, sometimes a hospice patient reaches a stable period in the illness and has no
   further skilled needs or the patient is no longer homebound per Medicare
   home health care criteria. When this occurs, one option is to discharge the
   patient from Medicare home health agency reimbursement and maintain the
   patient on grant funds or other available resources. If the patient's status deteriorates and again meets the Medicare criteria, a new start of care is initiated on the HCFA form 485. Usually hospices continue volunteer support,
   nursing, and other services indicated during these periods of no reimbursement.

   The Medicare hospice benefit does not require that the patient be homebound or have identified skilled needs. Though it is a needed and viable
   program, the Medicare hospice benefit may not be indicated for all Medicare
   eligible beneficiaries. For further information on this benefit, please refer to
   HCFA Hospice Manual 21.

   Should the patient's status deteriorate and increased personal care be
   needed, obtain a telephone order for the increased service, noting frequency
   and estimating the duration.

Obtain a telephone order for all medication and treatment changes of the medical regimen and document these in the clinical record.

Unless the patient is in a hospice insurance program, some insurers will not pay for a skilled nurse visit made at death if the patient is dead when the nurse arrives at the home. From a Medicare home care perspective, the visit at the time of death may be covered when the orders and clinical record document assessment of the patient's status or signs of death/life or state law allows pronouncement of death by a nurse.

Document patient deterioration

Document dehydration, dehydrating

Document patient change or instability

Document pain, other symptoms not controlled

Document status after acute episode of _____ (specify)

Document positive urine, sputum, etc. culture; patient started on _____ (specify ordered antibiotic therapy)

Document patient impacted; impaction removed manually per physician's orders

Document RN in frequent communication with physician regarding _____ (specify)

Document febrile at _____, pulse change at _____, irr., irr.

Document change noted in _____

Document bony prominences red, opening

Document RN contacted physician regarding _____ (specify)

Document marked SOB

Document alteration in mental status

Document medications being adjusted, regulated, or monitored

Document unable to perform own ADL, personal care

Document all interdisciplinary team meetings and communications in the POC and in the progress notes of the clinical record

All hospice team members should have input into the POC and document their interventions and goals

Document in the clinical notes the clear progression and symptomatology and interventions that demonstrate the interventions and overall management of the patient with pain

Document when/if the patient has respiratory changes, shortness of breath, exacerbation of conditions, dysphagia, changes in pain, and other symptoms and that they are identified and resolved

Remember that the clinical documentation is key to measuring compliance for quality and reimbursement purposes. Care coordination, timely verbal and initial physician orders, and assessment and addressing of spiritual and psychosocial needs should be ongoing and documented in the patient's clinical record

The documentation should support that all hospice care supports comfort and dignity while meeting patient/family needs

The documentation should include ongoing assessment and management of pain and other symptoms and the anticipation and prevention of secondary symptoms such as constipation

It is important to note that all team members, including nurses and social workers, should assess, identify, and "hear" spiritual needs that the patient/family want to be addressed. These spiritual issues are key to the provision of quality hospice care and cannot be addressed effectively and promptly by the spiritual counselor only

Document clearly symptoms, clinical changes, and assessment findings related to pain and patient care

Document patient changes, symptoms, and clinical information identified from visits and team conferences that support hospice care and a limited life expectancy

Clearly support in the documentation the rationale that supports/explains the progression of the illness from the chronic to terminal stages

Document mentation, behavioral, and/or cognitive changes

Document dysphagia, weight loss, increased shortness of breath, dyspnea, infection, sepsis, new or changed medications, etc.

Document any skin changes (e.g., inflamed, painful, weeping skin or infusion site[s])

Document when the patient is actively dying, deteriorating, progressing toward death

Remember that the "litmus test" of care coordination rests on the quality of the clinical documentation by all team members. Review one of your patient's clinical records and ask yourself the following: "If I was unable to give a verbal report/update on this patient, would a peer be able to pick up and provide the same level of care and know (from the documentation) the current orders, medications, and other details that contribute to effective hospice care?"

This patient population usually has many clinical changes that should be documented. These include weight loss and multiple and changed medication regimens with varying routes. Side effects to the drug regimen should be observed, noted, documented, and reported

Document coordination of services or consultation of the other members of the IDT

Document communications and care coordination with other care providers, such as skilled nursing facility or nursing home staff, inpatient team members, and hired caregivers

Your assessments, observations, and clinical findings assist in painting a picture to support coverage and documentation requirements for hospice care

Document any hospitalizations and changed clinical findings

Document patient changes, symptoms, psychosocial issues impacting the care, information gathered at the patient/family visits and during team meetings

The documentation should reflect ongoing effects of the terminal condition, the patient's/family's difficulty with care or coping, and the continued desire for hospice care

10. **Resources for hospice care and practice**

For more information and standards related to infusion, contact the Intravenous Nurses Society at (617) 489-5205.

Infusion

P.O. Box 3066

Langhorne, PA 19047-9396

Intravenous Nurses Certification Corporation (INCC)
Fresh Pond Square
10 Fawcett St.
Cambridge, MA 02138
(617) 441-3008
National Home Infusion Association
205 Daingerfield Rd.
Alexandria, VA 22314
(703) 549-3740

LUNG CARE (END STAGE)

1. **General considerations**

   Patients and their family members may be referred to hospice care after long battles with chronic obstructive pulmonary diseases (COPDs) such as asthma, bronchitis, and tuberculosis. Care is directed toward controlling and reducing the symptoms of the specific lung pathology. Supportive and skillful care is directed toward comfort and relief of coughing, shortness of breath, feelings of tightness and dyspnea, and other complaints and problems.

2. **Needs for visit**

   Physician order for hospice care, specific to the hospice program's admission criteria and policies

   Standard precautions supplies

   Vital signs equipment for baseline assessment

   Other supplies or equipment, based on physician orders

3. **Safety considerations**

   Infection control/standard precautions

   Night-light

   Disposal of soiled tissues and used respiratory supplies

   Avoidance of environmental respiratory irritants

   Oxygen safety precautions

   Bathroom safety supports, including shower bench, tub rails

   Activity pacing

   Protective skin measures

   Identification and report of any skin problems

   Fall precautions/protocol

   Multiple medications (e.g., side effects, interactions, safe storage)

   Stairway precautions/handrail on stairs

   Pacing considerations

   Symptoms that necessitate immediate reporting/assistance

   The phone number of whom to call with a care problem

   Supportive and well-fitting, nonslip shoes

   Safety for home medical equipment (e.g., wheelchair, walker)

   Smoke detector and fire evacuation plan

   Others, based on the patient's unique condition and environment

4. **Potential diagnoses and codes**

Airway obstruction, chronic	496
Asthma	493.90
Bronchiolitis	466.19
Bronchitis, acute	466.0
Bronchitis	490
Chronic ischemic heart disease	414.9
Congestive heart failure	428.0
COPD	496
Cor pulmonale	416.9

Dehydration	276.5
Emphysema	492.8
Hemoptysis	786.3
Hypertension	401.9
Influenza with pneumonia	487.0
Interstitial emphysema	518.1
Left heart failure	428.1
Lung cancer	162.9
Lung disease	518.89
Metastases, general	199.1
Orthostatic hypotension	518.89
Peripheral vascular disease	443.9
Pleural effusion	511.9
Pneumonia	486
Pneumonia aspiration	507.0
Pneumonia, *Pneumocystis carinii*	042 and 136.3
Pneumonia with influenza	487.0
Protein-caloric malnutrition	263.9
Pulmonary edema	514
Pulmonary fibrosis	515
Respirator, dependence	V46.1
Respiratory failure	518.81
Tracheal bronchus disease	519.1
Tuberculosis (lung)	011.90
Tuberculosis, bronchial	012.2
Tuberculosis, bronchus	011.0
Ventilator, dependence on	V46.1

5. **Associated nursing diagnoses**
   Activity intolerance
   Activity intolerance, risk for
   Airway clearance, ineffective
   Anxiety
   Aspiration, risk for
   Body temperature, altered, risk for
   Breathing pattern, ineffective
   Cardiac output, decreased
   Caregiver role strain
   Caregiver role strain, risk for
   Communication, impaired verbal
   Coping, ineffective family: compromised
   Family processes, altered
   Fatigue
   Fear
   Fluid volume deficit, risk for
   Fluid volume excess
   Gas exchange, impaired
   Grieving, anticipatory
   Home maintenance management, impaired
   Infection, risk for

Knowledge deficit (disease process, drug regimen, and management)
Loneliness, risk for
Management of therapeutic regimen (individuals), ineffective
Mobility, impaired physical
Noncompliance (specify)
Nutrition altered: less than body requirements
Oral mucous membrane, altered
Pain
Pain, chronic
Parenting, altered
Protection, altered
Role performance, altered
Self-care deficit, bathing/hygiene
Self-care deficit, dressing/grooming
Self-care deficit, feeding
Self-care deficit, toileting
Sexuality patterns, altered
Social interaction, impaired
Spiritual distress (distress of the human spirit)
Spiritual well-being, potential for enhanced
Swallowing, impaired
Tissue perfusion, altered (cardiopulmonary)
Ventilation, inability to sustain spontaneous

6. **Skills and services identified**

   • *Hospice nursing*

     a. *Comfort and symptom control*
        Complete initial assessment of all systems of patient with
        _____ admitted to hospice for _____ (specify)
        Presentation of hospice philosophy and services
        Explain patient rights and responsibilities
        Observation and assessment of patient with TB for presence/absence of
           productive cough, fever, night sweats, weight loss, chest pain, cough,
           and other symptoms
        Comprehensive assessment of patient with COPD admitted for
           _____ (specify)
        Skilled evaluation and all systems assessment of the patient with COPD
        Observation and complete systems assessment of the patient with
           asthma
        Observation and assessment of patient with end stage lung disease on
           multiple medications, admitted to hospice with increasing shortness
           of breath, complaints of dyspnea, poor activity tolerance, and on
           oxygen therapy _____ hours a day (specify)
        Observation and assessment of patient with restrictive lung disease ad-
           mitted to hospice with significant weight loss, on steroids and mul-
           tiple bronchodilators
        Assess patient, family, and caregiver wishes and expectations regarding
           care
        Assess patient, family, and caregiver resources available for care

Provision of volunteer support to patient and family

Teach family or caregiver physical care of patient

Assess pain and other symptoms, including site, duration, characteristics, and relief measures

Observation and assessment of pain and other symptoms to be managed within parameters of disease process

Teaching and training of family caregivers related to disease and infection-control procedures

Monitoring of respiratory and other systems

Evaluate lung sounds, and assess amount, site(s), wheezing, rhonchi, etc.

Teach patient or caregiver to identify and avoid specific factors that precipitate an exacerbation (asthma attack)

Teach patient or caregiver how to use aerosol inhalers or treatments at home

Assess signs and symptoms of CHF

Assess vital signs, including pain, q visit

Evaluate sites and amount of edema

Assess respiratory and cardiovascular statuses

Assess need for chest PT

Pain assessment and management q visit

Teach patient effective coughing, deep breathing, and pursed lip or diaphragmatic breathing

Teach other pulmonary treatment as indicated

Assess breath and lung sounds

Teach patient, family, and caregiver use of nebulizer therapy

Postural drainage as ordered

Pain assessment and management for cough and chest pain

Respiratory rate and lung sounds assessed for improvement or deterioration

Evaluate sites and amount of edema

Teach patient correct use and techniques of inhalers

RN to monitor respiratory rate and pattern

RN to evaluate for presence or absence of cough and its frequency, character, and sputum production

Teach use of home peak flow meter

RN to assess patient's pain or other symptoms q visit to identify need for change, addition, or other plan or dose adjustment

Ongoing skilled observation and assessment of wheezing, cough, dyspnea, shortness of breath, and other symptoms

Effective management of pain and prevention of secondary symptoms

RN to provide and teach effective oral care and comfort measures

Teaching and training regarding the home environment and care needed

Intervention of symptoms directed toward comfort and palliation

Observation and assessment, communication with physician related to signs and symptoms of continuing decompensation, increased symptoms, pain, discomfort, and shortness of breath and measures to alleviate and control

Teach caregiver/patient use of pain assessment tool/scale and reporting mechanism(s)

Teach patient/family about realistic expectations of disease process

Teach care of dying and signs/symptoms of impending death

Presence and support

Other interventions, based on patient/family needs

b. *Safety and mobility considerations*

Patient provided with home safety information and instruction related to _____ and documented in the clinical record

Teach about safe oxygen or nebulizer therapy use in the home setting

Teach family about safety of patient in home

Teach energy conservation techniques

RN to teach energy conservation techniques and controlled breathing exercises

Teach patient, family, and caregiver safe, effective oxygen therapy at home

Teach about copious secretions and their safe disposal

Other interventions, based on patient/family needs

c. *Emotional/spiritual considerations*

Psychosocial assessment of patient and family regarding disease and prognosis

Provide emotional support to patient and family

Assess patient and family coping skills

Provide emotional support to patient and family

Psychosocial aspects of pain control (e.g., depression) assessed and acknowledged with team support/intervention

Ongoing acknowledgment of spirituality and related concerns of patient/family

Other interventions, based on patient/family needs

d. *Skin care*

Teach patient, family, or caregiver about proper body alignment and positioning in bed to prevent skin tears from shearing skin

Observation and skilled assessment of areas for possible breakdown, including heels, hips, elbows, ankles, and other pressure-prone areas

Teach caregiver about patient's skin care needs, including the need for frequent position changes, appropriate pressure pads and mattresses, and the prevention of breakdown

Other interventions, based on patient/family needs

e. *Elimination considerations*

RN to teach caregiver daily care of catheter

RN to evaluate the patient's bowel patterns and need for stool softeners, laxatives, and dietary adjustments and to develop bowel management plan

Other interventions, based on patient/family needs

f. *Hydration/nutrition*

Assessment of nutrition and hydration status of patient at risk for poor nutritional status with severe lung disease

Assess nutrition/hydration status

Teach ordered diet regimen of _____ (specify)

Nutrition/hydration supported by offering patient's choice of favorite or desired foods or liquids

Nutrition/hydration maintained by offering patient high-protein diet and foods of choice as tolerated

Teach patient and family to expect decreased nutritional and fluid intake as disease progresses

Other interventions, based on patient/family needs

g. *Therapeutic/medication regimens*

Medication management of patient on multiple medications; assess for side effects and compliance

Teach patient or caregiver new medication regimen

Obtain sputum culture as indicated q _____

Venipuncture as ordered q _____

RN to assess the patient's response to treatments and interventions and report changes, unfavorable responses, or reactions to the physician

Medication management and response to medications and side effects

Teach about and observe for steroid side effects

Nonpharmacological interventions, such as progressive muscle relaxation, imagery, positive visualization, music, massage and touch, and humor therapy of patient's choice implemented

Medication review and management including drug/drug and drug/food interactions

RN to instruct in pain-control measures and medications

Teach patient and caregiver use of PCA pump

Other interventions, based on patient/family needs

h. *Other considerations*

Assess progression of disease process

RN to assess the patient's response to treatments and interventions and to report to the physician changes, unfavorable responses, or reactions

Other interventions, based on patient/family needs

- **Home health aide or certified nursing assistant**
  Effective and safe personal care
  Safe ADL assistance and support
  Observation and reporting
  Respite care and active listening skills
  Meal preparation
  Homemaker services
  Comfort care
  Other duties

- **Hospice social worker**
  Psychosocial assessment of patient and family/caregiver, including adjustment to long-term illness and its implications
  Identification of optimal coping strategies
  Financial assessment and counseling regarding food acquisition, ability to prepare, and costs of needed medications
  Intervention/support related to terminal illness and loss
  Emotional/spiritual support
  Depression/fear assessed
  Facilitate communication among patient, family, and hospice team

Referral/linkage to community services and resources as indicated
Grief counseling and intervention/support related to illness/loss
Patient/caregiver counseling and support
Identification of caregiver role strain necessitating respite/relief measures/
    support
Obtain resources to enable patient to remain in the home
Identification of illness-related psychiatric condition necessitating care

- *Volunteer(s)*
  Support, friendship, companionship, and presence
  Comfort and dignity maintained/provided for patient and family
  Errands and transportation
  Advocacy and respite
  Other services, based on interdisciplinary team recommendations and
      patient/caregiver needs

- *Spiritual counselor*
  Spiritual assessment and care
  Counseling, intervention, and support related to that dimension of life
      related to life's meaning (consistent with patient's beliefs)
  Support, listening, and presence
  Participation in sacred or spiritual rituals or practices
  Other supportive care, based on patient's/family's needs and belief
      systems

- *Dietitian/nutritional counseling*
  Assessment of patient with decreased intake, weight loss, anorexia, and
      increased shortness of breath (e.g., "don't feel like eating")
  Supportive counseling with patient/family indicating that patient will have
      a decreased appetite and usually at some point may not eat/drink
  Assessment and recommendations for swallowing difficulties
  Teaching and support of family members and caregivers
  Support and care with food and nourishment as desired by patient
  Evaluation/management of nutritional deficits and needs
  Encourage nutritional supplements and snacks to increase protein and fat
      intake with moderate/low carbohydrate intake
  Food and dietary recommendations incorporate patient choice and wishes

- *Occupational therapist*
  Evaluation of ADLs, functional mobility
  Assess for need for adaptive equipment and assistive devices
  Safety assessment of patient's environment and ADLs
  Assessment for energy conservation training
  Assessment of upper extremity function, retraining motor skills

- *Physical therapist*
  Evaluation
  Safety assessment of patient's environment
  Safe transfer training or bed mobility exercises
  Pain assessment/reduction factors
  Strengthening exercises/program
  Assessment of gait safety and home safety measures

Instruct/supervise caregiver and volunteers with regard to home exercise program for conditioning and strength

Assistive, adaptive devices and evaluation of equipment and teaching

- **Bereavement counselor**

  Assessment of the needs of the bereaved family and friends

  Support and intervention, based on assessment and ongoing findings

  Presence and counseling

  Supportive visits, follow-up, and other interventions (e.g., mailings, calls)

  Other services related to bereavement work and support

- **Pharmacist**

  Evaluation of hospice patient on multiple medications (nebulizer, inhalers, antibiotics, steroids, aminophylline, etc.) for possible food/drug and drug/drug interactions

  Medication monitoring regarding therapeutic levels and dosages

  Pain consult and input into interdisciplinary plan of care related to pain control, dyspnea, and need for palliation and symptom management

  Assessment of medication regimen and plan for safety and compliance

- **Music, massage, art, or other therapies or services**

  Evaluation and intervention based on patient's and caregiver's unique wishes and needs that support care, comfort, and death in the setting of the patient's choice

  Assessment plan to engage patient and support comfort, quality, enjoyment, and dignity

7. **Outcomes for care**

- **Hospice nursing**

  Death with dignity, and symptoms controlled in setting of patient/family choice

  Optimal comfort, support, and dignity provided throughout illness

  Planned and effective bowel program, as evidenced by regular bowel movements and patient/family report of no problems

  Death with maximum comfort through effective symptom control with specialized hospice support

  Patient and caregiver able to list adverse drug reactions/problems with medication regimen and whom to call for follow-up and resolution

  Dyspnea, pain, and other symptoms managed/controlled in setting of patient/family choice (e.g., patient/family report ability to eat, sleep, speak more clearly with pacing)

  Patient's/family's privacy, independence, and choices supported with respect and maintained through death

  Enhancement and support of quality of life

  Effective symptom relief and control (e.g., a peaceful and comfortable death at home, some enjoyment of life)

  Maximizing the patient's quality of life (e.g., alert and pain free or as patient wishes)

  Pharmacological and nonpharmacological interventions, such as localized heat application, positioning, use of fan for dyspnea (if desired), relaxation methods, and music

Patient cared for and family supported through death with physical, psychosocial, spiritual, and other concerns/needs acknowledged/ addressed

Patient- and family-centered hospice care provided based on the patient's/ family's unique situation and needs

Infection control and palliation

Grief/bereavement expression and support provided

Patient is pain free by next _____ visit

Caregiver demonstrates ability to manage pain, where applicable

Patient maintains comfort and dignity throughout illness

Patient and caregiver verbalize satisfaction with care

Educational tools/plans incorporated in daily care, and patient/caregiver verbalizes understanding of safe, needed care

Patient and family will decide on care, interventions, and evaluation

Caregiver effective in care management and knows whom to call for questions/concerns

Patient will express satisfaction with hospice support received and will experience increased comfort

Patient will be made comfortable at home through death in accordance with the patient's wishes

Effective pain control and symptom control verbalized by patient

Patient and family verbalize understanding of and adhere to care and medication regimens

Patient and caregiver supported through patient's death

Comfort maintained through course of care

Patient and family receive hospice support and care, and family members and friends are able to spend quality time with the patient

Caregiver able and verbalizes comfort with role and understands when to call hospice team members

Patient supported through and receives the maximum benefit from palliative chemotherapy and radiation with minimal complications

Patient and caregiver list adverse reactions, potential complications, signs/ symptoms of infection (e.g., sputum change, chest congestion)

Comfort maintained through death with dignity

Pain effectively managed, and patient verbalizes comfort

Patient has stable respiratory status with patent airway and decreased dyspnea

Patient is protected from injury, has stable respiratory status, and is compliant with medication, safety, and care regimens

Comfort and individualized intervention of patient with immobility/ bedbound status (e.g., skin, urinary, musculature, vascular)

Spiritual and psychosocial needs met (specify) as defined by patient and caregiver throughout course of care

Patient and caregiver demonstrate necessary disposal of secretions using infection-control procedure taught

Compliance to care program as evidenced by observation and demonstration during nurse's and other team members' visits

Patient states pain is _____ on 0-10 scale by next visit

Patient and caregiver demonstrate appropriate back-up or "rescue" therapies for breakthrough pain or other symptoms (e.g., dyspnea)

- *Home health aide or certified nursing assistant*
  Effective hygiene, personal care, and comfort
  ADL assistance and ambulation
  Safe environment maintained

- *Hospice social worker*
  Problem identified and addressed, with patient/caregiver linked with appropriate support services and plan of care successfully implemented
  Patient and caregiver cope adaptively with illness and death
  Adaptive adjustment to changed body and body image
  Psychosocial support and counseling offered to patient/caregivers experiencing loss and grief
  Caregiver system assessed, and development of stable caregiver plan facilitated

- *Volunteer(s)*
  Comfort, respite, companionship, and friendship extended to patient/family
  Support provided as defined by the needs of the patient/caregiver
  Patient and family supported by team with care, comfort, and companionship

- *Spiritual counseling*
  Spiritual support offered and provided as defined by needs of patient/caregiver
  Provision of spiritual support and care based on the assessed and ongoing needs of the patient and family
  Spiritual support offered, and patient and family needs met
  Patient and family express relief of symptoms of spiritual suffering

- *Dietitian/nutritional counseling*
  Family and caregiver integrate recommendations into nutrition teaching (where appropriate)
  Patient and caregiver know when to call for nutrition- and hydration-related questions/concerns
  Nutrition/hydration per patient's choices
  Caregiver integrates recommendations into daily meal planning
  Patient and family verbalize comprehension of changing nutritional needs

- *Occupational therapist*
  Maximize independence in ADLs for patient/caregiver
  Optimal function maintained/attained
  Patient and caregiver demonstrate ADL program for maximum safety
  Patient and caregiver demonstrate energy conservation techniques
  Splints used to maintain functional joint position
  Patient and caregiver demonstrate ADL program for maximum safety and independence
  Patient and caregiver demonstrate maximum independence with ADL, adaptive techniques, and assistive devices
  Patient and caregiver demonstrate maximum safety in ADL and functional mobility
  Patient and caregiver demonstrate effective use of energy conservation techniques

Verbalization/demonstration of improved functional activity level and enhanced quality of life
Patient and caregiver demonstrate effective use of diaphragmatic breathing
to reduce shortness of breath and relaxation techniques to help in pain/
symptom management

- *Physical therapist*
  Prevention of complications
  Home exercise and upper extremity program taught to caregiver
  Optimal strength, mobility, and function maintained/achieved
  Compliance with home exercise program by _____ (specify
  date)

- *Bereavement counselor*
  Grief support services provided to patient and family
  Well-being and resolution process of grief initiated and followed through
  bereavement services

- *Pharmacist*
  Multiple drug regimen reviewed for food/drug and drug/drug interactions in
  patient on multiple meds
  Stability and safety in complex medication regimen with maximum benefit
  to patient
  Effective pain, dyspnea, and symptom control and symptom management
  as reported by patient/caregiver
  Lab reports reviewed for therapeutic dosages and effective patient response

- *Music, massage, art, or other therapies or services*
  Therapeutic massage/touch effective for patient as self-reported or observed
  by caregivers/family
  Improved muscle tone, relaxation, and/or sleep
  Patient comfortable and relaxed (e.g., sleeping) after massage
  Music therapy intervention based on assessment to decrease pain percep-
  tion and provide emotional expression and support
  Maintenance of comfort and physical, psychosocial, and spiritual health
  Holistic health maintained and comfort achieved through _____
  (specify modality)

8. **Patient, family, and caregiver educational needs**
   Educational needs are the care regimens that contribute to safe and effective
   care at home between the hospice team's visits.
   These include the following:
   The basic tenets of hospice and the availability of support 24 hours a day, 7
   days a week
   Home safety assessment and counseling
   The patient's medication regimen
   Safe and proper body mechanics to promote patient comfort and prevent
   caregiver safety problems
   Other teaching specific to the patient's and family's unique needs
   Support groups available to patient's family, such as the hospice program's
   "Caregiver Support Group" meetings for family members and friends of
   the patient

Anticipated disease progression

Safe, effective inhaler or metered dose unit use

Safe, effective oxygen therapy use at home

The importance of diet, rest, and exercise

Other teaching specific to the patient's and caregiver's unique medical and
other identified needs

The prevention of infections and avoidance of stress and other "triggers" for
the individual patient. These can include environmental factors such as
pollens, smoke, animals, dust, and chemicals

Effective hand-washing techniques, tissue/sputum disposal, and other aspects
of infection control

Other teaching specific to the patient and caregiver, based on their unique
needs

9. **Specific tips for quality and reimbursement**

Document any variances to expected outcomes. There are many models of
hospice programs. Those that are home health agency–based must work
within the framework of the Medicare home care program. For example,
sometimes a hospice patient reaches a stable period in the illness and has no
further skilled needs or the patient is no longer homebound per Medicare
home health care criteria. When this occurs, one option is to discharge the
patient from Medicare home health agency reimbursement and maintain the
patient on grant funds or other available resources. If the patient's status deteriorates and again meets the Medicare criteria, a new start of care is initiated on the HCFA form 485. Usually hospices continue volunteer support,
nursing, and other services indicated during these periods of no reimbursement.

The Medicare hospice benefit does not require that the patient be homebound or have identified skilled needs. Though it is a needed and viable
program, the Medicare hospice benefit may not be indicated for all Medicare-
eligible beneficiaries. For further information on this benefit, please refer to
HCFA Hospice Manual 21.

Should the patient's status deteriorate and increased personal care be
needed, obtain a telephone order for the increased service, noting frequency
and estimating the duration.

Obtain a telephone order for all medication and treatment changes of the
medical regimen and document these in the clinical record.

Unless the patient is in a hospice insurance program, some insurers will
not pay for a skilled nurse visit that is made at death if the patient is dead
when the nurse arrives at the home. From a Medicare home care perspective,
the visit at the time of death may be covered when the orders and clinical
record document assessment of the patient's status or signs of death/life or
state law allows pronouncement of death by a nurse.

Document patient deterioration

Document dehydration, dehydrating

Document patient change or instability

Document pain, other symptoms not controlled

Document status after acute episode of _____ (specify)

Document positive urine, sputum, etc. culture; patient started on
_____ (specify ordered antibiotic therapy)

Document patient impacted; impaction removed manually

Document RN in frequent communication with physician regarding
_____ (specify)

Document febrile at _____, pulse change at _____, irr.,
irr.

Document change noted in _____

Document bony prominences red, opening

Document RN contacted physician regarding _____ (specify)

Document marked SOB

Document alteration in mental status

Document medications being adjusted, regulated, or monitored

Document unable to perform own ADLs, personal care

Document all interdisciplinary team meetings and communications in the
POC and in the progress notes of the clinical record

All hospice team members should have input into the POC and document
their interventions and goals

Document changes to the plan of care, such as medications, services, frequency, communication, and concurrence of other team members

Document coordination of services or consultation of the other members of
the IDT

Document communications and care coordination with other care providers,
such as skilled nursing facility or nursing home staff, inpatient team
members, and hired caregivers

Document all abnormal breath and lung sounds heard

Obtain a telephone order for any POC changes, and document these
changes

These patients are usually sick, so be objective and document what the
patient looks like (frail, pale, poor intake, SOB, unable to do ADLs, etc.)

Document patient's continued poor activity level because of SOB

Document the ordered rate of oxygen flow, mode, and specific hours needed

Discuss patient at case conference with physical therapy, occupational
therapy, home health aide, and other ordered services

Document any increased SOB

Document any change, including medications, on the POC

Document RN contacted physician regarding _____ (specify)

Document RN in frequent communications with physician regarding
_____ (specify)

Document febrile at _____ or tachycardia at _____,
irr., irr.

New onset (any symptom)

Document patient deteriorating or progressing well

Document dehydration, dehydrating

Document stable, unstable

Document pain uncontrolled, any other symptom not controlled

Document positive sputum culture; physician started patient on
_____ (specify ordered medication)

Document medications being regulated

Document bony prominences, red or opening skin sites

Document care coordination among the interdisciplinary team members, such
as phone calls, case conferences, or team meetings

Phone calls to physicians for changes in the patient's condition; obtaining orders for a change on the plan of care or requesting an increase in the visit frequency needs physician orders

Document all abnormalities, such as fever, tachycardia, rales, wheezing, and rhonchi

Document the instability of the patient; document any edema, SOB, medication reaction, further acute episodes, pulse irregularities

Obtain a telephone order to change the visit frequency or make any changes to the POC

Often these patients have other medical problems, specifically cardiac, that impede progress; document these problems also

Document medications changed or medications being regulated on the daily visit note or record

Document RN contacted physician regarding _____

Document in the clinical notes the clear progression and symptomatology and interventions that demonstrate the interventions and overall management of the patient with end stage lung disease

Document when/if the patient has respiratory changes, shortness of breath, exacerbation of conditions, dysphagia, pain, and other symptoms and that they are identified and resolved

Remember that the clinical documentation is key to measuring compliance for quality and reimbursement purposes. Care coordination, timely verbal and initial physician orders, and assessment and addressing of spiritual and psychosocial needs should be clearly documented in the patient's clinical record

The documentation should support that all hospice care supports comfort and dignity while meeting patient/family needs

The documentation should include the ongoing assessment and management of pain and other symptoms and the anticipation and prevention of secondary symptoms such as constipation

It is important to note that all team members, including nurses and social workers, should assess, identify, and "hear" spiritual needs that the patient/family want to be addressed. These spiritual issues are key to the provision of quality hospice care and cannot be addressed effectively and promptly by the spiritual counselor only

Document clearly symptoms, clinical changes, and assessment findings that support the end stage of the lung process

Document patient changes, symptoms, and clinical information identified from visits and team conferences that support hospice care and a limited life expectancy

Clearly support in the documentation the rationale that supports/explains the progression of the illness from the chronic to terminal stages

Document mentation, behavioral, and/or cognitive changes

Document dysphagia, weight loss, increased shortness of breath, dyspnea, infection, sepsis, new or changed medications, etc.

Document any skin changes (e.g., inflamed, painful, weeping skin site[s])

Document when the patient is actively dying, deteriorating, progressing toward death

Remember that the "litmus test" of care coordination rests on the quality of the clinical documentation completed by all team members. Review one of your patient's clinical records and ask yourself the following: "If I was unable to give a verbal report/update on this patient, would a peer be able to pick up and provide the same level of care and know (from the documentation) the current orders, including specific medications and other details that contribute to effective hospice care?"

This patient population usually has many clinical changes that should be documented. These include weight loss, dyspnea, and multiple and changed medication regimens with varying routes, including nebulizer therapy, steroids, antibiotics, varying bronchodilators such as aminophylline. Some patients have cardiac side effects to the drug regimen that should be observed, noted, documented, and reported (e.g., patient has ascites, is cyanotic, has severe finger clubbing noted on admission, has peripheral edema). All these clinical findings are examples that assist in painting a picture to support coverage and documentation requirements for hospice care

Document any hospitalizations and changed clinical findings.

In the clinical documentation, paint the picture of the patient with end stage lung disease. The patient may be very short of breath and have poor or no activity tolerance or energy. This is the kind of clinical documentation specificity that clearly shows why the hospice team was called in at this point along the patient's illness continuum and supports coverage and documentation requirements of an insurance provider, such as Medicare.

For this and other noncancer diagnoses, document clearly the symptoms and clinical and assessment findings that support the end stage of the chronic illness process

Document patient changes, symptoms, and psychosocial issues impacting the care, including information gathered at the patient/family visits and during team meetings

The documentation should reflect ongoing effects of the terminal condition, the patient's/family's difficulty with care or coping, and the continued desire for hospice care.

10. **Resources for hospice care and practice**
    The American Lung Association publishes the *Asthma Handbook* and can be reached at 1-800-232-5864.

    Another helpful resource is the NHO's second edition of *Medical Guidelines for Determining Prognoses in Selected Non-Cancer Diseases*. Call NHO at 1-703-243-5900 for more information.

PAIN CARE

1. **General considerations**

   It has been said that the most frequently identified nursing diagnosis or patient problem may be pain. It is important to remember that patients (and family members providing the direct care) are the experts on their pain, their histories, and often even the necessary relief measures. This information can be most easily elicited during completion of the pain assessment tool. Once asked, hospice patients will readily assess and discuss their pain perceptions.

   Hospice nurses are becoming the experts in this area, and experienced clinicians develop accepted assessment tools, protocols for medication titration, and overall pain management. For effective pain management, efforts of the entire hospice team must be directed toward comfort and validation or verbalization of relief, when possible. Part Seven provides pain assessment and management resources for your review and information. See also Figure 4-1 (p. 165) and Box 4-1 (p. 171) for information on cancer-related pain.

2. **Needs for visit**

   Physician order for hospice care, specific to the hospice program's admission criteria and policies

   Standard precautions/supplies

   Vital signs equipment for baseline assessment

   Other supplies or equipment, based on physician orders

3. **Safety considerations**

   Infection control/standard precautions

   Night-light

   Extra caution on slippery surfaces

   Removal of scatter rugs

   Tub rail, grab bars for bathroom safety

   Supportive and nonskid shoes

   Handrail on stairs

   Fall precautions/protocol

   Protective skin measures

   Identification and report of any skin problems

   Smoke detector and fire evacuation plan

   Assistance with ambulation

   Others, based on the patient's unique condition and environment

4. **Potential diagnoses and codes**

   Pain can come from any cause, source, or diagnosis. Please refer to the other care guidelines for specific diagnosis codes such as cancer, depression, and any other section that is appropriate for your patient's pain problems.

5. **Associated nursing diagnoses**

   Activity intolerance

   Activity intolerance, risk for

   Anxiety

   Body image disturbance

   Caregiver role strain

Caregiver role strain, risk for
Constipation
Coping, family: potential for growth
Coping, ineffective family: disabling
Coping, ineffective individual: disabling
Family processes, altered
Fatigue
Fear
Grieving, anticipatory
Home maintenance management, impaired
Hopelessness
Infection, risk for
Injury, risk for
Knowledge deficit (pain management)
Mobility, impaired physical
Oral mucous membrane, altered
Noncompliance (specify)
Pain
Pain, chronic
Powerlessness
Role performance, altered
Self-care deficit, bathing/hygiene
Self-care deficit, dressing/grooming
Self-care deficit, feeding
Self-care deficit, toileting
Self-esteem disturbance
Sensory/perceptual alterations (specify) (visual, auditory, kinesthetic, gustatory, tactile, olfactory)
Sexual dysfunction
Sexuality patterns, altered
Sleep pattern, disturbance
Social interaction, impaired
Spiritual distress (distress of the human spirit)
Spiritual well-being, potential for enhanced
Thought processes, altered
Tissue perfusion, altered (specify)

6. **Skills and services identified**

- *Hospice nursing*

   a. *Comfort and symptom control*
      Comprehensive initial assessment of systems in patient with pain for baseline information
      Presentation of hospice philosophy and services
      Explain patient rights and responsibilities
      Observation and assessment of patient with _____ (specify) on multiple medications, admitted to hospice with increasing shortness of breath and pain
      Assess patient, family, and caregiver wishes and expectations regarding care
      Assess patient, family, and caregiver resources available for care

Provision of volunteer support to patient and family

Teach family or caregiver physical care of patient

Pain assessment and management q visit, including source/type of pain (e.g., cancer pain, infection, pathological fracture, and other medical problems such as cardiac or arthritis pain)

RN to provide and teach effective oral care and comfort measures

Assess pain and other symptoms, including site, duration, characteristics, and relief measures

RN to assess patient's pain q visit to identify need for change, addition, or other plan or dose adjustment

RN to assess all aspects of pain, including site(s), character, description, relation to activity or position, type of pain (constant, spontaneous, episodic), and other factors patient identifies

RN to teach patient and caregivers about the importance of and rationale for round-the-clock schedule of analgesia for continuous pain

Teach patient how to use the standardized pain scale

Teach patient how to rate pain using the scale of 0-10 or other scale specific to the patient's ability

Assist patient in establishing goals for relief

Evaluate pain in relation to other symptoms, including fatigue, confusion, constipation, depression, and SOB

RN to evaluate need for noninvasive methods of pain control, including heat or cold applications and a transcutaneous electrical nerve stimulation (TENS) unit

Assess pain, and evaluate pain management's effectiveness

Teach care of bedridden patient

Measure vital signs, including pain, q visit

Assess cardiovascular, pulmonary, and respiratory status

Teach caregiver care of weak, terminally ill patient

Comfort measures of backrub and hand or other therapeutic massage

Teach patient/family use of standardized form/tool to use between hospice team members' visits (and for care coordination between team members)

Teach patient/family principles of effective pain management

Observation and assessment, communication with physician related to signs and symptoms of continuing decompensation and increased symptoms, pain, discomfort, and shortness of breath, and measures to alleviate and control

Effective management of pain and prevention of secondary symptoms

Interventions of symptoms directed toward comfort and palliation

Teach caregiver/patient use of pain assessment tool/scale and reporting mechanism(s)

Teach patient and family about realistic expectations of disease process

Teach care of dying and signs/symptoms of impending death

Presence and support

Other interventions, based on patient/family needs

b. *Safety and mobility considerations*

Provide caregiver with home safety information and instruction related to _____ and documented in the clinical record

Assess relationship of pain to increased safety risks, such as falls, in the home; counsel regarding safety and precautions

Other interventions, based on patient/family needs

c. *Emotional/spiritual considerations*

Psychosocial assessment of patient and family regarding disease and prognosis

RN to provide emotional support to patient and family

RN to evaluate for emotional distress and other factors having an impact on pain

Assess mental status and sleep disturbance changes

Assess for and manage plans for psychosocial and/or spiritual pain (e.g., all pain, anxiety, interpersonal distress)

Assessment and care/support related to depression, changed body image concerns, fever, mouth sores/ulcers, complaints of extreme tiredness, and dry/cracking skin in patient receiving palliative chemotherapy

Psychosocial aspects of pain control (e.g., depression, others) assessed and acknowledged with team support/intervention

Ongoing acknowledgment of spirituality and related concerns of patient/ family

Other interventions, based on patient/family needs

d. *Skin care*

Assess skin integrity

Observation and evaluation of wound and surrounding skin

Evaluate patient's need for equipment, including supplies to decrease pressure, alternating pressure mattress, gel foam seat cushion, and heel and elbow protectors

RN to teach patient regarding care of irradiated skin sites

Teach patient, family, or caregiver about proper body alignment and positioning in bed to prevent skin tears from shearing skin

Observe and apply skilled assessment of areas for possible breakdown, including heels, hips, elbows, ankles, and other pressure-prone areas

Teach caregiver regarding skin care needs, including the need for frequent position changes, appropriate pressure pads and mattresses, and the prevention of breakdown

Other interventions, based on patient/family needs

e. *Elimination considerations*

RN to develop bowel management plan

Assess amount and frequency of urinary output

RN to evaluate the patient's bowel patterns and need for stool softeners, laxatives, dietary adjustments, and to develop bowel management plan

Teaching and ongoing assessment regarding prevention and early identification of constipation and its correction/resolution

Initiate bowel management program per hospice physician

Implement bowel assessment and management program

Teach patient, family, and aide the importance of observing and noting bowel movements between scheduled nursing visits

Obtain patient history related to norms for bowel movements to date (e.g., "all my life I go only every other day")

Consider stool softeners, and offer laxative of choice, Fleet's Enemas
   prn, and other methods per patient wishes and physician's orders
Other interventions, based on patient/family needs

f. *Hydration/nutrition*
   Assess nutrition/hydration statuses
   Nutrition/hydration supported by offering patient's choice of favorite or
      desired foods or liquids
   Nutrition/hydration maintained by offering patient high-protein diet and
      foods of choice as tolerated
   Assessment and plan related to anorexia/cachexia, tube feedings,
      difficulty/painful swallowing, and/or transitional feedings (e.g., TPN
      to oral)
   Teach patient and family to expect decreased nutritional and fluid intake
      as disease progresses
   Assessment and interventions/plan related to patient/family complaints
      of dry mouth, with painful chewing, difficulty speaking, and denture
      fit concerns after radiation and surgery
   Other interventions, based on patient/family needs

g. *Therapeutic/medication regimens*
   Monitor for signs/symptoms of narcotic overdose and treat as appropri-
      ate (e.g., following established protocols)
   RN to implement nonpharmacological interventions with medication
      schedule, including therapeutic massage, hypnosis, distraction,
      imagery, progressive muscle relaxation, humor, music therapies, and
      biofeedback
   Administer antiemetic on round-the-clock basis to control nausea caused
      by narcotic analgesia ordered for continuous pain
   Patient taught about and provided with educational materials regarding
      pain medication and side effects
   RN to titrate the dose to achieve patient pain relief with minimal side
      effects (per the range noted in the physician orders)
   RN to assess the patient's response to therapeutic treatments and inter-
      ventions and to report any changes or unfavorable responses to the
      physician
   Medication assessment and management q visit
   Teach new pain- and symptom-control medication regimen
   Teach patient and caregiver use of PCA pump
   Nonpharmacological interventions such as progressive muscle relax-
      ation, imagery, positive visualization, music, massage and touch, and
      humor therapy of patient's choice implemented
   RN to instruct in pain control measures and medications
   Teach about and observe side effects of palliative chemotherapy, includ-
      ing constipation, anemia, and fatigue
   Venipuncture q _____ (specify ordered frequency) for moni-
      toring platelet count
   Teaching of patient/family, including medications, pain management
      program, strength, type, actions, times, and compliance tips
   Encourage family/caregivers to give the patient medications on the
      schedule per physician orders

Medications changed using equianalgesic conversion tables/physician orders (e.g., from oral morphine to an equianalgesic dose of transdermal fentanyl)

RN to instruct in the use of breakthrough or "rescue" dosing of pain medication

Other interventions, based on patient/family needs

h. *Other considerations*

Assess progression of disease process

RN to assess the patient's response to treatments and interventions and to report to the physician changes, unfavorable responses, or reactions

Other interventions, based on patient/family needs

- *Home health aide or certified nursing assistant*

Effective and safe personal care

Safe ADL assistance and support

Observation and reporting

Report patient complaints of unrelieved, new, or changed pain

Respite care and active listening skills

Meal preparation

Homemaker services

Comfort care

Other duties

- *Hospice social worker*

Psychosocial assessment of patient and family/caregiver, including adjustment to illness, pain, and its implications

Identification of optimal coping strategies

Financial assessment and counseling regarding food acquisition, ability to prepare, and costs of needed medications

Intervention/support related to terminal illness and loss

Emotional/spiritual support

Depression/fear assessed

Facilitate communication among patient, family, and hospice team

Referral/linkage to community services and resources as indicated

Grief counseling and intervention/support related to illness/loss

Patient/caregiver counseling and support

Identification of caregiver role strain necessitating respite/relief measures/ support

For patients who live alone with no support system (e.g., able, available, willing caregiver[s]): obtain resources to enable patient to remain in home setting

Identification of illness-related psychiatric condition necessitating support and care/intervention

Evaluate impact of pain on quality of life

- *Volunteer(s)*

Support, friendship, companionship, and presence

Comfort and dignity maintained/provided for patient and family

Errands and transportation

Advocacy and respite

Other services, based on interdisciplinary team recommendations and patient/caregiver needs

- *Spiritual counselor*
  Spiritual assessment and care
  Counseling, intervention, and support related to that dimension of life related to life's meaning (consistent with patient's beliefs)
  Support, listening, and presence
  Participation in sacred or spiritual rituals or practices
  Other supportive care, based on patient's/family's needs and belief systems

- *Dietitian/nutritional counseling*
  Assessment of patient with decreased intake, weight loss, anorexia, and pain
  Supportive counseling with patient/family indicating that patient will have a decreased appetite and possible inability to eat/drink
  Assessment and recommendations for swallowing difficulties, nausea, vomiting, and constipation associated with pain medications
  Teaching and support of family members and caregivers
  Support and care with food and nourishment as desired by patient
  Evaluation/management of nutritional deficits and needs
  Encourage nutritional supplements and snacks to increase protein and caloric intake
  Food and dietary recommendations incorporate patient choice and wishes

- *Occupational therapist*
  Evaluation of ADL and functional mobility
  Assess for need for adaptive equipment and assistive devices
  Safety assessment of patient's environment and ADLs
  Assessment for energy conservation training
  Assessment of upper extremity function, retraining motor skills, and/or splinting for contracture(s)

- *Physical therapist*
  Evaluation
  Safety assessment of patient's environment
  Safe transfer training or bed mobility in patient with pain
  Pain assessment/reduction factors
  Strengthening exercises/program
  Assessment of gait safety and home safety measures
  Instruct/supervise caregiver and volunteers on home exercise program for conditioning and strength
  Assistive, adaptive devices and evaluation of equipment and teaching

- *Speech-language pathologist*
  Evaluation for speech/swallowing problems
  Food texture recommendations
  Alternate functional communication

- *Bereavement counselor*
  Assessment of the needs of the bereaved family and friends
  Support and intervention, based on assessment and ongoing findings
  Presence and counseling

Supportive visits, follow-up, and other interventions (e.g., mailings, calls)

Other services related to bereavement work and support

- *Pharmacist*

  Evaluation of hospice patient with constipation on cathartics, stool softeners, and other medications for possible food/drug and drug/drug interactions

  Medication monitoring regarding therapeutic levels and dosages

  Pain consult and input into interdisciplinary plan of care related to pain
  control, palliation, and symptom management

  Assessment of medication regimen and plan for pain relief and safety

- *Music, massage, art, or other therapies or services*

  Evaluation and intervention based on patient's and caregiver's unique
  wishes and needs that support care, comfort, and death in the setting of
  the patient's choice

  Assessment plan to engage patient and support comfort, quality, enjoyment,
  dignity, and pain/symptom relief

  Pet therapy (including patient's pet, if available) and therapeutic intervention

7. **Outcomes for care**

- *Hospice nursing*

  Pain and symptoms managed/controlled in setting of patient/family choice
  (e.g., patient/family report ability to eat, sleep, speak with pacing)

  Planned and effective bowel program, as evidenced by regular bowel
  movements and patient/family report of comfort

  Death with dignity, and pain/symptoms controlled in setting of patient/
  family choice

  Optimal comfort, support, and dignity provided throughout illness

  Death with maximum comfort through effective symptom control with specialized hospice support

  Patient and caregiver able to list adverse drug reactions and problems with
  medication regimen and whom to call for follow-up and resolution

  Spiritual and psychosocial needs met (specify) as defined by patient and
  caregiver throughout course of care

  Patient's/family's privacy, independence, and choices supported with
  respect and maintained through death

  Enhancement and support of quality of life

  Effective pain and other symptom relief and control (e.g., a peaceful and
  comfortable death at home, some enjoyment of life)

  Maximizing the patient's quality of life (e.g., alert and pain free or as
  patient wishes)

  Pharmacological and nonpharmacological interventions, such as localized
  heat application, positioning, relaxation methods, and music

  Patient cared for and family supported through death, with physical, psychosocial, spiritual, and other concerns/needs acknowledged/addressed

  Patient- and family-centered hospice care provided based on the patient's/
  family's unique situation and needs

  Infection control and palliation

Grief/bereavement expression and support provided

Patient is protected from injury, has stable respiratory status, and is compliant with medication, safety, and care regimens

Comfort and individualized intervention of patient with immobility/bedbound status (e.g., skin, urinary, musculature, vascular)

Patient and caregiver verbalize satisfaction with care

Educational tools/plans incorporated in daily care, and patient and caregiver verbalize understanding of safe, needed care

Patient will decide on care, interventions, and evaluation

Caregiver effective in care management and knows whom to call for questions/concerns

Patient will express satisfaction with hospice support received and will experience increased comfort

Patient will be made comfortable at home through death in accordance with the patient's wishes

Effective pain control and symptom control verbalized by patient

Patient verbalizes understanding of and adheres to care and medication regimens

Patient and caregiver supported through patient's death

Comfort maintained through course of care

The patient and family receive hospice support and care, and family members and friends are able to spend quality time with the patient

Caregiver able and verbalizes comfort with role and understands when to call hospice team members

Patient supported through and receives the maximum benefit from palliative chemotherapy and radiation with minimal complications

Patient and caregiver list adverse reactions, potential complications, and signs/symptoms of infection (e.g., sputum change, chest congestion)

Comfort maintained through death with dignity

Pain effectively managed, and patient verbalizes comfort

Patient has stable respiratory status with patent airway (e.g., no dyspnea, infection free)

Patient will decide on care and pain intervention and evaluation

Patient will experience increased comfort and pain control through self-report and _____ (specify parameters)

Patient will have palliative care and comfort maintained through death

Patient and caregiver knowledgeable about side effects (e.g., constipation) and interventions needed

Control of pain and other symptoms that affect daily function, quality of life, and ability to interact with friends/family

Teaching related to safety, medications, and self-care successful as demonstrated by patient's verbalization and (specify measurable parameters)

Effective pain control and symptom relief by _____ (specify date)

Patient and caregiver knowledgeable about pain regimen, relief measures, and care for optimal relief/control

Early detection and intervention of problems related to patients with immobility/bedbound status (e.g., skin, urinary, musculature, vascular, others)

Patient/caregiver demonstrates appropriate back-up or "rescue" therapies
for breakthrough pain or other symptoms (e.g., dyspnea)
Caregiver demonstrates ability to manage pain, where applicable
Patient maintains comfort and dignity throughout illness
Patient states pain is at _____ on 0-10 scale by next visit.

- *Home health aide or certified nursing assistant*
Effective hygiene, personal care, and comfort
ADL assistance
Safe environment maintained

- *Hospice social worker*
Problem identified and addressed, with patient/caregiver linked with appro-
priate support services and plan of care successfully implemented
Patient and caregiver cope adaptively with illness and death
Adaptive adjustment to changed body and body image
Psychosocial support and counseling offered to patient/caregivers experi-
encing loss and grief
Caregiver system assessed, and development of stable caregiver plan facili-
tated

- *Volunteer(s)*
Comfort, companionship, and friendship extended to patient/family
Support provided as defined by the needs of the patient/caregiver
Patient and family supported by team with care, comfort, and companion-
ship
Advocacy and respite

- *Spiritual counseling*
Spiritual support offered and provided as defined by needs of patient/
caregiver
Provision of spiritual support and care as based on the assessed and
ongoing needs of the patient and family
Spiritual support offered, and patient and family needs met
Participation in sacred or spiritual rituals or practices
Patient and family express relief of symptoms of spiritual suffering
Support, listening, and presence
Intervention and support provided related to that dimension of life related
to life's meaning (consistent with patient's beliefs)

- *Dietitian/nutritional counseling*
Family and caregiver integrate recommendations into nutrition teaching and
daily meal planning
Patient and caregiver know whom to call for nutrition/hydration concerns
Patient and family verbalize comprehension of changing nutritional needs

- *Occupational therapist*
Patient and caregiver demonstrate maximum independence with ADL,
adaptive techniques, and assistive devices
Patient and caregiver demonstrate maximum safety in ADL and functional
mobility
Patient and caregiver demonstrate effective use of energy conservation
techniques

Verbalization/demonstration of improved functional activity level and enhanced quality of life

Patient and caregiver demonstrate effective use of diaphragmatic breathing to reduce shortness of breath and relaxation techniques to help in pain/symptom management

Patient and caregiver demonstrate correct use of exercise and splints for maximum upper extremity function and joint position

- *Physical therapist*
  Prevention of complications
  Home exercise and upper extremity program taught to caregiver
  Optimal strength, mobility, function maintained/achieved
  Pain management program effective as verbalized by patient/caregiver

- *Speech-language pathologist*
  Communication method implemented, and patient able to be understood as self-reported or reported by family/caregivers
  Safe swallowing and functional communication
  Recommended lists of foods/textures for safety and patient choice

- *Bereavement counselor*
  Support services related to grief provided to patient and family
  Well-being and resolution process of grief initiated and followed through bereavement services

- *Music, massage, art, or other therapies or services*
  Therapeutic massage/touch effective for patient as self-reported or observed by caregivers/family
  Improved relaxation (relief from pain) and/or sleep
  Patient comfortable and relaxed (e.g., sleeping) after massage
  Music therapy intervention based on assessment to decrease pain perception and provide emotional expression and support
  Maintenance of comfort and physical, psychosocial, and spiritual health
  Holistic health maintained and comfort achieved through _____ (specify modality)
  Patient has pet's presence as desired—in all care sites, when possible

8. **Patient, family, and caregiver educational needs**
   Educational needs are the care regimens that contribute to safe and effective care at home between the hospice team's visits.
   These include the following:
   The basic tenets of hospice and the availability of support 24 hours a day, 7 days a week
   Home safety assessment and counseling
   The patient's medication regimen
   Safe and proper body mechanics to promote patient comfort and prevent caregiver safety problems
   Anticipated disease progression
   Support groups available to patient's family, such as the hospice program's "Caregiver Support Group" meetings for family members and friends of the patient
   Other teaching specific to the patient's and family's unique needs
   Importance of all aspects of the pain-control regimen (e.g., timing)

9. **Specific tips for quality and reimbursement**

Unless the patient is in a hospice insurance program, some insurers will not pay for a skilled nurse visit made at death if the patient is dead when the nurse arrives at the home. From a Medicare home care perspective, the visit at the time of death may be covered when the orders and clinical record document assessment of the patient's status or signs of death/life or state law allows pronouncement of death by a nurse.

Document patient deterioration

Document dehydration, dehydrating

Document patient change or instability

Document pain, other symptoms not controlled

Document status after acute episode of _____ (specify)

Document positive urine, sputum, etc. culture; patient started on _____ (specify ordered antibiotic therapy)

Document patient impacted; impaction removed manually per physician's orders

Document RN in frequent communication with physician regarding _____ (specify)

Document febrile at _____, pulse change at _____, irr., irr.

Document change noted in _____

Document bony prominences red, opening

Document RN contacted physician regarding _____ (specify)

Document marked SOB

Document alteration in mental status

Document medications being adjusted, regulated, or monitored

Document unable to perform own ADLs, personal care

Document all interdisciplinary team meetings and communications in the POC and in the progress notes of the clinical record

All hospice team members involved should have input into the POC and document their interventions and goals

Document any variances to expected outcomes. There are many models of hospice programs. Those that are home health agency–based must work within the framework of the Medicare home care program. For example, sometimes a hospice patient reaches a stable period in the illness and has no further skilled needs or the patient is no longer homebound per Medicare home health care criteria. When this occurs, one option is to discharge the patient from Medicare home health agency reimbursement and maintain the patient on grant funds or other available resources. If the patient's status deteriorates and again meets the Medicare criteria, a new start of care is initiated on the HCFA form 485. Usually hospices continue volunteer support, nursing, and other services indicated during these periods of no reimbursement.

The Medicare hospice benefit does not require that the patient be homebound or have identified skilled needs. Though it is a needed and viable program, the Medicare hospice benefit may not be indicated for all Medicare-eligible beneficiaries. For further information on this benefit, please refer to HCFA Hospice Manual 21.

Should the patient's status deteriorate and increased personal care be needed, obtain a telephone order for the increased service, noting frequency and estimating the duration.

Obtain a telephone order for all medication and treatment changes of the medical regimen and document these in the clinical record.

The nursing skills used primarily in the area of pain and other symptom management will be (1) observation and assessment; (2) management and evaluation of the patient's POC; (3) administration of medications, depending on the patient's unique medical condition; and (4) teaching and training activities related to the medication regimen, side effects, and safe and effective administration of medication.

Examples of teaching or training activities may be, for example, teaching the patient and family the use of the PCA pump, safe administration of medication, and care of the bedbound patient.

Document all care provided, including that related to pain management and the patient response to those interventions. Document any changes to the POC and physician communications, and obtain orders for any changes. Document changes or alterations to the POC and the patient's response to the changed interventions. The documentation should reflect the learning accomplishments of the patient/family including side effects and adverse reaction information.

Document in the clinical notes the clear progression and symptomatology and interventions that demonstrate the interventions and overall management of the patient with pain

Document when/if the patient has respiratory changes, shortness of breath, exacerbation of conditions, dysphagia, changes in pain, and other symptoms and that they are identified and resolved

Remember that the clinical documentation is key to measuring organizational compliance for quality and reimbursement purposes. Care coordination, timely verbal and initial physician orders, and assessment and addressing of spiritual and psychosocial needs should be ongoing and documented in the patient's clinical record

The documentation should support that all hospice care supports comfort and dignity while meeting patient/family needs

The documentation should include ongoing assessment and management of pain and other symptoms and the anticipation and prevention of secondary symptoms such as constipation

It is important to note that all team members, including nurses and social workers, should assess, identify, and "hear" spiritual needs that the patient/family want to be addressed. These spiritual issues are key to the provision of quality hospice care and cannot be addressed effectively and promptly by the spiritual counselor only

Document clearly symptoms, clinical changes, and assessment findings related to pain and patient care

Document patient changes, symptoms, and clinical information identified from visits and team conferences that support hospice care and a limited life expectancy

Clearly support in the documentation the rationale that supports/explains the progression of the illness from the chronic to terminal stages

Document mentation, behavioral, and/or cognitive changes

Document dysphagia, weight loss, increased shortness of breath, dyspnea, infection, sepsis, new or changed medications, etc.

Document any skin changes (e.g., inflamed, painful, weeping skin site[s])

Document when the patient is actively dying, deteriorating, and progressing toward death

Remember that the "litmus test" of care coordination rests on the quality of the clinical documentation by all team members. Review one of your patient's clinical records and ask yourself the following: "If I was unable to give a verbal report/update on this patient, would a peer be able to pick up and provide the same level of care and know (from the documentation) the current orders, medications, and other details that contribute to effective hospice care?"

This patient population usually has many clinical changes that should be documented. These include weight loss and multiple and changed medication regimens with varying routes. Side effects to the drug regimen should be observed, noted, documented, and reported

Document changes to the plan of care, such as medications, services, frequency, communication, and concurrence of other team members

Document communications and care coordination with other care providers, such as skilled nursing facility or nursing home staff, inpatient team members, and hired caregivers

Your assessments, observations, and clinical findings assist in painting a picture to support coverage and documentation requirements for hospice care

Document any hospitalizations and changed clinical findings

Document patient changes, symptoms, psychosocial issues impacting the care, and information gathered at the patient/family visits and during team meetings

The documentation should reflect ongoing effects of the terminal condition, the patient's/family's difficulty with care or coping, and the continued desire for hospice care

Document coordination of services and consultations with the other members of the IDG

10. **Resources for hospice care and practice**

The Mayday Pain Resource Center is a clearinghouse for information and resources to improve the quality of pain management and can be reached at 1-818-359-8111, ext. 3829. The Roxane Pain Institute provides informational booklets and articles on pain management and can be reached at 1-800-335-9100 or via e-mail at http://www. roxane.com/roxane/pri (no period at the end).

Available free from the Agency for Health Care Policy and Research (AHCPR) are three resources: *Clinical Practice Guideline Number 9: Management of Cancer Pain, Quick Reference Guide for Clinicians: Management of Cancer Pain: Adults,* and *Consumer's Guide: Management of Cancer Pain.* The patient guides are available in English and Spanish, and all can be ordered by calling 1-800-358-9295.

Get Relief From Cancer Pain is a pamphlet available from the National Cancer Institute's Cancer Information Service. Call 1-800-4-CANCER (1-800-422-6237).

Questions and Answers About Pain Control is a 76-page booklet available free from the National Cancer Institute's Cancer Information Service. Call 1-800-4-CANCER (1-800-422-6237).

Many drug companies provide easily carried equianalgesic charts; contact the representatives, who are usually very willing to help clinicians and share resources.

PROSTATE CANCER CARE

1. **General considerations**

   Many patients with prostate cancer have a long history of curative-focused care interventions such as surgery, radiation, and chemotherapy. The hospice team interventions focus on care and comfort, while providing support to the patient and the family.

   Please refer to "Cancer Care," "Pain Care," and "Supportive Care" should these sections also pertain to your patient.

2. **Needs for visit**

   Physician order for hospice care, specific to the hospice program's admission criteria and policies

   Standard precautions supplies

   Vital signs equipment for baseline assessment

   Other supplies or equipment, based on physician orders

3. **Safety considerations**

   Infection control/standard precautions

   Night-light

   Extra caution on slippery surfaces

   Removal of scatter rugs

   Tub rail, grab bars for bathroom safety

   Supportive and nonskid shoes

   Handrail on stairs

   Fall precautions/protocol

   Phone number of person to call with a care or pain problem

   Supportive and well-fitting, nonslip shoes

   Equipment safety for home medical equipment (e.g., wheelchair, walker)

   Protective skin measures

   Identification and report of any skin problems

   Smoke detector and fire evacuation plan

   Assistance with ambulation

   Others, based on the patient's unique condition and environment

4. **Potential diagnoses and codes**

Adenocarcinoma, metastatic	199.1
Attention to other artificial opening of urinary tract	V55.6
Bladder cancer	188.9
Bone metastasis	198.5
Cancer of the prostate	185
Fracture, pathological	733.10
Incontinence of feces	787.6
Incontinence of urine	788.30
Kidney, cancer of the (renal)	189.0
Pain, low back	724.2
Pressure ulcer	707.0
Prostate, cancer of	185

Prostatectomy (TURP) (surgical)	60.2
Prostatitis	601.9
Rectosigmoid, cancer of	154.0
Rectum, cancer of the	154.1
Renal cell cancer, metastatic	198.0
Urinary tract infection	599.0

5. **Associated nursing diagnoses**
   Activity intolerance
   Activity intolerance, risk for
   Adjustment, impaired
   Airway clearance, ineffective
   Anxiety
   Aspiration, risk for
   Body image disturbance
   Body temperature, altered, risk for
   Bowel incontinence
   Breathing pattern, ineffective
   Cardiac output, decreased
   Caregiver role strain
   Caregiver role strain, risk for
   Constipation
   Coping, ineffective family: compromised
   Decisional conflict (treatments)
   Denial, ineffective
   Diarrhea
   Family processes, altered
   Fatigue
   Fear
   Grieving, anticipatory
   Home maintenance management, impaired
   Incontinence, total
   Infection, risk for
   Injury, risk for
   Knowledge deficit (disease and management)
   Mobility, impaired physical
   Nutrition, altered: less than body requirements
   Oral mucous membrane, altered
   Pain
   Pain, chronic
   Parenting, altered
   Protection, altered
   Role performance, altered
   Self-care deficit, bathing/hygiene
   Self-care deficit, dressing/grooming
   Self-care deficit, feeding
   Self-care deficit, toileting
   Sensory/perceptual alterations (specify) (visual, auditory, kinesthetic, gustatory, tactile, olfactory)
   Sexual dysfunction

Skin integrity, impaired
Skin integrity, impaired, risk for
Sleep pattern disturbance
Social interaction, impaired
Spiritual distress (distress of the human spirit)
Spiritual well-being, potential for enhanced
Thought processes, altered
Tissue integrity, impaired
Urinary elimination, altered
Urinary retention

6. **Skills and services identified**

   • *Hospice nursing*

     a. *Comfort and symptom control*
        Skilled observation and complete systems assessment of the patient with prostate cancer admitted to hospice
        Presentation of hospice philosophy and services
        Explain patient rights and responsibilities
        Assess patient, family, and caregiver wishes and expectations regarding care
        Assess patient, family, and caregiver resources available for care
        Assess pain and other symptoms, including site, duration, characteristics, and relief measures
        Provision of volunteer support to patient and family
        Teach family or caregiver physical care of patient
        RN to provide and teach effective oral care and comfort measures
        Teach care of bedridden patient
        Measure vital signs and pain q visit
        Assess cardiovascular, pulmonary, and respiratory statuses
        Oxygen on at _____ liter per _____ (specify physician orders)
        Pain assessment and management
        RN to assess patient's pain or other symptoms q visit to identify need for change, addition, or other plan or dose adjustment
        RN to teach patient and caregiver about disease process and management
        Comfort measures of backrub and hand or other therapeutic massage
        Teach caregiver or family care of weak, terminally ill patient
        Observation, assessment, and supportive care to patient and family
        Teach patient/family use of standardized form/tool to use between hospice team members' visits (and for care coordination between team members)
        Supportive care and scopolamine patches as ordered per physician orders
        Teach patient/family principles of effective pain management
        Effective management of pain and prevention of secondary symptoms
        Interventions of symptoms directed toward comfort and palliation
        Pain assessment and management q visit, including source of pain (e.g., cancer pain, infection, pathological fracture, other medical problems such as cardiac or arthritis pain)

Observation and assessment, communication with physician related to signs and symptoms of continuing decompensation and increased symptoms, pain, discomfort, and shortness of breath, and measures to alleviate and control

Teach patient and family about realistic expectations of disease process

Teach care of dying and signs/symptoms of impending death

Presence and support

Other interventions, based on patient/family needs

b. *Safety and mobility considerations*

Provide caregiver with home safety information and instruction related to _____ (specify) and documented in the clinical record

Teach family regarding safety of patient in home

Teach family regarding energy conservation techniques

Teach family regarding home safety and fall precautions

Other interventions, based on patient/family needs

c. *Emotional/spiritual considerations*

Psychosocial assessment of patient and family regarding disease and prognosis

RN to provide emotional support to patient and family

Assess mental status and sleep disturbance changes

Observation of patient for neuropsychiatric complications of illness, including confusion, depression, and anxiety

RN to provide support and intervention for depression

Teach patient/family about depression and signs/symptoms of exacerbation that necessitate more intervention

Assess for and manage plans for psychosocial and/or spiritual pain (e.g., all pain, anxiety, interpersonal and other distress)

Observation and assessment of mental status changes/complaints of depression in new hospice patient with cancer of the prostate

Psychosocial aspects of pain control (e.g., depression) assessed and acknowledged with team support/intervention

Ongoing acknowledgment of spirituality and related concerns of patient/family

Other interventions, based on patient/family needs

d. *Skin care*

RN to teach patient regarding irradiated skin sites

Teach caregiver regarding patient's skin care needs, including the need for frequent position changes, appropriate pressure pads and mattresses, and the prevention of breakdown

Pressure ulcer care as indicated

Assess skin integrity q visit

Observation and evaluation of wound and surrounding skin

Evaluate patient's need for equipment, including supplies to decrease pressure, alternating pressure mattress, gel foam seat cushion, and heel and elbow protectors

Teach family to perform dressing between RN visits, specifically

_____

Teach patient, family, or caregiver about proper body alignment and positioning in bed to prevent skin tears from shearing skin

Observe and apply skilled assessment of areas for possible breakdown, including heels, hips, elbows, ankles, and other pressure-prone areas

Other interventions, based on patient/family needs

e. *Elimination considerations*

Assess bowel regimen, and implement program as needed

RN to assess patient's bowel patterns and need for stool softeners, laxatives, and dietary adjustments, and to develop bowel management plan

Assess amount and frequency of urinary output

Teach catheter care to caregiver

Check for and remove impaction as needed

Condom catheter or indwelling catheter care as ordered

Observation and complete systems assessment of patient with an indwelling catheter

RN to change catheter every 4 weeks and to make 3 prn visits for catheter problems, including patient complaints, signs and symptoms of infection, and other factors necessitating evaluation and possible catheter change

RN to teach caregiver daily care of catheter

Teaching and ongoing assessment for prevention and early identification of constipation and its correction/resolution

Initiate bowel management program per physician

Implement bowel assessment management program

Teach patient, family, and aide the importance of observing and noting bowel movements between scheduled nursing visits

Obtain patient history related to norms for bowel movements to date (e.g., "all my life I go only every other day")

Bowel management program of stool softeners, laxative of choice, Fleet's Enemas prn, and other methods per patient wishes and physician orders

Other interventions, based on patient/family needs

f. *Hydration/nutrition*

Assess nutrition and hydration statuses

Diet counseling for patient with anorexia

RN to teach family about patient's need for small, high-calorie meals of his or her choice

Nutrition/hydration supported by offering patient's choice of favorite or desired foods or liquids

Nutrition/hydration maintained by offering patient high-protein diet and foods of choice as tolerated

Other interventions, based on patient/family needs

g. *Therapeutic/medication regimens*

Teach new pain or symptom control medication regimen

Teach new medications and effects

Assess for electrolyte imbalance

Teach and observe regarding side effects of chemotherapy, including constipation, anemia, and fatigue

Medication review, education, and management

Assess the patient's response to therapeutic treatments and interventions, and report any changes or unfavorable responses to the physician

Ongoing observation, assessment, and intervention related to side effects of therapy, including fever, dry skin, mouth pain/sores/ulcers, extreme tiredness, and depression due to symptoms and poor energy level

Teach patient and caregiver use of PCA pump

Nonpharmacological interventions such as progressive muscle relaxation, imagery, positive visualization, music, massage and touch, and humor therapy of patient's choice

Teaching of patient/family, including medications, management program, strength, type, actions, times, and compliance tips

Encourage family/caregivers to give the patient medications on the schedule and around the clock

Medications changed using equianalgesic conversion tables/physician orders (e.g., from oral morphine to an equianalgesic dose of transdermal fentanyl)

Nonpharmacological or other interventions, including relaxation, hot/cold therapy, biofeedback, distraction, guided imagery, humor, music therapy, acupuncture, TENS technology, hypnosis, and massage

Other interventions, based on patient/family needs

h. *Other considerations*

Assess progression of disease process

RN to assess the patient's response to treatments and interventions and to report to the physician changes, unfavorable responses, or reactions

Other interventions, based on patient/family needs

- **Home health aide or certified nursing assistant**

Effective and safe personal care

Safe ADL assistance and support

Respite care and active listening skills

Observation and reporting

Meal preparation

Homemaker services

Comfort care

Other duties

- **Hospice social worker**

Psychosocial assessment of patient and family/caregiver, including adjustment to illness and its implications

Identification of optimal coping strategies

Financial assessment and counseling regarding food acquisition, ability to prepare, and costs of needed medications

Intervention/support related to terminal illness and loss

Emotional/spiritual support

Depression/fear assessed

Facilitate communication among patient, family, and hospice team

Referral/linkage to community services and resources as indicated

Grief counseling and intervention/support related to illness/loss

Patient/caregiver counseling and support

Identification of caregiver role strain necessitating respite/relief measures/support

For patients who live alone with no support system (e.g., able, available, willing caregiver[s]): obtain resources to enable patient to remain in home

Identification of illness-related psychiatric condition necessitating care

- *Volunteer(s)*

Support, friendship, companionship, and presence

Comfort and dignity maintained/provided for patient and family

Advocacy and respite

Errands and transportation

Other services, based on interdisciplinary team recommendations and patient/caregiver needs

- *Spiritual counselor*

Spiritual assessment and care

Counseling, intervention, and support related to that dimension of life related to life's meaning (consistent with patient's beliefs)

Support, listening, and presence

Participation in sacred or spiritual rituals or practices

Other supportive care, based on patient/family needs and belief systems

- *Dietitian/nutritional counseling*

Supportive counseling with patient/family indicating that patient will have a decreased appetite and possible inability to eat/drink

Assessment and recommendations for swallowing difficulties

Teaching and support of family members and caregivers

Evaluation/management of nutritional deficits and needs

Food and dietary recommendations incorporate patient choice and wishes

- *Occupational therapist*

Evaluation of ADL and functional mobility

Assess for need for adaptive equipment and assistive devices

Safety assessment of patient's environment and ADLs

Assessment for energy conservation training

Teach compensatory techniques

- *Physical therapist*

Evaluation

Safety assessment of patient's environment

Safe transfer training or bed mobility exercises

Pain assessment/reduction factors

Strengthening exercises/program

Assessment of gait safety and home safety measures

Instruct/supervise caregiver and volunteers on home exercise program for conditioning and strength

Assistive, adaptive devices and evaluation of equipment and teaching

- *Speech-language pathologist*

Evaluation for speech/swallowing problems

Food texture recommendations

Alternate functional communication

- *Bereavement counselor*

  Assessment of the needs of the bereaved family and friends

  Support and intervention, based on assessment and ongoing findings

  Presence and counseling

  Supportive visits, follow-up, and other interventions (e.g., mailings, calls)

  Other services related to bereavement work and support

- *Pharmacist*

  Evaluation of hospice patient with constipation on cathartics, stool soften-
      ers, and other medications for possible food/drug and drug/drug interac-
      tions

  Medication monitoring regarding therapeutic levels and dosages

  Pain consult and input into interdisciplinary plan of care related to pain
      control, palliation, and symptom management

  Assessment of medication regimen and plan for safety and compliance

- *Music, massage, art, or other therapies or services*

  Evaluation and intervention based on patient's and caregiver's unique
      wishes and needs that support care, comfort, and death in the setting of
      the patient's choice

  Assessment plan to engage patient and support comfort, quality, enjoyment,
      and dignity

  Pet therapy (including patient's pet, if available) and therapeutic interven-
      tion

7. **Outcomes for care**

- *Hospice nursing*

  Patient and caregiver verbalize satisfaction with care

  Patient will decide on care and pain intervention and evaluation

  Patient will experience increased comfort and pain control through self-
      report (specify parameters)

  Patient will have palliative care and comfort maintained through death

  Patent and infection-free catheter

  Patient and caregiver knowledgeable about side effects (e.g., constipation)
      and interventions needed

  Control of pain and other symptoms that affect daily function, quality of
      life, and ability to interact with friends/family

  Teaching related to safety, medications, catheter, and self-care successful as
      demonstrated by patient's verbalization (specify measurable parameters)

  Effective pain control and symptom relief by _____ (specify
      date)

  Patient and caregiver knowledgeable about pain regimen, relief measures,
      and care for optimal relief/control

  Early detection and intervention of problems related to patients with
      immobility/bedbound status

  Patient is protected from injury, has stable respiratory status, and is compli-
      ant with medication, safety, and care regimens

  Comfort and individualized intervention of patient with immobility/
      bedbound status (e.g., skin, urinary, musculature, vascular)

  Spiritual and psychosocial needs met (specify) as defined by patient and
      caregiver throughout course of care

Educational tools/plans incorporated in daily care, and patient/caregiver verbalizes understanding of safe, needed care

Patient will decide on care, interventions, and evaluation of care processes

Caregiver is effective in care management, verbalizes changes, and knows whom to call for questions/concerns

Patient will express satisfaction with hospice support received and will experience increased comfort

Patient will be made comfortable at home through death in accordance with the patient's wishes

Effective pain control and symptom control verbalized by patient

Patient verbalizes understanding of and adheres to care and medication regimens

Patient and caregiver supported through patient's death

Comfort maintained through course of care

The patient and family receive hospice support and care, and family members and friends are able to spend quality time with the patient

Caregiver able and verbalizes comfort with role and understands when to call hospice team members

Patient supported through and receives the maximum benefit from palliative chemotherapy and radiation with minimal complications

Patient and caregiver list adverse reactions, potential complications, signs/symptoms of infection (e.g., sputum change, chest congestion)

Comfort maintained through death with dignity

Pain effectively managed, and patient verbalizes comfort

Comfort through death with support and care of hospice team

Mental distress, depression, and fear of dying addressed throughout care by hospice team

Family able to care for and support patient

Patient and caregiver can verbalize symptoms, changes, or accelerations that necessitate call to physician

Patient and family demonstrate compliance with medication regimen and other therapeutic interventions

Patient demonstrates stabilization and increased or enhanced coping skills related to functioning and depression

Pain and symptoms managed/controlled in setting of patient/family choice (e.g., patient/family report ability to eat, sleep, speak with pacing)

Planned and effective bowel program, as evidenced by regular bowel movements and patient/family report of comfort

Death with dignity, and pain/symptoms controlled in setting of patient/family choice

Optimal comfort, support, and dignity provided throughout illness

Death with maximum comfort through effective symptom control with specialized hospice support

Patient and caregiver able to list adverse drug reactions/problems with medication regimen and whom to call for follow-up and resolution

Patient's/family's privacy, independence, and choices supported with respect and maintained through death

Enhancement and support of quality of life

Effective symptom relief and control (e.g., a peaceful and comfortable
  death at home, depression controlled, some enjoyment of life)

Maximizing the patient's quality of life (e.g., alert and pain free or as
  patient wishes)

Pharmacological and nonpharmacological interventions, such as localized
  heat application, biofeedback, massage, positioning, relaxation methods,
  and music

Patient and caregiver demonstrate appropriate back-up or "rescue" therapies
  for breakthrough pain or other symptoms (e.g., dyspnea)

Patient cared for and family supported through death with physical, psychosocial, spiritual, and other concerns/needs acknowledged/addressed

Patient- and family-centered hospice care provided based on the patient's/
  family's unique situation and needs

Infection control and palliation through death in setting of patient's choice

Grief/bereavement expression and support provided

Patient is pain free by next _____ visit

Caregiver demonstrates ability to manage pain, where applicable

Patient maintains comfort and dignity throughout illness

Other outcomes/goals, based on the patient condition with input from the
  hospice team and patient and family

- *Home health aide or certified nursing assistant*
  Effective hygiene, personal care, and comfort maintained
  ADL assistance
  Safe environment maintained

- *Hospice social worker*
  Problem identified and addressed, with patient/caregiver linked with appro-
    priate support services and plan of care successfully implemented
  Patient and caregiver cope adaptively with illness and death
  Adaptive adjustment to changed body and body image
  Psychosocial support and counseling offered to patient/caregivers experi-
    encing loss and grief
  Caregiver system assessed, and development of stable caregiver plan facili-
    tated

- *Volunteer(s)*
  Comfort, companionship, and friendship extended to patient/family
  Support and respite provided as defined by the needs of the patient/
    caregiver
  Patient and family supported by team with care, comfort, and companion-
    ship

- *Spiritual counseling*
  Spiritual support offered and provided as defined by needs of patient/
    caregiver
  Provision of spiritual support and care as based on the assessed and
    ongoing needs of the patient and family
  Spiritual support offered, and patient and family needs met
  Participation in sacred or spiritual rituals or practices
  Patient and family express relief of symptoms of spiritual suffering
  Support, listening, and presence

- *Dietitian/nutritional counseling*

  Family and caregiver integrate recommendations into daily meal planning (when appropriate)

  Patient and caregiver know whom to call for nutrition- and hydration-related questions/concerns

  Nutrition/hydration per patient choices

  Caregiver integrates recommendations into daily meal planning

  Patient and family verbalize comprehension of changing nutritional needs

- *Occupational therapist*

  Patient and caregiver demonstrate maximum independence with ADLs, adaptive techniques, and assistive devices

  Patient and caregiver demonstrate maximum safety in ADL and functional mobility

  Patient and caregiver demonstrate effective use of energy conservation techniques

  Verbalization/demonstration of improved functional activity level and enhanced quality of life

  Patient and caregiver demonstrate effective use of diaphragmatic breathing to reduce shortness of breath and relaxation techniques to help in pain/symptom management

- *Physical therapist*

  Prevention of complications

  Home exercise and upper extremity program taught to caregiver

  Optimal strength, mobility, and function maintained/achieved

  Compliance with home exercise program by _____ (date)

  Comfort measures of backrub or hand or other therapeutic massage

- *Speech-language pathologist*

  Communication method implemented, and patient able to be understand as self-reported or reported by family/caregivers

  Safe swallowing and functional communication

  Recommended lists of food/textures for safety and patient choice

- *Bereavement counselor*

  Grief support services provided to patient and family

  Well-being and resolution process of grief initiated and followed through bereavement services

- *Pharmacist*

  Regimen for bowel regimen successful as self-reported by patient and in update at team meeting

  Multiple drug regimen reviewed for food/drug and drug/drug interactions in patient on multiple medications

  Stability and safety in complex medication regimen, with maximum benefit to patient

  Effective pain and symptom control and management as reported by patient/caregiver

- *Music, massage, art, or other therapies or services*

  Therapeutic massage/touch effective for patient as self-reported or observed by caregivers/family

Improved muscle tone, relaxation, and/or sleep

Patient comfortable and relaxed (e.g., sleeping) after massage

Music therapy intervention based on assessment to decrease pain perception and provide emotional expression and support

Maintenance of comfort and physical, psychosocial, and spiritual health

Holistic health maintained and comfort achieved through _____ (specify modality)

Patient has pet's presence as desired—in all care sites, when possible

8. **Patient, family, and caregiver educational needs**

Educational needs are the care regimens that contribute to safe and effective care at home between the hospice team's visits. These include the following:

The basic tenets of hospice and the availability of support 24 hours a day, 7 days a week

Home safety assessment and counseling

The patient's medication regimen

Safe and proper body mechanics to promote patient comfort and prevent caregiver safety problems

Support groups available to patient's family, such as the hospice program's "Caregiver Support Group" meetings for family members and friends of the patient

Anticipated disease progression

The availability of adequate pain relief measures

The need for keeping records related to and assessing for constipation

The safe use of oxygen therapy at home

The therapeutic and palliative value of nonpharmacological comfort measures, such as positioning, massage, progressive muscle relaxation, and other interventions of patient choice

The patient's medications and their relationship to each other

The importance of round-the-clock analgesia

Teach patient management of hair loss

The importance of medical follow-up

Care of the catheter, changing bags, and signs of catheter problems

The availability of support and hospice programs, if appropriate

Teach about the prevention of infection and the signs and symptoms of infection

Other teaching specific to the patient's and caregiver's needs

9. **Specific tips for quality and reimbursement**

Document any variances to expected outcomes. There are many models of hospice programs. Those that are home health agency–based must work within the framework of the Medicare home care program. For example, sometimes a hospice patient reaches a stable period in the illness and has no further skilled needs or the patient is no longer homebound per Medicare home health care criteria. When this occurs, one option is to discharge the patient from Medicare home health agency reimbursement and maintain the patient on grant funds or other available resources. If the patient's status deteriorates and again meets the Medicare criteria, a new start of care is initiated on the HCFA form 485. Usually hospices continue volunteer support,

nursing, and other services indicated during these periods of no reimbursement.

The Medicare hospice benefit does not require that the patient be homebound or have identified skilled needs. Though it is a needed and viable program, the Medicare hospice benefit may not be indicated for all Medicare-eligible beneficiaries. For further information on this benefit, please refer to HCFA Hospice Manual 21.

Should the patient's status deteriorate and increased personal care be needed, obtain a telephone order for the increased service, noting frequency and estimating the duration.

Obtain a telephone order for all medication and treatment changes of the medical regimen, and document these in the clinical record.

Document changes to the plan of care such as medications, services, frequency, communication, and concurrence of other team members

Document coordination of services or consultation of the other members of the IDT

Unless the patient is in a hospice insurance program, some insurers will not pay for a skilled nurse visit that is made at death if the patient is dead when the nurse arrives at the home. From a Medicare home care perspective, the visit at the time of death may be covered when the orders and clinical record document assessment of the patient's status or signs of death/life or state law allows pronouncement of death by a nurse.

Document patient deterioration

Document dehydration, dehydrating

Document patient change or instability

Document pain, other symptoms not controlled

Document status after acute episode of _____ (specify)

Document positive urine, sputum, etc. culture; patient started on _____ (specify ordered antibiotic therapy)

Document patient impacted; impaction removed manually per physician's orders

Document RN in frequent communication with physician regarding _____ (specify)

Document febrile at _____, pulse change at _____, irr., irr.

Document change noted in _____

Document bony prominences red, opening

Document RN contacted physician regarding _____ (specify)

Document marked SOB

Document alteration in mental status

Document medications being adjusted, regulated, or monitored

Document unable to perform own ADLs, personal care

Document all interdisciplinary team meetings and communications in the POC and in the progress notes of the clinical record

All hospice team members should have input into the POC and document their interventions and goals

Document all patient changes in the clinical record

Document an exacerbation of symptoms

Document unstable, not stable

Document urine culture obtained and the results

Document RN in communication with physician regarding _____
(specify)

Document any POC change in the documentation and obtain orders for all
changes

Document the coordination of care and communications among/between disciplines

Document communications and care coordination with other care providers,
such as skilled nursing facility or nursing home staff, inpatient team
members, and hired caregivers

Document in the clinical notes the clear progression and symptomatology and
interventions that demonstrate the interventions and overall management
of the patient with pain

Document when/if the patient has respiratory changes, shortness of breath,
exacerbation of conditions, dysphagia, changes in pain, and other symptoms and that they are identified and resolved

Remember that the clinical documentation is key to measuring compliance
for quality and reimbursement purposes. Care coordination, timely verbal
and initial physician orders, and assessment and addressing of spiritual
and psychosocial needs should be ongoing and documented in the patient's clinical record

The documentation should support that all hospice care supports comfort and
dignity while meeting patient/family needs

The documentation should include ongoing assessment and management of
pain and other symptoms and the anticipation and prevention of secondary symptoms such as constipation

It is important to note that all team members, including nurses and social
workers, should assess, identify, and "hear" spiritual needs that the
patient/family want to be addressed. These spiritual issues are key to the
provision of quality hospice care and cannot be addressed effectively and
promptly by the spiritual counselor only

Document clearly symptoms, clinical changes, and assessment findings
related to pain and patient care

Document weight loss, increased shortness of breath, dyspnea, infection,
sepsis, new or changed medications, etc.

Document any skin changes (e.g., inflamed, painful, weeping skin site[s])

Remember that the "litmus test" of care coordination rests on the quality of
the clinical documentation by all team members. Review one of your patient's clinical records and ask yourself the following: "If I was unable to
give a verbal report/update on this patient's/family's course of care,
would a peer be able to pick up and provide the same level of care and
know (from the documentation) the current orders, medications, and other
details that contribute to effective hospice care?"

This patient population usually has many clinical changes that should be
documented. These include weight loss and multiple and changed medication regimens with varying routes. Side effects to the drug regimen should
be observed, noted, documented, and reported

Your assessments, observations, and clinical findings assist in painting a
picture to support coverage and documentation requirements for hospice
care

Document any hospitalizations and changed clinical findings

Document patient changes, symptoms, and psychosocial issues impacting the patient and family and plan of care

Document patient changes, symptoms, and clinical information identified from visits and team conferences that support hospice care and a limited life expectancy

Clearly support in the documentation the rationale that supports/explains the progression of the illness from the chronic to terminal stages

Document mentation, behavioral, and/or cognitive changes

Document dysphagia, weight loss, increased shortness of breath, dyspnea, infection, sepsis, new or changed medications, etc.

Document any skin changes (e.g., inflamed, painful, weeping skin site[s])

Document when the patient is actively dying, deteriorating, or progressing toward death

10. **Resources for hospice care and practice**

The National Institutes of Health's National Cancer Institute offers *What You Need to Know About Prostate Cancer, Caring for the Patient with Cancer at Home,* and other information. Call the Cancer Information Service at 1-800-4-CANCER. The American Foundation for Urologic Disease can be reached at 1-410-727-2908 and maintains a network of prostate cancer survivor organizations and services and initiates prostate cancer advocacy programs.

The American Cancer Society has support groups such as "I Can Cope" and other programs. To locate the chapter nearest your patient, call 1-800-ACS-2345.

Facts on Prostate Cancer can be obtained from the American Cancer Society by calling 1-800-ACS-2345.

RENAL DISEASE CARE (END STAGE)

1. **General conditions**

   Patients with renal disease, or ESRD, may have a long history of multiple surgeries and treatment interventions related to access sites such as shunts and sometimes transplants and infections, with the devastating cycle of rejection. Other care problems may include DM, CVA, hypertension, and skin care problems. Some patients choose to discontinue dialysis because of illness, whereas others may be referred to hospice because of more acute kidney or other health problems. Please refer to "Bedbound Care," "Cardiac Care (End Stage)," or "Pain Care" should these sections also pertain to your patient.

2. **Needs for visit**

   Physician order for hospice care, specific to the hospice program's admission criteria policies

   Standard precautions supplies

   Vital signs equipment for baseline assessment

   Other supplies or equipment, based on physician orders

3. **Safety considerations**

   Infection control/standard precautions

   Night-light

   Protective skin measures

   Identification and report of any skin problems

   Tub rail, grab bars for bathroom safety

   Supportive and nonskid shoes

   Cardiac/diabetes/bleeding precautions based on medication regimen(s)

   Fall precautions/protocol

   The phone number and name of person to call with a care problem

   Safety for home medical equipment (e.g., wheelchair, walker)

   Smoke detector and fire evacuation plan

   Others, based on the patient's unique condition and environment

4. **Potential diagnoses and codes**

Acute myocardial infarction	410.92
Acute pyelonephritis	590.10
Acute renal failure	584.9
Anemia	285.9
Angina pectoris	413.9
Ascites	789.5
Benign prostatic hypertrophy	600
Bronchitis, acute	466.0
CAPD (continuous ambulatory peritoneal dialysis)	54.98
Chronic ischemic heart disease	414.9
Chronic renal failure	585
Cirrhosis of the liver	571.5
Congestive heart failure	428.0

Constipation	564.0
Convulsions	780.3
COPD	496
Coronary artery disease (CAD)	414.00
CVA	436
Debility	799.3
Decubitus ulcer (pressure ulcer)	707.0
Dehydration	276.5
Diabetes mellitus, with complications, adult	250.90
Diabetes mellitus, with complications, juv.	250.91
Diabetic nephropathy	250.41 and 583.81
Emphysema	492.8
Gastritis	535.50
Glomerulonephritis	583.9
Heart disease, chronic ischemic	414.9
Heart failure	428.9
Heart failure, left	428.1
Hemiplegia	342.9
Hepatitis	573.3
Hepatitis B	070.30
Hepatitis (viral)	070.9
Hypercalcemia	275.4
Hyperosmolality	276.0
Hypertension	403.91
Hypoglycemia	251.2
Hypopotassemia	276.8
Kidney, cancer of the (renal)	189.0
Kidney transplant (S/P)	V42.0
Kidney transplant (surgical)	55.69
Liver disorder	573.9
Lung disease	518.89
Malaise and fatigue	780.7
Malnutrition	263.9
Myocardial infarction	410.92
Nephrosclerosis	403.91
Nephrotic syndrome	581.9
Neuropathy	357.2
Obesity	278.0
Peptic ulcer	533.90
Pericardial effusion	423.9
Pericarditis	423.9
Peripheral neuropathy	357.4
Peripheral vascular disease	443.9
Peritonitis	567.9
Pneumonia	486
Postoperative infection	998.5
Postoperative wound disruption	998.3
Pressure ulcer	707.0
Protein-caloric malnutrition	263.9

Psychosis	294.8
Pyelonephritis	590.80
Renal cell cancer, metastatic	198.0
Renal failure, chronic	585
Renal polycystic disease	753.12
Renal transplant (surgical)	50.59
Retention of urine	788.20
Septicemia	038.9
Shunt, arteriovenous	V45.1
Shunt, infected	996.62
Shunt, peritoneovascular	54.94
Shunt revision (surgical)	39.42
Skin eruptions, nonspecific	782.1
Stomach ulcer	531.90
Systemic lupus erythematosus	710.0
Tubular necrosis (acute)	584.5
Urinary retention	788.20
Wound debridement	86.28
Wound dehiscence	998.3

5. **Associated nursing diagnoses**
   Activity intolerance
   Anxiety
   Body image disturbance
   Bowel incontinence
   Cardiac output, decreased
   Caregiver role strain
   Caregiver role strain, risk for
   Constipation
   Coping, family: potential for growth
   Coping, ineffective family: compromised
   Coping, ineffective family: disabling
   Coping, ineffective individual
   Diarrhea
   Family processes, altered
   Fatigue
   Fear
   Fluid volume deficit, risk for
   Fluid volume excess
   Gas exchange, impaired
   Health maintenance, altered
   Home maintenance management, impaired
   Hopelessness
   Infection, risk for
   Injury, risk for
   Knowledge deficit (related to renal disease and care)
   Management of therapeutic regimen (individuals), ineffective
   Mobility, impaired physical
   Noncompliance (specify)

Nutrition, altered: less than body requirements
Nutrition, altered: more than body requirements
Oral mucous membrane, altered
Pain
Pain, chronic
Peripheral neurovascular dysfunction, risk for
Powerlessness
Protection, altered
Self-care deficit, bathing/hygiene
Self-care deficit, dressing/grooming
Self-care deficit, feeding
Self-care deficit, toileting
Sensory/perceptual alterations (specify) (visual, auditory, kinesthetic, gustatory, tactile, olfactory)
Sexual dysfunction
Skin integrity, impaired
Skin integrity, impaired, risk for
Sleep patterns, altered
Spiritual distress (distress of the human spirit)
Spiritual well-being, potential for enhanced
Thought processes, altered
Tissue perfusion, altered (renal)
Urinary elimination, altered

6. **Skills and services identified**

   • *Hospice nursing*

      a. *Comfort and symptom control*
         Comprehensive assessment of cardiovascular and all other systems in patient with impaired renal function admitted to hospice for _____ (specify)
         Observation and assessment of the patient with RF problem necessitating care
         Presentation of hospice philosophy and services
         Explain patient rights and responsibilities
         Assess patient, family, and caregiver wishes and expectations regarding care
         Assess patient, family, and caregiver resources available for care
         Assess pain and other symptoms, including site, duration, characteristics, and relief measures
         Provision of volunteer support to patient and family
         Teach family or caregiver physical care of patient
         RN to provide and teach effective oral care and comfort measures
         Teach signs and symptoms of bleeding and precautions
         RN to teach patient and caregiver self-observational and care skills (e.g., TPR, I and O, BP, weight, and record keeping)
         Report changes, including signs and symptoms, to physician
         Monitor for signs and symptoms of infection
         Teach about effective oral hygiene measures
         Monitor blood pressure and other vital signs

Oxygen on at _____ liter per _____ (specify physician orders)

Assess progression of disease process

Identify and monitor pain, symptoms, and relief measures

Teach caregiver or family care of weak, terminally ill patient

RN to instruct in pain-control measures and medications

Teach patient/family use of standardized form/tool to use between hospice team members' visits (and for care coordination between team members)

Teach patient/family principles of effective pain management

Observation and assessment, communication with physician related to signs and symptoms of continuing decompensation and increased symptoms, pain, discomfort, and shortness of breath, and measures to alleviate and control

Effective management of pain and prevention of secondary symptoms

Interventions of symptoms directed toward comfort and palliation

Pain assessment and management q visit, including source of pain (e.g., cancer pain, infection, pathological fracture, other medical problems, such as cardiac or arthritis pain)

RN to assess patient's pain or other symptoms q visit to identify need for change, addition, or other plan or dose adjustment

Teach caregiver/patient use of pain assessment tool/scale and reporting mechanism(s)

Observation, assessment, and comfort measures of neuropathy, encephalopathy, and edema

Teach patient and family about realistic expectations of disease process

Teach care of dying and signs/symptoms of impending death

Presence and support

Other interventions, based on patient/family needs

b. *Safety and mobility considerations*

Provide caregiver with home safety information and instruction related to _____ and documented in the clinical record

Teach family about safety of patient in home

Teach family about energy conservation techniques

Other interventions, based on patient/family needs

c. *Emotional/spiritual considerations*

Psychosocial assessment of patient and family regarding disease and prognosis

RN to provide emotional support to patient and family

Assess mental status and sleep disturbance changes

Observation and assessment of mental status changes/complaints of depression

Observation of patient for neuropsychiatric complications of illness, including confusion, depression, and anxiety

RN to provide support and intervention for depression

Teach patient/family about depression and signs/symptoms of exacerbation that necessitate more intervention

Psychosocial aspects of pain control (e.g., depression) assessed and acknowledged with team support/intervention

Assess for and manage plans for psychosocial and/or spiritual pain (e.g., all pain, anxiety, interpersonal and other distress)

Ongoing acknowledgment of spirituality and related concerns of patient/family

Other interventions, based on patient/family needs

d. *Skin care*

Teach caregiver wound care regimen

Assessment of dressing and teaching to patient and caregiver about subclavian access

Teach application of topical lotion to pruritic areas

Assessment of infection shunt, graft, or fistula sites

Teach caregiver patient's skin care needs, including the need for frequent position changes, appropriate pressure pads and mattresses, and the prevention of breakdown

Pressure ulcer care as indicated

Assess skin integrity

Observation and evaluation of wound and surrounding skin

Evaluate patient's need for equipment, including supplies to decrease pressure, alternating pressure mattress, gel foam seat cushion, and heel and elbow protectors

Teach family to perform dressing between RN visits, specifically

---

Teach patient, family, or caregiver about proper body alignment and positioning in bed to prevent skin tears from shearing skin

Observe and apply skilled assessment of areas for possible breakdown, including heels, hips, elbows, ankles, and other pressure-prone areas

Other interventions, based on patient/family needs

e. *Elimination considerations*

Assess bowel regimen, and implement program as needed

Monitor bowel patterns and need for stool softeners, laxatives, and dietary adjustments, and develop bowel management plan

Catheterize patient for residual urine

Assess amount and frequency of urinary output

Teach catheter care to caregiver

RN to teach caregiver daily care of catheter

Teaching and ongoing assessment for the prevention and early identification of constipation and its correction/resolution

Implement bowel assessment and management program

Teach patient, family, and aide the importance of observing and noting bowel movements between scheduled nursing visits

Obtain patient history related to norms for bowel movements to date (e.g., "all my life I go only every other day")

Consider stool softeners, and offer laxative of choice, Fleet's Enemas prn, and other methods per patient wishes and physician orders

Other interventions, based on patient/family needs

f. *Hydration/nutrition*

Monitoring/reporting of fluid changes in patient (e.g., weight increase, edema, shortness of breath)

RN to teach patient and caregiver nutrition and hydration regimen

Instruct about diet (e.g., low protein with fluid or other specified dietary orders and restrictions as specified by physician)

Nutrition/hydration supported by offering patient's choice of favorite or desired foods or liquids

Other interventions, based on patient/family needs

g. *Therapeutic/medication regimens*

Administer epoetin (EPO) sq _____ (specify dose and frequency)

Venipuncture to monitor patient's hematocrit related to anemia and EPO therapy

RN to assess for complications of new medication therapy

Obtain venipuncture as ordered q _____ (specify frequency)

Teach new medications and effects

Assess for electrolyte imbalance

Teach patient and caregiver use of PCA pump

Nonpharmacological interventions such as progressive muscle relaxation, imagery, positive visualization, music, massage and touch, and humor therapy of patient's choice

RN to assess the patient's response to therapeutic treatments and interventions, and to report any changes or unfavorable responses to the physician

Teaching of patient/family, including medications, the management program, strength, type, actions, times, and compliance tips

Encourage family/caregivers to give the patient medications on the schedule and around-the-clock

Medications changed using equianalgesic conversion tables/physician orders (e.g., from oral morphine to an equianalgesic dose of transdermal fentanyl)

Other interventions, based on patient/family needs

h. *Other considerations*

Assess progression of disease process

RN to assess the patient's response to treatments and to report to the physician changes, unfavorable responses, or reactions

Other interventions, based on patient/family needs

- *Home health aide or certified nursing assistant*

Effective and safe personal care

Safe ADL assistance and support

Respite care and active listening skills

Observation and reporting

Meal preparation

Homemaker services

Comfort care

Other duties

- *Hospice social worker*

Psychosocial assessment of patient and family/caregiver, including adjustment to long-term illness and its implications

Identification of optimal coping strategies

Financial assessment and counseling regarding food acquisition, ability to prepare, and costs of needed medications

Intervention/support related to terminal illness and loss
Emotional/spiritual support
Depression/fear assessed
Facilitate communication among patient, family, and hospice team
Referral/linkage to community services and resources as indicated
Grief counseling and intervention/support related to illness/loss
Patient/caregiver counseling and support
For patients who live alone with no support system (e.g., able, available, willing caregiver[s]): obtain resources to enable patient to remain in the home
Identification of illness-related psychiatric condition necessitating care

- *Volunteer(s)*
Support, friendship, companionship, and presence
Advocacy and respite comfort and dignity maintained/provided for patient and family
Errands and transportation
Other services, based on interdisciplinary team recommendations and patient/caregiver needs

- *Spiritual counselor*
Spiritual assessment and care
Counseling, intervention, and support related to that dimension of life related to life's meaning (consistent with patient's beliefs)
Support, listening, and presence
Participation in sacred or spiritual rituals or practices
Other supportive care, based on patient/family needs and belief systems

- *Dietitian/nutritional counseling*
Assessment of patient with decreased intake, weight loss, anorexia, and increased shortness of breath (e.g., "don't feel like eating")
Supportive counseling with patient/family indicating that patient will have a decreased appetite and possible inability to eat/drink
Assessment and recommendations for swallowing difficulties
Assessment related to specialized medical nutritional supplements
Teaching and support of family members and caregivers
Support and care with food and nourishment as desired by patient
Evaluation/management of nutritional deficits and needs
Encourage nutritional supplements and snacks to increase protein and caloric intake
Food and dietary recommendations incorporate patient choice and wishes

- *Occupational therapist*
Evaluation of ADLs and functional mobility
Assess need for adaptive equipment and assistive devices
Safety assessment of patient's environment and ADLs
Assessment for energy conservation training
Assessment of upper extremity function, retraining motor skills

- *Physical therapist*
Evaluation
Safety assessment of patient's environment

Safe transfer training or bed mobility exercises

Pain assessment/reduction factors

Strengthening exercises/program

Assessment of gait safety and home safety measures

Instruct/supervise caregiver and volunteers on home exercise program for conditioning and strength

Assistive, adaptive devices and evaluation of equipment and teaching

- *Speech-language pathologist*

  Evaluation for speech/swallowing problems

  Food texture recommendations

  Alternate functional communication

- *Bereavement counselor*

  Assessment of the needs of the bereaved family and friends

  Support and intervention, based on assessment and ongoing findings

  Presence and counseling

  Supportive visits, follow-up, and other interventions (e.g., mailings, calls)

  Other services related to bereavement work and support

- *Pharmacist*

  Evaluation of hospice patient with constipation on cathartics, stool softeners, and other medications for possible food/drug and drug/drug interactions

  Medication monitoring regarding therapeutic levels and dosages

  Pain consult and input into interdisciplinary plan of care related to pain control, palliation, and symptom management

  Assessment of medication regimen and plan for safety and compliance

- *Music, massage, art, or other therapies or services*

  Evaluation and intervention based on patient's and caregiver's unique wishes and needs that support care, comfort, and death in the setting of the patient's choice

  Assessment plan to patient and support comfort, quality, enjoyment, and dignity

  Pet therapy (including patient's pet, if available) and therapeutic intervention

7. **Outcomes for care**

- *Hospice nursing*

  Symptoms controlled in setting of patient/family choice

  Effective pain relief and control (e.g., a peaceful and comfortable death)

  Mental distress, depression, and fear of dying addressed throughout care by hospice team

  Patient and family able to care for and support patient

  Patient and caregiver can verbalize symptoms, changes, or accelerations that necessitate call to physician

  Patient and family demonstrate compliance with medication regimen and other therapeutic interventions

  Patient demonstrates stabilization and increased or enhanced coping skills related to functioning and depression

Pain and symptoms managed/controlled in setting of patient/family choice (e.g., patient/family report ability to eat, sleep, speak with pacing)

Planned and effective bowel program, as evidenced by regular bowel movements and patient/family report of comfort

Death with dignity, and pain/symptoms controlled in setting of patient/family choice

Optimal comfort, support, and dignity provided throughout illness

Death with maximum comfort through effective symptom control with specialized hospice support

Patient and caregiver able to list adverse drug reactions/problems with medication regimen and whom to call for follow-up and resolution

Patient's/family's privacy, independence, and choices supported with respect and maintained through death

Enhancement and support of quality of life

Effective symptom relief and control (e.g., a peaceful and comfortable death at home, depression controlled, some enjoyment of life)

Maximizing the patient's quality of life (e.g., alert and pain free or as patient wishes)

Pharmacological and nonpharmacological interventions, such as localized heat application, biofeedback, massage, positioning, relaxation methods, and music

Patient cared for and family supported through death with physical, psychosocial, spiritual, and other concerns/needs acknowledged/addressed

Patient- and family-centered hospice care provided based on the patient's/family's unique situation and needs

Patient/caregiver verbalizes satisfaction with care

Patient will decide on care, interventions, and evaluation

Patient will experience increased comfort and pain control through self-report (specify parameters)

Patient will have palliative care and comfort maintained through death

Patent and infection-free catheter and other care sites

Skin integrity maintained or improved

Patient and caregiver knowledgeable about side effects (e.g., constipation) and interventions needed

Control of pain and other symptoms that affect daily function, quality of life, and ability to interact with friends/family

Patient and caregiver knowledgeable about and compliant with renal care regimen, relief measures, and care for optimal control

Early detection and intervention regarding problems of patients with immobility/bedbound status (e.g., skin, urinary, musculature, vascular)

Educational tools/plans incorporated in daily care, and patient/caregiver verbalizes understanding of safe, needed care

Patient will decide on care, interventions, and evaluation

Caregiver effective in care management and knows whom to call for questions/concerns

Patient will express satisfaction with hospice support received and will experience increased comfort

Patient will be made comfortable at home through death in accordance with the patient's wishes

Effective pain control and symptom control verbalized by patient

Patient verbalizes understanding of and adheres to care and medication regimens

Patient and caregiver supported through patient's death

Comfort maintained through course of care

The patient and family receive hospice support and care, and family members and friends are able to spend quality time with the patient

Caregiver able and verbalizes comfort with role and understands when to call hospice team members

Patient supported through and receives the maximum benefit from palliative chemotherapy and radiation with minimal complications

Patient/caregiver lists adverse reactions, potential complications, signs/symptoms of infection (e.g., sputum change, chest congestion)

Comfort maintained through death with dignity

Pain effectively managed, and patient verbalizes comfort

Patient states pain is _____ on 0-10 scale by next visit

Patient/caregiver demonstrates appropriate back-up or "rescue" therapies for breakthrough pain or other symptoms (e.g., dyspnea)

Infection control and palliation

Grief/bereavement expression and support provided

Patient is pain free by next _____ visit

Caregiver demonstrates ability to manage pain, where applicable

Patient maintains comfort and dignity throughout illness

- ***Home health aide or certified nursing assistant***
  Effective hygiene, personal care, and comfort
  ADL assistance
  Safe environment maintained

- ***Hospice social worker***
  Problem identified and addressed, with patient/caregiver linked with appropriate support services and plan of care successfully implemented
  Patient and caregiver cope adaptively with illness and death
  Adaptive adjustment to changed body and body image
  Psychosocial support and counseling offered to patient/caregivers experiencing loss and grief
  Resources identified, community linkage as appropriate for patient/family
  Caregiver system assessed, and development of stable caregiver plan facilitated

- ***Volunteer(s)***
  Comfort, respite, companionship, and friendship extended to patient/family
  Support provided as defined by the needs of the patient/caregiver
  Patient and family supported by team with care, comfort, and companionship

- ***Spiritual counseling***
  Spiritual support offered and provided as defined by needs of patient/caregiver
  Provision of spiritual support and care based on the assessed and ongoing needs of the patient and family
  Spiritual support offered, and patient and family needs met
  Patient and family express relief of symptoms of spiritual suffering

Support, listening, and presence
Participation in sacred or spiritual rituals or practices

- ***Dietitian/nutritional counseling***
  Family and caregiver integrate recommendations into nutrition teaching (where appropriate)
  Patient and caregiver know whom to call for nutrition- and hydration-related questions/concerns
  Nutrition/hydration per patient choices
  Caregiver integrates recommendations into daily meal planning
  Patient and family verbalize comprehension of changing nutritional needs

- ***Occupational therapist***
  Patient and caregiver demonstrate maximum independence with ADLs, adaptive techniques, and assistive devices
  Patient and caregiver demonstrate maximum safety in ADLs and functional mobility
  Patient and caregiver demonstrate effective use of energy conservation techniques
  Verbalization/demonstration of improved functional activity level and enhanced quality of life
  Patient and caregiver demonstrate effective use of diaphragmatic breathing to reduce shortness of breath and relaxation techniques to help in pain/symptom management
  Patient and caregiver demonstrate correct use of exercise

- ***Physical therapist***
  Prevention of complications
  Home exercise and upper extremity program taught to caregiver
  Optimal strength, mobility, and function maintained/achieved
  Compliance with home exercise program

- ***Speech-language pathologist***
  Communication method implemented, and patient able to be understand as self-reported or reported by family/caregivers
  Safe swallowing and functional communication
  Recommended lists of food textures for safety and patient choice

- ***Bereavement counselor***
  Support services related to grief provided to patient and family
  Well-being and resolution process of grief initiated and followed through bereavement services

- ***Pharmacist***
  Bowel regimen successful as self-reported by patient/family and in update at team meeting
  Multiple drug regimen reviewed for food/drug and drug/drug interactions in patient on multiple medications
  Stability and safety in complex medication regimen, with maximum benefit to patient
  Effective pain and symptom control and management as reported by patient/caregiver

- *Music, massage, art, or other therapies or services*
  Therapeutic massage/touch effective for patient as self-reported or observed by caregivers/family
  Improved muscle tone, relaxation, and/or sleep
  Patient comfortable and relaxed (e.g., sleeping) after massage
  Music therapy intervention based on assessment to decrease pain perception and provide emotional expression and support
  Maintenance of comfort and physical, psychosocial, and spiritual health
  Holistic health maintained and comfort achieved through _____ (specify modality)
  Patient has pet's presence as desired—in all care sites, when possible

8. **Patient, family, and caregiver educational needs**
  Educational needs are the care regimens that contribute to safe and effective care at home between the hospice team's visits. These include the following:
  The basic tenets of hospice and the availability of support 24 hours a day, 7 days a week
  Home safety assessment and counseling
  The patient's medication regimen
  Anticipated disease progression
  Safe and proper body mechanics to promote patient comfort and prevent caregiver safety problems
  Support groups available to patient's family, such as the hospice program's "Caregiver Support Group" meetings for family members and friends of the patient
  Other teaching specific to the patient's and family's unique needs

9. **Specific tips for quality and reimbursement**
  Document any variances to expected outcomes. There are many models of hospice programs. Those that are home health agency–based must work within the framework of the Medicare home care program. For example, sometimes a hospice patient reaches a stable period in the illness and has no further skilled needs or the patient is no longer homebound per Medicare home health care criteria. When this occurs, one option is to discharge the patient from Medicare home health agency reimbursement and maintain the patient on grant funds or other available resources. If the patient's status deteriorates and again meets the Medicare criteria, a new start of care is initiated on the HCFA form 485. Usually hospices continue volunteer support, nursing, and other services indicated during these periods of no reimbursement.
  The Medicare hospice benefit does not require that the patient be homebound or have identified skilled needs. Though it is a needed and viable program, the Medicare hospice benefit may not be indicated for all Medicare eligible beneficiaries. For further information on this benefit, please refer to HCFA Hospice Manual 21.
  Should the patient's status deteriorate and increased personal care be needed, obtain a telephone order for the increased service, noting frequency and estimating the duration.

Obtain a telephone order for all medication and treatment changes of the medical regimen, and document these in the clinical record.

Document the coordination occurring among team members based on the POC. Have the multidisciplinary conference notes reflected in the clinical record.

For Medicare home health patients, know that when a patient has end stage renal disease (ESRD), this is a special and separate Medicare benefit from home care. All dialysis-related care needs are to be provided by the dialysis center. Therefore the patients who are seen in home care usually have another medical problem separate from the ESRD or renal dialysis problems. These include hypertension and the monitoring and medication regulation that occurs, diabetes mellitus, CVA, wound care, insulin administration, and other problems not directly related to the dialysis condition.

Keep in mind that Medicare patients can receive care under both the ESRD and the home care benefit. The condition, though, should not be related to ESRD. Examples of covered care could include care of an abdominal access site or wounds or care not related to ESRD.

ESRD is usually not the principal diagnosis when completing the HCFA form 485. The principal diagnosis is the reason that skilled care is needed (e.g., the wound, DM, or hypertension). The documentation should reflect the actual care provided for the wound (e.g., hands-on care, teaching or observation, and assessment) and your patient's response to those care interventions.

Document coordination of services or consultation with the other members of the IDT

Document communications and care coordination with other care providers, such as skilled nursing facility or nursing home staff, inpatient team members, and hired caregivers

Document in the clinical notes the clear progression and symptomatology and interventions that demonstrate the interventions and overall management of the patient/family with end stage renal failure and attendant needs for hospice support

Document when/if the patient has respiratory changes, shortness of breath, exacerbation of conditions, pain, increased somnolence, and other symptoms and that they are identified and resolved

Remember that the clinical documentation is key to measuring compliance for quality reimbursement purposes. Care coordination, timely verbal and initial physician orders, and assessment and addressing of spiritual and psychosocial needs should be ongoing and documented in the patient's clinical record

The documentation should support that all hospice care supports comfort and dignity while meeting patient/family needs

The documentation should include ongoing assessment and management of pain and other symptoms and the anticipation and prevention of secondary symptoms such as constipation

It is important to note that all team members, including nurses and social workers, should assess, identify, and "hear" spiritual needs that the patient/family want to be addressed. These spiritual issues are key to the provision of quality hospice care and cannot be addressed effectively and promptly by the spiritual counselor only

Document clearly symptoms, clinical changes, and assessment findings related to pain and patient care

Document patient changes, symptoms, and clinical information identified from visits and team conferences that support hospice care and a limited life expectancy

Clearly support in the documentation the rationale that supports/explains the progression of the illness from the chronic to terminal stages

Document mentation, behavioral, and/or cognitive changes

Document changes in edema, increased shortness of breath, dyspnea, infection, sepsis, new or changed medications, etc.

Document any skin changes (e.g., inflamed, painful, weeping skin site[s])

Document when the patient is actively dying, deteriorating, and progressing toward death

Remember that the "litmus test" of care coordination rests on the quality of the clinical documentation by all team members. Review one of your patient's clinical records and ask yourself the following: "If I was unable to give a verbal report/update on this patient, would a peer be able to pick up and provide the same level of care and know (from the documentation) the current orders, medications, and other details that contribute to effective hospice care?"

Your assessments, observations, and clinical findings assist in painting a picture to support coverage and documentation requirements for hospice care

Document any hospitalizations and changed clinical findings

Document patient changes, symptoms, psychosocial issues impacting the care, and information gathered at the patient/family visits

Document changes to the plan of care, such as medications, services, frequency, communication, and concurrence of other team members

The documentation should reflect ongoing effects of the terminal condition, the patient's/family's difficulty with care or coping, and the continued desire for hospice care.

Unless the patient is in a hospice insurance program, some insurers will not pay for a skilled nurse visit that is made at death if the patient is dead when the nurse arrives at the home. From a Medicare home care perspective, the visit at the time of death may be covered when the orders and clinical record document assessment of the patient's status or signs of death/life or state law allows pronouncement of death by a nurse.

Document patient deterioration

Document dehydration, dehydrating

Document patient change or instability

Document pain, other symptoms not controlled

Document status after acute episode of _____ (specify)

Document positive urine, sputum, etc. culture; patient started on _____ (specify ordered antibiotic therapy)

Document patient impacted; impaction removed manually

Document RN in frequent communication with physician regarding _____ (specify)

Document febrile at _____, pulse change at _____, irr., irr.

Document change noted in _____
Document bony prominences red, opening
Document RN contacted physician regarding _____ (specify)
Document marked SOB
Document alteration in mental status
Document medications being adjusted, regulated, or monitored
Document unable to perform own ADLs, personal care
Document all interdisciplinary team meetings and communications in the
   POC and in the progress notes of the clinical record
All hospice team members should have input into the POC and document
   their interventions and goals

10. **Resources for hospice care and practice**
   For more information, contact the National Kidney Foundation at 1-800-622-
   9010 to order a General Public Materials Catalog, with information on
   kidney disease, related conditions, and organ donation.
     Various booklets are available, and *When Stopping Dialysis Treatment Is
   Your Choice* and *If You Choose Not To Start Dialysis Treatment* are patient
   education materials. There is also a text entitled *Initiation or Withdrawal of
   Dialysis in End Stage Renal Disease: Guidelines for the Health Care Team*
   that is a comprehensive review of policy considerations related to values,
   ethics, decision-making, and the dying process. These resources can be obtained by calling 1-800-622-9010.
     Another helpful resource is the NHO's second edition of *Medical Guide-
   lines for Determining Prognoses in Selected Non-Cancer Diseases.* Call NHO
   at 1-703-243-5900 for more information.

SUPPORTIVE CARE: CATHETER, FEEDING TUBE, AND OSTOMY CARE

1. **General considerations**

   Patients with these major alterations in "normal body functions" for eating and elimination, together with their families, will have significant feelings of loss and control. Body image adjustments and grief need to be acknowledged and incorporated into skillful hospice care.

2. **Needs for visit**

   Physician order for hospice care, specific to the hospice program's admission criteria and policies

   Standard precautions supplies

   Vital signs equipment for baseline assessment

   For catheter care: catheter and insertion supplies

   For feeding tube or enteral feeding care: related skin care supplies and nutritional supplements

   For ostomy care: ostomy bag, belts, and skin care supplies

   Other equipment, based on physician orders

3. **Safety considerations**

   Infection control/standard precautions

   Night-light

   Extra caution on slippery surfaces

   Removal of scatter rugs

   Tub rail, grab bars for bathroom safety

   Supportive and nonskid shoes

   Handrail on stairs

   Fall precautions/protocol

   Protective skin measures

   Identification and report of any skin problems

   Smoke detector and fire evacuation plan

   Assistance with ambulation

   Disposal of used catheters and related supplies

   Supervised medication administration

   Safety for home medical equipment (e.g., use, safe storage)

   Safe care of stoma/skin site

   The phone number and name of the person to call with a care problem

   Smoke detector and fire evacuation plan

   Others, based on the patient's unique condition and environment

4. **Potential diagnoses and codes**

   Catheter care

Attention to other artificial opening of urinary tract	V55.4
Bladder atony	596.4
Bladder repair (surgical)	57.89
Constipation	564.0

CVA	436
Cystoscopy (surgical)	57.32
Decubitus ulcer	707.0
Fitting and adjustment of urinary devices	V53.6
Hematuria	599.7
Hypertension	401.9
Impaction	560.30
Incontinence of urine	788.30
Indwelling Foley catheter	57.94
Neurogenic bladder	596.54
Pressure wound	707.0
Prostate, cancer of the	185
Suprapubic tube	57.18
Urinary incontinence	788.30
Urinary tract infection	599.0
Urinary retention	788.20
Vaginitis	616.10

Feeding tube care

Attention to gastrostomy	V55.1
CVA	436
Decubitus ulcer (pressure ulcer)	707.0
Dysphagia	787.2
Foley catheter	57.94
Gastrostomy (other)	43.19
Gastrostomy tube insertion	43.11
Hemiparesis	342.9
Nasogastric tube feeding	96.6
Nasogastric tube insertion	96.07
Paralysis agitans (Parkinson's)	332.0
Pneumonia	486
Pneumonia, aspiration	507.0
Pressure ulcer	707.0
Urinary incontinence	788.30

Ostomy care

Attention to colostomy	V55.3
Attention to cystostomy	V55.5
Attention to ileostomy	V55.2
Attention to other artificial opening of digestive tract	V55.4
Attention to other artificial opening of urinary tract	V55.6
Bladder cancer	188.9
Bowel obstruction	560.9
Bowel perforation	569.83
Bowel resection (surgical)	45.79
Cancer of the colon	153.9
Cancer of the rectosigmoid	154.0

Cancer of the rectum	154.1
Colectomy, sigmoid (surgical)	45.76
Colitis	558.9
Colitis, ulcerative	556.9
Colostomy (surgical)	46.10
Colostomy, attention to	V55.3
Cystostomy, attention to	V55.5
Diverticulitis	562.11
Enteritis, radiation	558.1
Hemicolectomy with colostomy	45.75 and 46.10
Ileostomy or other intestinal appliance, fitting and adjustment	V53.5
Ileostomy, attention to	V55.2
Metastases, general	199.1
Proctocolectomy (surgical)	45.79
Radiation enteritis	558.1
Rectum, cancer of the	154.1
Skin eruptions	782.1
Skin, excoriation of	919.8
Ulcerative colitis	556.9
Urinary devices, fitting and adjustment	V53.6
Wound evisceration	998.3

5. **Associated nursing diagnoses**

   Catheter care
   Body image disturbance
   Constipation
   Constipation, colonic
   Constipation, perceived
   Family processes, altered
   Incontinence, functional
   Incontinence, reflex
   Incontinence, stress
   Incontinence, total
   Incontinence, urge
   Infection, risk for
   Injury, risk for
   Mobility, impaired physical
   Pain
   Pain, chronic
   Self-care deficit, toileting
   Sexual dysfunction
   Sexuality patterns, altered
   Skin integrity, impaired, potential
   Spiritual distress (distress of the human spirit)
   Spiritual well-being, potential for enhanced
   Urinary elimination, altered
   Urinary retention

Feeding tube care
Aspiration, risk for
Body image disturbance
Bowel elimination, alteration in, diarrhea
Bowel incontinence
Caregiver role strain
Caregiver role strain, risk for
Comfort, alteration in, pain
Diarrhea
Family processes, altered
Fluid volume deficit, risk for
Infection, risk for
Injury, risk for
Knowledge deficit (care management)
Knowledge deficit, disease process
Nutrition, alteration in, actual
Nutrition, altered: less than body requirements
Nutrition, altered: more than body requirements
Oral mucous membrane, altered
Pain
Pain, chronic
Self-care deficit, feeding
Skin integrity, impaired, risk for
Skin integrity, impairment of actual, incision
Spiritual distress (distress of the human spirit)
Spiritual well-being, potential for enhanced
Swallowing, impaired

Ostomy care
Anxiety
Body image disturbance
Bowel incontinence
Caregiver role strain
Caregiver role strain, risk for
Constipation
Diarrhea
Family processes, altered
Fatigue
Fear
Fluid volume deficit, risk for
Infection, risk for
Injury, risk for
Grieving, anticipatory
Knowledge deficit (self-management and disease process)
Management of therapeutic regimen (individuals), ineffective
Nutrition, altered: less than body requirements
Pain
Pain, chronic
Self-care deficit (specify)
Skin integrity, impaired, risk for

Social interaction, impaired
Spiritual distress (distress of the human spirit)
Spiritual well-being, potential for enhanced
Tissue integrity, impaired
Tissue perfusion, altered (gastrointestinal)
Urinary elimination, altered

6. **Skills and services identified**

   • *Hospice nursing*

   Catheter care

   a. *Comfort and symptom control*
   Comprehensive assessment of patient admitted to hospice with
   _____ catheter, due to _____
   Observation and complete systems assessment of the patient with an
   indwelling catheter
   Document catheter (type, size, balloon size) inserted on
   _____ (specify date)
   Presentation of hospice philosophy and services
   Explain patient rights and responsibilities
   Assess patient, family, and caregiver wishes and expectations regarding
   care
   Assess patient, family, and caregiver resources available for care
   Provision of volunteer support to patient and family
   Teach family or caregiver physical care of patient
   RN to provide and teach effective oral care and comfort measures
   Assess pain and other symptoms, including site, duration, characteris-
   tics, and relief measures
   RN to assess patient's pain q visit to identify need for change, addition,
   or other plan or dose adjustment
   Change catheter number _____ French _____ cc q
   month
   Evaluate the patient for catheter complaints, and contact physician if
   necessary
   Obtain UA/C&S if symptoms of infection are present
   Maintain hydration fluid volumes as indicated
   Irrigate catheter with 30 cc NSS prn per physician orders
   Teach family indwelling catheter care, irrigation of catheter, S/S UTI,
   adequate hydration, skin care, change of drainage bag, and when to
   call nurse
   Teach family removal of catheter with syringe, how to change bag, and
   care and positioning of bag
   Assess amount, frequency of urinary drainage, intake, and output
   Pain assessment and management q visit
   Teach family reason for catheter (e.g., bladder atony, retention)
   RN to change catheter every 4 weeks and may make 3 prn visits for
   catheter problems, including patient complaints, signs and symptoms
   of infection, and other factors necessitating evaluation and possible
   catheter change

Assess pain, and evaluate pain management's effectiveness

Teach care of bedridden patient

Measure vital signs, including pain, q visit

Assess cardiovascular, pulmonary, and respiratory status

Teach caregivers symptom control and relief measures

Oxygen on at _____ liters per _____ (specify physician orders)

Identify and monitor pain, symptoms, and relief measures

Teach caregiver care of weak, terminally ill patient

Comfort measures of backrub and hand/other therapeutic massage

Observation and assessment related to signs/symptoms of urinary infection

Teaching and training about symptoms/changes that necessitate notification of nurse

Observation, assessment, and supportive care to patient and family

Teach patient/family use of standardized form/tool to use between hospice team members' visits (and for care coordination between team members)

Supportive care and scopolamine patches as ordered per physician orders

Teach patient/family principles of effective pain management

Observation and assessment, communication with physician related to signs and symptoms of continuing decompensation, increased symptoms, pain, discomfort, shortness of breath, and measures to alleviate and control

Effective management of pain and prevention of secondary symptoms

Teach family and caregiver signs and changes to report to nurse and physician

Interventions of symptoms directed toward comfort and palliation

Teach patient and family about realistic expectations of disease process

Teach care of dying and signs/symptoms of impending death

Presence and support

Other interventions, based on patient/family needs

b. *Safety and mobility considerations*

Provide caregiver/family with home safety information and instruction related to _____ and documented in the clinical record

Teach family regarding safety of patient in home

Other interventions, based on patient/family needs

c. *Emotional/spiritual considerations*

Psychosocial assessment of patient and family regarding disease and prognosis

RN to provide emotional support to patient and family

Assess mental status and sleep disturbance changes

Observation and assessment of mental status changes/complaints of depression in new hospice patient with catheter

Observation of patient for neuropsychiatric complications of illness, including confusion, depression, and anxiety

RN to provide support and intervention/referral for depression

Teach patient/family about depression and signs/symptoms of exacerbation that require more intervention

Assess for and manage plans for psychosocial and/or spiritual pain (e.g., all pain, anxiety, interpersonal and other distress)

Psychosocial aspects of pain control (e.g., depression, other) assessed and acknowledged with team support/intervention

Ongoing acknowledgment of spirituality and related concerns of patient/family

Other interventions, based on patient/family needs

d. *Skin care*

Maintain skin integrity, and teach care of the immobilized patient, if indicated

Pressure ulcer care as indicated

Observation and evaluation of wound and surrounding skin

Evaluate patient's need for equipment, including supplies to decrease pressure, alternating pressure mattress, gel foam seat cushion, and heel and elbow protectors

RN to teach patient about care of irradiated skin sites

Maintain skin integrity, and teach care of the immobilized patient as indicated

Teach patient, family, or caregiver about proper body alignment and positioning in bed to prevent skin tears from shearing skin

Observe and apply skilled assessment of areas for possible breakdown, including heels, hips, elbows, ankles, and other pressure-prone areas

Teach caregiver regarding skin care needs, including the need for frequent position changes, appropriate pressure pads and mattresses, and the prevention of breakdown

Other interventions, based on patient/family needs

e. *Elimination considerations*

Assess bowel regimen, and implement program as needed

Assess amount and frequency of urinary output

RN to evaluate the patient's bowel patterns and need for stool softeners, laxatives, and dietary adjustments, and to develop bowel management plan

Check for and remove impaction as needed

Condom catheter or indwelling catheter as indicated

Teaching and ongoing assessment for the prevention and early identification of constipation and its correction/resolution

Implement bowel assessment management program

Teach patient, family, and aide the importance of observing and noting bowel movements between scheduled nursing visits

Obtain patient history related to norms for bowel movements to date (e.g., "all my life I go only every other day")

Bowel management program of stool softeners, laxative of choice, Fleet's Enemas prn, and other methods per patient wishes and physician orders

Teach catheter care to caregiver

RN to teach caregiver daily care of catheter

RN to change catheter (specify type, size) q _____ (specify ordered frequency)

RN to change catheter every 4 weeks and may make 3 prn visits for catheter problems, including patient complaints, signs and symptoms of infection, and other factors necessitating evaluation and possible catheter change

Observation and complete systems assessment of patient with an indwelling catheter

Other interventions, based on patient/family needs

f. *Hydration/nutrition*

Assess nutrition/hydration status

Teach feeding-tube care to family

Nutrition/hydration supported by offering patient's choice of favorite or desired foods or liquids

Nutrition/hydration maintained by offering patient high-protein diet and foods of choice as tolerated

Teach patient and family to expect decreased nutritional and fluid intake as disease progresses

Other interventions, based on patient/family needs

g. *Therapeutic/medication regimens*

Medication management related to antibiotics and food/drug and drug/drug interactions

RN to assess the patient's response to therapeutic treatments and interventions and report any changes or unfavorable responses to the physician

Medication assessment and management q visit

Teach new medication and effects

Assess for electrolyte imbalance

Teach patient and caregiver use of PCA pump

Nonpharmacological interventions such as progressive muscle relaxation imagery, positive visualization, music, massage and touch, and humor therapy of patient's choice implemented

Teach and observe regarding side effects of palliative chemotherapy, including constipation, anemia, and fatigue

Teaching of patient/family, including medications, management program, strength, type, actions, times, and compliance tips

Encourage family/caregivers to give the patient medications on the schedule and around the clock

RN to instruct in pain control measures and medications

Medications changed using equianalgesic conversion tables/physician orders (e.g., from oral morphine to an equianalgesic dose of transdermal fentanyl)

Nonpharmacological or other interventions of relaxation, hot/cold therapy, biofeedback, distraction, guided imagery, humor, music therapy, acupuncture, TENS technology, hypnosis, massage, or others as patient and family wish

Other interventions, based on patient/family needs

h. *Other considerations*

Assess disease process progression

RN to assess the patient's response to treatments and interventions and to report to the physician any changes, unfavorable responses, or reactions

Other interventions, based on patient/family needs

Feeding tube care

a. *Comfort and symptom control*

Skilled observation and systems assessment of patient with feeding tube _____ (specify type, site) due to _____ (specify)

Comprehensive assessment of patient with G tube

Observation, assessment, and supportive care to patient with feeding tube _____ (specify type) and family

Presentation of hospice philosophy and services

Explain patient rights and responsibilities

Assess patient, family, and caregiver wishes and expectations regarding care

Assess patient, family, and caregiver resources available for care

Provision of volunteer support to patient and family

Teach family or caregiver physical care of patient

RN to provide and teach effective oral care and comfort measures

Assess pain and other symptoms, including site, duration, characteristics, and relief measures

RN to assess patient's pain q visit to identify need for change, addition, or other plan or dose adjustment

Measure vital signs

Teach family or caregiver about enteral feeding

Teach about equipment for feeding, preparation, and storage of feeding

Teach patient and caregiver protocols of changing feeding bags and administration tubing per physician orders

RN to observe q visit for leaking, movement, discomfort, or other change

Instruct patient and family in jejunostomy or other tube feedings

RN/enterostomal therapist to evaluate patient and peristomal skin to identify nursing care needs

Teach the importance of verifying the tube's placement before every feeding

Teach family mouth and oral hygiene care

Teach caregiver regarding irrigation with water or per protocol

Teach family observational skills, including record keeping of intake and output, nutritional solution or supplement, and rate, frequency, amount, and time of ordered feedings

Pain assessment and management q visit

Monitor for complications, including diarrhea

Teach care of feeding tube (PEG or PEJ)

Change nasogastric tube q _____ (specify physician orders)

Teach family or caregiver gastrostomy feeding

Teach family or caregiver equipment care and preparation

Teach Dobhoff tube care, including _____ (specify)

Teach use of kangaroo pump to family or caregiver

Weigh daily or weekly per physician order(s)

Monitor amount and sites of edema

Assess gastric tube for proper placement and patency, and teach patient or family

Cleanse gastric tube site q _____ with hydrogen peroxide and water

Teach family or caregiver care of gastric tube

Administer and teach feedings at three-fourths strength at _____ cc/hr

Assess respiratory and cardiovascular statuses

Gastric tube feedings of _____ in 24 hours at _____ cc/hr

Change and reinsert tube prn, per physician orders

Teach patient/family use of standardized form/tool to use between hospice team members' visits (and for care coordination between team members)

Supportive care and scopolamine patches per physician orders

Teach patient/family principles of effective pain management

Observation and assessment, communication with physicians related to signs and symptoms of continuing decompensation, increased symptoms, pain, discomfort, shortness of breath, and measures to alleviate and control

Effective management of pain and prevention of secondary symptoms

Pain assessment and management q visit, including source of pain (e.g., neuropathy, phantom pain, claudication, infection, and other problems such as cardiac or arthritis pain)

Oxygen on at _____ liters per _____ (specify physician orders)

Identify and monitor pain, symptoms, and relief measures

Teach caregiver care of weak, terminally ill patient

Comfort measures of backrub and hand or other therapeutic massage

Assess pain, and evaluate pain management's effectiveness

Teach care of bedridden patient

Measure vital signs, including pain, q visit

Assess cardiovascular, pulmonary, and respiratory status

Teach caregivers symptom control and relief measures

Interventions of symptoms directed toward comfort and palliation

Teach patient and family about realistic expectations of disease process

Teach care of dying and signs/symptoms of impending death

Presence and support

Other interventions, based on patient/family needs

b. *Safety and mobility considerations*

Provide caregiver/family with home safety information and instruction related to _____ and documented in the clinical record

Teach regarding elevated position of head in bed for safety

Teach family regarding safety of patient in home

Other interventions, based on patient/family needs

c. *Emotional/spiritual considerations*

Psychosocial assessment of patient and family regarding disease and prognosis

RN to provide emotional support to patient and family

Assess mental status and sleep disturbance changes

Observation and assessment of mental status and changes/complaints of depression in new hospice patient

Observation of patient for neuropsychiatric complications of illness, including confusion, depression, and anxiety

RN to provide support and intervention/referral for depression

Teach patient/family about depression and signs/symptoms of exacerbation that require more intervention

Assess for and manage plans for psychosocial and/or spiritual pain (e.g., all pain, anxiety, interpersonal and other distress)

Psychosocial aspects of pain control (e.g., depression, other) assessed and acknowledged with team support/intervention

Ongoing acknowledgment of spirituality and related concerns of patient/family

Other interventions, based on patient/family needs

d. *Skin care*

Wound care to abdominal site

Pressure ulcer care as indicated

Assess skin integrity

Observation and evaluation of wound and surrounding skin

Evaluate patient's need for equipment, including supplies to decrease pressure, alternating pressure mattress, gel foam seat cushion, and heel and elbow protectors

RN to teach patient about care of irradiated skin sites

Teach patient, family, or caregiver about proper body alignment and positioning in bed to prevent skin tears from shearing skin

Teach family to perform dressing changes between RN visits

Observe areas for possible breakdown, including heels, hips, elbows, ankles, and other pressure-prone areas

Teach caregiver about skin care needs, including the need for frequent position changes, appropriate pressure pads and mattresses, and the prevention of breakdown

Other interventions, based on patient/family needs

e. *Elimination considerations*

Assess bowel regimen, and implement program as needed

Observation and assessment of patient's bowel patterns

Teaching and ongoing assessment for the prevention and early identification of constipation and its correction/resolution

Initiate bowel management program per physician

Implement bowel assessment management program

Teach patient, family, and aide the importance of observing and noting bowel movements between scheduled nursing visits

Obtain patient history related to norms for bowel movements to date (e.g., "all my life I go only every other day")

Bowel management program of stool softeners, offer laxative of choice,
Fleet's Enemas prn, and other methods per patient wishes and physician orders

Assess amount and frequency of urinary output

RN to evaluate the patient's bowel patterns and need for stool softeners,
laxatives, and dietary adjustments and to develop bowel management
plan

RN to teach daily catheter care

Assess bowel regimen, and implement program as needed

Check for and remove impaction as needed

Condom catheter or indwelling catheter as indicated

Other interventions, based on patient/family needs

f. *Hydration/nutrition*

Teach and monitor for signs of dehydration and diarrhea

Assess nutrition/hydration status

Diet counseling for patient with anorexia

Nutrition/hydration supported by offering patient's choice of favorite or
desired foods or liquids

Nutrition/hydration maintained by offering patient high-protein diet and
foods of choice as tolerated

Teach patient and family to expect decreased nutritional and fluid intake
as disease progresses

Teach feeding-tube care to family

Other interventions, based on patient/family needs

g. *Therapeutic/medication regimens*

RN to assess the patient's response to therapeutic treatments and interventions and to report to the physician any changes or unfavorable
responses

Teaching of patient/family, including medications and the management
program (e.g., strength, type, actions, times, compliance tips)

Encourage family/caregivers to give the patient medications on the
schedule and around the clock

Medications changed using equianalgesic conversion tables/physician
orders (e.g., from oral morphine to an equianalgesic dose of transdermal fentanyl)

Nonpharmacological or other interventions of relaxation, hot/cold
therapy, biofeedback, distraction, guided imagery, humor, music
therapy, acupuncture, TENS technology, hypnosis, massage, or others
as patient and family wish

Teach about and observe side effects of palliative chemotherapy, including constipation, anemia, and fatigue

Teach new medication and effects

RN to instruct in pain control measures and medications

Assess for electrolyte imbalance

Teach patient and caregiver use of PCA pump

Nonpharmacological interventions such as progressive muscle relaxation
imagery, positive visualization, music, massage and touch, and
humor therapy of patient's choice implemented

Teach new pain and symptom control medication regimen

Medication assessment and management
Other interventions, based on patient/family needs

h. *Other considerations*
Assess disease process progression
RN to assess the patient's response to treatments and interventions and
    to report to the physician any changes, unfavorable responses, or
    reactions
Other interventions, based on patient/family needs

Ostomy care

a. *Comfort and symptom control*
Skilled observation and systems assessment of patient with a
    _____ (specify) ostomy due to _____
    (specify)
Comprehensive assessment of patient with ostomy
Presentation of hospice philosophy and services
Explain patient rights and responsibilities
Assess patient, family, and caregiver wishes and expectations regarding
    care
Assess patient, family, and caregiver resources available for care
Provision of volunteer support to patient and family
Teach family or caregiver physical care of patient
RN to provide and teach effective oral care and comfort measures
Assess pain and other symptoms, including site, duration, characteris-
    tics, and relief measures
RN to assess patient's pain q visit to identify need for change, addition,
    or other plan or dose adjustment
Teach ostomy care
Adjust size of karaya seal
Teach patient modification of appliance to preserve wound integrity
Closely assess stoma and wound progress
Help patient find best ostomy equipment and supplies, based on patient
    needs and price
Teach regarding irrigation procedure(s)
Consult with enterostomal therapist for review of care and care planning
Assess for allergy to sealant or appliances
Teach patient to be prepared for "accidents" and have cosmetic bag with
    supplies, one of each appliance used, and small plastic bag for dis-
    posal of soiled materials
ET nurse consultant contacted for care and care plan review
Comfort measures of backrub and hand or other therapeutic massage
Assess pain, and evaluate pain management's effectiveness
Teach care of bedridden patient
Measure vital signs, including pain, q visit
Assess cardiovascular, pulmonary, and respiratory status
Teach caregivers symptom control and relief measures
Oxygen on at _____ liters per _____ (specify physician orders)
Identify and monitor pain, symptoms, and relief measures
Teach caregiver care of weak, terminally ill patient

Teach patient/family use of standardized form/tool to use between hospice team members' visits (and for care coordination between team members)

Observation, assessment, and supportive care to patient and family

Teach patient/family principles of effective pain management

Effective management of pain and prevention of secondary symptoms

Observation and assessment, communication with physician related to signs and symptoms of continuing decompensation, increased symptoms, pain, discomfort, shortness of breath, and measures to alleviate and control

Teach caregiver/patient use of pain assessment tool/scale and reporting mechanism(s)

Interventions directed toward comfort and palliation of symptoms

Teach patient and family about realistic expectations of disease process

Teach care of dying and signs/symptoms of impending death

Presence and support

Other interventions, based on patient/family needs

b. *Safety and mobility considerations*

Provide caregiver and family with home safety information and instruction related to _____ and documented in the clinical record

Teach family regarding safety of patient in home

Teach patient and family regarding energy conservation techniques

Other interventions, based on patient/family needs

c. *Emotional/spiritual considerations*

Psychosocial assessment of patient and family regarding disease and prognosis

Document emotional or physical barriers to learning or coping (e.g., severe arthritis of hands)

RN to provide emotional support to patient and family

Assess mental status and sleep disturbance changes

Observation and assessment of mental status and changes/complaints of depression in new hospice patient with ostomy

Observation of patient for neuropsychiatric complications of illness, including confusion, depression, and anxiety

RN to provide support and intervention/referral for depression

Teach patient/family about depression and signs/symptoms of exacerbation that require more intervention

Assess for and manage plans for psychosocial and/or spiritual pain (e.g., all pain, anxiety, interpersonal and other distress)

Psychosocial aspects of pain control (e.g., depression) assessed and acknowledged with team support/intervention

Assessment and care/support related to depression, changed body image concerns, fever, mouth sores/ulcers, complaints of extreme tiredness, and dry/cracking skin in patient receiving palliative chemotherapy

Ongoing acknowledgment of spirituality and related concerns of patient/family

Other interventions, based on patient/family needs

d. *Skin care*

Instruct patient regarding skin care and air-dry procedures

Teach about skin care to protect from irritation and infection

Pressure ulcer care as indicated

Assess skin integrity

Teach family to perform dressing between RN visits

Observation and evaluation of wound and surrounding skin

Evaluate patient's need for equipment, including supplies to decrease pressure, alternating pressure mattress, gel foam seat cushion, and heel and elbow protectors

RN to teach patient about care of irradiated skin sites

Teach patient, family, or caregiver about proper body alignment and positioning in bed to prevent skin tears from shearing skin

Observe and apply skilled assessment of areas for possible breakdown, including heels, hips, elbows, ankles, and other pressure-prone areas

Teach caregiver about skin care needs, including the need for frequent position changes, appropriate pressure pads and mattresses, and the prevention of breakdown

Other interventions, based on patient/family needs

e. *Elimination considerations*

Assess bowel regimen, and implement program as needed

Check for and remove impaction as needed

Condom catheter or indwelling catheter as indicated

Assess amount and frequency of urinary output

RN to evaluate the patient's bowel patterns and need for stool softeners, laxatives, and dietary adjustments and to develop bowel management plan

RN to teach daily catheter care

Teach patient, family, and aide the importance of observing and noting bowel movements between scheduled nursing visits

Obtain patient history related to norms for bowel movements to date (e.g., "all my life I go only every other day")

Teaching and ongoing assessment for the prevention and early identification of constipation and its correction/resolution

Implement bowel assessment management program

Bowel management program of stool softeners, laxative of choice, Fleet's Enemas prn, and other methods per patient wishes and physician orders

Observation and complete systems assessment of the patient with an indwelling catheter

RN to change catheter every 4 weeks and to make 3 prn visits for catheter problems, including patient complaints, signs and symptoms of infection, and other factors necessitating evaluation and possible catheter change

Other interventions, based on patient/family needs

f. *Hydration/nutrition*

Teach patient about avoidance of gas-producing foods such as cauliflower, cabbage, beans, cucumbers, and onions

Teach about appropriate diet

Assess nutrition/hydration status

Diet counseling for patient with anorexia

Nutrition/hydration supported by offering patient's choice of favorite or
desired foods or liquids

Nutrition/hydration maintained by offering patient high-protein diet and
foods of choice as tolerated

Teach patient and family to expect decreased nutritional and fluid intake
as disease progresses

Teach feeding-tube care to family

Assessment and plan related to anorexia/cachexia, tube feedings,
difficulty swallowing, and/or transitional feedings (e.g., TPN to
oral)

Assessment and interventions/plan related to patient/family complaints
of dry mouth, with painful chewing, difficulty speaking, and denture
fit concerns after radiation and surgery

Other interventions, based on patient/family needs

g. *Therapeutic/medication regimens*

RN to assess the patient's response to therapeutic treatments and interventions, and to report any changes or unfavorable responses to the
physician

Teach and observe regarding side effects of palliative chemotherapy,
including constipation, anemia, and fatigue

Teach new pain and symptom control medication regimen

Medication assessment and management

Venipuncture q _____ (specify ordered frequency) for monitoring platelet count

Obtain venipuncture as ordered q _____ (specify ordered
frequency)

Teach about new medication and effects

RN to instruct in pain control measures and medications

Assess for electrolyte imbalance

Teach patient and caregiver use of PCA pump

Teaching of patient/family, including medications and the management
program (e.g., strength, type, actions, times, and compliance tips)

Encourage family/caregivers to give the patient medications on the
schedule and around the clock

Medications changed using equianalgesic conversion tables/physician
orders (e.g., from oral morphine to an equianalgesic dose of transdermal fentanyl)

Nonpharmacological or other interventions of relaxation, hot/cold
therapy, biofeedback, distraction, guided imagery, humor, music
therapy, acupuncture, TENS technology, hypnosis massage, or others
as patient and family wish

Nonpharmacological interventions such as progressive muscle relaxation
imagery, positive visualization, music, massage and touch, and
humor therapy of patient's choice implemented

Other interventions, based on patient/family needs

h. *Other considerations*
   Assess disease process progression
   RN to assess the patient's response to treatments and interventions and
      to report to the physician any changes, unfavorable responses, or
      reactions
   Other interventions, based on patient/family needs

- *Home health aide or certified nursing assistant*
   Effective and safe personal care
   Safe ADL assistance and support
   Observation and reporting
   Respite care and active listening skills
   Meal preparation
   Homemaker services
   Comfort care
   Other duties

- *Hospice social worker*
   Psychosocial assessment of patient and family/caregiver, including adjust-
      ment to illness and its implications
   Identification of optimal coping strategies
   Financial assessment and counseling regarding food acquisition, ability to
      prepare, and costs of needed medications
   Intervention/support related to terminal illness and loss
   Emotional/spiritual support
   Depression/fear assessed
   Facilitate communication among patient, family, and hospice team
   Referral/linkage to community services and resources as indicated
   Grief counseling and intervention/support related to illness/loss
   Patient/caregiver counseling and support
   For patients who live alone with no support system (e.g., able, available,
      willing caregiver[s]): identify/review possible resources to enable
      patient to remain in home
   Identification of illness-related psychiatric condition necessitating care
   Caregiver system assessed, and development of stable caregiver plan facili-
      tated
   Identification of caregiver role strain necessitating respite/relief measures/
      support

- *Volunteer(s)*
   Support, friendship, companionship, and presence
   Comfort and dignity maintained/provided for patient and family
   Errands and transportation
   Advocacy and respite
   Other services, based on interdisciplinary team recommendations and
      patient/caregiver needs

- *Spiritual counselor*
   Spiritual assessment and care
   Counseling, intervention, and support related to that dimension of life
      related to life's meaning (consistent with patient's beliefs)

Support, listening, and presence
Participation in sacred or spiritual rituals or practices
Other supportive care, based on patient's/family's needs and belief systems
Patient and family express relief of symptoms of spiritual suffering

- *Dietitian/nutritional counseling*
  Assessment of patient with decreased intake, weight loss, anorexia, and
      increased shortness of breath (e.g., "don't feel like eating")
  Supportive counseling with patient/family indicating that patient may have
      a decreased appetite and usually at some point may not eat/drink
  Assessment and recommendations for swallowing difficulties
  Teaching and support of family members and caregivers
  Support and care, with food and nourishment as desired by patient
  Evaluation/management of nutritional deficits and needs
  Encourage nutritional supplements and snacks to increase protein and
      caloric intake
  Food and dietary recommendations incorporate patient choice and wishes
  Patient and family verbalize comprehension of changing nutritional needs

- *Occupational therapist*
  Evaluation of ADL and functional mobility
  Assess for need for adaptive equipment and assistive devices
  Safety assessment of patient's environment and ADL
  Assessment for energy conservation training
  Assessment of upper extremity function, retraining motor skills

- *Physical therapist*
  Evaluation
  Assessment of patient's environment for safety
  Safe transfer training or bed mobility exercises
  Pain assessment/reduction factors
  Strengthening exercises/program
  Assessment of gait safety and home safety measures
  Instruct/supervise caregiver and volunteers on home exercise program for
      conditioning and strength
  Assistive, adaptive devices and evaluation of equipment and teaching

- *Speech-language pathologist*
  Evaluation for speech/swallowing problems
  Food texture recommendations
  Alternate functional communication

- *Bereavement counselor*
  Assessment of the needs of the bereaved family and friends
  Support and intervention, based on assessment and ongoing findings
  Presence and counseling
  Supportive visits, follow-up, and other interventions (e.g., mailings, calls)
  Other services related to bereavement work and support

- *Pharmacist*
  Evaluation of hospice patient with constipation on cathartics, stool soften-
      ers, and other medications for possible food/drug, drug/drug interactions
  Medication monitoring regarding therapeutic levels and dosages

Pain consult and input into interdisciplinary plan of care related to pain control, palliation, and symptom management

Assessment of medication regimen and plan for safety and compliance

- *Music, massage, art, or other therapies or services*

  Evaluation and intervention based on patient's and caregiver's unique wishes and needs that support care, comfort, and death in the setting of the patient's choice

  Assessment plan to engage patient and support comfort, quality, enjoyment, and dignity

  Pet therapy (including patient's pet, if available) and therapeutic intervention

7. **Outcomes for care**

- *Hospice nursing*

  Catheter care

  Patient and caregiver verbalize satisfaction with care

  Infection-free, patent urinary catheter

  No skin breakdown, and family able to provide care as taught

  Support and care from hospice team facilitate patient to die as he/she wishes (setting, symptoms controlled, etc.)

  Mental distress, depression, and fear of dying addressed throughout care by hospice team

  Patient and family able to care for and support patient

  Patient and caregiver can verbalize symptoms, changes, or accelerations that necessitate call to physician

  Patient and family demonstrate compliance with medication regimen and other therapeutic interventions

  Patient demonstrates stabilization and increased or enhanced coping skills related to functioning and depression

  Pain and symptoms managed/controlled in setting of patient/family choice (e.g., patient/family report ability to eat, sleep, speak with pacing)

  Planned and effective bowel program, as evidenced by regular bowel movements and patient/family report of comfort

  Death with dignity, and pain/symptoms controlled in setting of patient/family choice

  Optimal comfort, support, and dignity provided throughout illness

  Death with maximum comfort through effective symptom control with specialized hospice support

  Patient and caregiver able to list adverse drug reactions/problems with medication regimen and whom to call for follow-up and resolution

  Patient's/family's privacy, independence, and choices supported with respect and maintained through death

  Enhancement and support of quality of life

  Effective symptom relief and control (e.g., a peaceful and comfortable death at home, depression controlled, some enjoyment of life)

  Maximizing the patient's quality of life (e.g., alert and pain free or as patient wishes)

Pharmacological and nonpharmacological interventions such as localized heat application, biofeedback, massage, positioning, relaxation methods, and music

Patient cared for and family supported through death, with physical, psychosocial, spiritual and others concerns/needs acknowledged/addressed

Patient- and family-centered hospice care provided based on the patient's/family's unique situation and needs

Infection control and palliation

Grief/bereavement expression and support provided

Patient is pain free by next _____ visit

Caregiver demonstrates ability to manage pain, where applicable

Patient maintains comfort and dignity throughout illness

Educational tools/plans incorporated in daily care, and patient/caregiver verbalizes understanding of safe, needed care

Patient will decide on care, interventions, and evaluation

Caregiver effective in care management and knows whom to call for questions/concerns

Patient will express satisfaction with hospice support received and will experience increased comfort

Patient will be made comfortable at home through death in accordance with the patient's wishes

Effective pain control and symptom control verbalized by patient

Patient verbalizes understanding of and adheres to care and medication regimens

Patient and caregiver supported through patient's death

Comfort maintained through course of care

The patient and family receive hospice support and care, and family members and friends are able to spend quality time with the patient

Caregiver able and verbalizes comfort with role and lists when to call hospice team members

Patient supported through and receives the maximum benefit from palliative chemotherapy and radiation with minimal complications

Patient and caregiver list adverse reactions, potential complications, signs/symptoms of infection (e.g., sputum change, chest congestion)

Comfort maintained through death with dignity

Pain effectively managed, and patient verbalizes comfort

Patient has stable respiratory status with patent airway

Patient is protected from injury, has stable respiratory status, and is compliant with medication, safety, and care regimens

Comfort and individualized intervention of patient with immobility/bedbound status (e.g., skin, urinary, musculature, vascular)

Spiritual and psychosocial needs met (specify) as defined by patient and caregiver throughout course of care

Other outcomes/goals, based on the patient condition with input from the hospice team and patient and family

Feeding-tube care

Patent tube with correct placement, and skin site infection free

Adherence to POC as demonstrated and verbalized by caregiver and demonstrated by patient findings by _____ (specify date)

Caregiver effective in care management and knows whom to call for questions/concerns

Patient verbalizes understanding of and adheres to medication regimens

Patient and caregiver verbalize satisfaction with care

Educational tools/plans incorporated in daily care, and patient/caregiver verbalizes understanding of safe, needed care

Patient and caregiver compliant with medications and tube-feeding schedules as demonstrated to visiting team members

Support and care from hospice through symptom-controlled death

Mental distress, depression, and fear of dying addressed throughout care by hospice team

Patient and family able to care for and support patient

Patient and caregiver can verbalize symptoms, changes, or accelerations that necessitate call to physician

Patient and family demonstrate compliance with medication regimen and other therapeutic interventions

Patient demonstrates stabilization and increased or enhanced coping skills related to functioning and depression

Pain and symptoms managed/controlled in setting of patient/family choice (e.g., patient/family report ability to eat, sleep, speak with pacing)

Planned and effective bowel program, as evidenced by regular bowel movements and patient/family report of comfort

Death with dignity, and pain/symptoms controlled in setting of patient/ family choice

Optimal comfort, support, and dignity provided throughout illness

Death with maximum comfort through effective symptom control with specialized hospice support

Patient and caregiver able to list adverse drug reactions/problems with medication regimen and whom to call for follow-up and resolution

Patient's/family's privacy, independence, and choices supported with respect and maintained through death

Enhancement and support of quality of life

Effective symptom relief and control (e.g., a peaceful and comfortable death at home, depression controlled, some enjoyment of life)

Maximizing the patient's quality of life (e.g., alert and pain free or as patient wishes)

Pharmacological and nonpharmacological interventions such as localized heat application, biofeedback, massage, positioning, relaxation methods, and music

Patient cared for and family supported through death, with physical, psychosocial, spiritual, and other concerns/needs acknowledged/ addressed

Patient- and family-centered hospice care provided based on the patient's/ family's unique situation and needs

Infection control and palliation

Grief/bereavement expression and support provided

Patient is pain free by next _____ visit

Caregiver demonstrates ability to manage pain, where applicable

Patient maintains comfort and dignity throughout illness

Patient and caregiver verbalize satisfaction with care

Educational tools/plans incorporated in daily care, and patient and caregiver verbalize understanding of safe, needed care

Patient will decide on care, interventions, and evaluation

Caregiver effective in care management and knows whom to call for questions/concerns

Patient will express satisfaction with hospice support received and will experience increased comfort

Patient will be made comfortable at home through death in accordance with the patient's wishes

Effective pain control and symptom control verbalized by patient

Patient verbalizes understanding of and adheres to care and medication regimens

Patient and caregiver supported through patient's death

Comfort maintained through course of care

Patient and family receive hospice support and care, and family members and friends are able to spend quality time with the patient

Caregiver able and verbalizes comfort with role and lists when to call hospice team members

Patient supported through and receives the maximum benefit from palliative chemotherapy and radiation with minimal complications

Patient and caregiver list adverse reactions, potential complications, signs/symptoms of infection (e.g., sputum change, chest congestion)

Comfort maintained through death with dignity

Patient is protected from injury, has stable respiratory status, and is compliant with medication, safety, and care regimens

Comfort and individualized intervention of patient with immobility/bedbound status (e.g., skin, urinary, musculature, vascular)

Spiritual and psychosocial needs met (specify) as defined by patient and caregiver throughout course of care

Other outcomes/goals, based on the patient condition with input from the hospice team and patient and family

Ostomy care

Patient and caregiver verbalize satisfaction with care

Educational tools/plans incorporated in daily care, and patient/caregiver verbalize understanding of safe, needed care

Stoma site and incision free of signs/symptoms of infection

Patient and caregiver effective in providing skin care

Patient able to care for ostomy through self-report and demonstration

Patient and caregiver effective in care management and know whom to call for questions/concerns

Patient verbalizes understanding of and adheres to pain and other medication regimens

Patient and caregiver demonstrate understanding of care and associated regimens

Support and care from hospice through symptom-controlled death

Mental distress, depression, and fear of dying addressed throughout care by hospice team

Patient and family able to care for and support patient

Patient and caregiver can verbalize symptoms, changes, or accelerations that necessitate call to physician

Patient and family demonstrate compliance with medication regimen and other therapeutic interventions

Patient demonstrates stabilization and increased or enhanced coping skills related to functioning and depression

Pain and symptoms managed/controlled in setting of patient/family choice (e.g., patient and family report ability to eat, sleep, speak with pacing)

Planned and effective bowel program, as evidenced by regular bowel movements and patient/family report of comfort

Death with dignity, and pain/symptoms controlled in setting of patient/family choice

Optimal comfort, support, and dignity provided throughout illness

Death with maximum comfort through effective symptom control with specialized hospice support

Patient and caregiver able to list adverse drug reactions/problems with medication regimen and whom to call for follow-up and resolution

Patient's/family's privacy, independence, and choices supported with respect and maintained through death

Enhancement and support of quality of life

Effective symptom relief and control (e.g., a peaceful and comfortable death at home, depression controlled, some enjoyment of life)

Maximizing the patient's quality of life (e.g., alert and pain free or as patient wishes)

Pharmacological and nonpharmacological interventions such as localized heat application, biofeedback, massage, positioning, relaxation methods, and music

Patient cared for and family supported through death, with physical, psychosocial, spiritual, and other concerns/needs acknowledged/addressed

Patient- and family-centered hospice care provided based on the patient's/family's unique situation and needs

Infection control and palliation

Grief/bereavement expression and support provided

Patient is pain free by next _____ visit

Caregiver demonstrates ability to manage pain, where applicable

Patient maintains comfort and dignity throughout illness

Patient and caregiver verbalize satisfaction with care

Educational tools/plans incorporated in daily care, and patient and caregiver verbalize understanding of safe, needed care

Patient will decide on care, interventions, and evaluation

Caregiver effective in care management and knows whom to call for questions/concerns

Patient will express satisfaction with hospice support received and will experience increased comfort

Patient will be made comfortable at home through death in accordance with the patient's wishes

Effective pain control and symptom control verbalized by patient

Patient verbalizes understanding of and adheres to care and medication regimens

Patient and caregiver supported through patient's death

Comfort maintained through course of care

Patient and family receive hospice support and care, and family members and friends are able to spend quality time with the patient

Caregiver able and verbalizes comfort with role and lists when to call hospice team members

Patient supported through and receives the maximum benefit from palliative chemotherapy and radiation with minimal complications

Patient and caregiver list adverse reactions, potential complications, signs/symptoms of infection (e.g., sputum change, chest congestion)

Comfort maintained through death with dignity

Pain effectively managed, and patient verbalizes comfort

Patient has stable respiratory status with patent airway

Patient and caregiver demonstrate appropriate back-up or "rescue" therapies for breakthrough pain or other symptoms (e.g., dyspnea)

Patient is protected from injury, has stable respiratory status, and is compliant with medication, safety, and care regimens

Comfort and individualized intervention of patient with immobility/bedbound status (e.g., skin, urinary, musculature, vascular)

Spiritual and psychosocial needs met (specify) as defined by patient and caregiver throughout course of care

Other outcomes/goals, based on the patient condition with input from the hospice team and patient and family

- ***Home health aide or certified nursing assistant***
  Effective hygiene, personal care, and comfort
  ADL assistance
  Safe environment maintained
  Advocacy and respite

- ***Hospice social worker***
  Problem identified and addressed, with patient/caregiver linked with appropriate support services and plan of care successfully implemented
  Patient and caregiver cope adaptively with illness and death
  Adaptive adjustment to changed body and body image
  Psychosocial support and counseling offered to patient/caregivers experiencing loss and grief

- ***Volunteer(s)***
  Comfort, companionship, and friendship extended to patient/family
  Support provided as defined by the needs of the patient/caregiver
  Patient and family supported by team with care, comfort, and companionship

- ***Spiritual counseling***
  Spiritual support offered and provided as defined by needs of patient/caregiver
  Provision of spiritual support and care as based on the assessed and ongoing needs of the patient and family
  Spiritual support offered, and patient and family needs met
  Support, listening, and presence

- *Dietitian/nutritional counseling*

    Family and caregiver integrate recommendations into nutrition teaching (where appropriate)

    Patient and caregiver know whom to call for nutrition- and hydration-related questions/concerns

    Nutrition/hydration per patient's choices

    Caregiver integrates recommendations into daily meal planning

- *Occupational therapist*

    Patient and caregiver demonstrate maximum independence with ADLs, adaptive techniques, and assistive devices

    Patient and caregiver demonstrate maximum safety in ADLs and functional mobility

    Patient and caregiver demonstrate effective use of energy conservation

    Verbalization/demonstration of improved functional activity level and enhanced quality of life

    Patient and caregiver demonstrate effective use of diaphragmatic breathing to reduce shortness of breath and relaxation techniques to help in pain/symptom management

    Patient and caregiver demonstrate correct use of exercise and splints for maximum upper extremity function and joint position

- *Physical therapist*

    Prevention of complications

    Home exercise and upper extremity program taught to caregiver

    Optimal strength, mobility, and function maintained/achieved

    Compliance with home exercise program by _____ (specify date)

- *Speech-language pathologist*

    Communication method implemented, and patient able to be understood as self-reported or reported by family/caregivers

    Safe swallowing and functional communication

    Recommended lists of foods/textures for safety and patient choice

- *Bereavement counselor*

    Support services related to grief provided to patient and family

    Well-being and resolution process of grief initiated and followed through bereavement services

- *Pharmacist*

    Regimen for bowel regimen successful as self-reported by patient and in update at team meeting

    Multiple drug regimen reviewed for food/drug and drug/drug interactions in patient on multiple medications

    Stability and safety in complex medication regimen, with maximum benefit to patient

    Effective pain and symptom control and symptom management as reported by patient/caregiver

    Other outcomes/goals, based on the patient's condition, with input from the hospice team and patient and family

- *Music, massage, art, or other therapies or services*

    Therapeutic massage/touch effective for patient as self-reported or observed by caregivers/family

    Improved muscle tone, relaxation, and/or sleep

    Patient comfortable and relaxed (e.g., sleeping) after massage

    Music therapy intervention based on assessment to decrease pain perception and provide emotional expression and support

    Maintenance of comfort and physical, psychosocial, and spiritual health

    Patient has pet's presence as desired—in all care sites, when possible

    Holistic health maintained and comfort achieved through _____ (specify modality)

8. **Patient, family, and caregiver educational needs**

    Educational needs are the care regimens that contribute to safe and effective care at home between the hospice team's visits. These include the following:

    The basic tenets of hospice and the availability of support 24 hours a day, 7 days a week

    Home safety assessment and counseling

    Anticipated disease progression

    The patient's medication regimen

    Safe and proper body mechanics to promote patient comfort and avoid caregiver safety problems

    Other teaching specific to the patient's and family's unique needs

    Support groups available to patient's family, such as the hospice program's "Caregiver Support Group" meetings for family members and friends of the patient

    Catheter care

    The symptoms of a urinary tract or other infection that necessitate calling the RN or physician

    The importance of keeping the bag below the patient's waist or lower than the catheter insertion site

    Skin care and hygiene regimens in the patient with an indwelling catheter

    Aspects of infection control, including effective hand washing and catheter site care and the importance of keeping the bag off the floor

    Safety issues that the caregiver needs to be aware of in safely caring for the homebound patient

    Other specific teaching as needed based on the patient's unique medical condition and the caregiver's needs

    Feeding-tube care

    Peristomal skin site care routines

    Teach caregiver all aspects of the particular tube (e.g., teach care of percutaneous gastrostomy tube)

    Teach about continuous infusion or other ordered method of administration

    All aspects of safe enteral feeding preparation and delivery

    Teach effective hand washing and infection control techniques, including safe storage of feedings and care and changing of supplies

    Other information that this patient and family need to know to function safely and effectively

Ostomy care

Care of ostomy, including bag changes, skin care, and signs and symptoms to
   report

Teach patient/family observational skills regarding skin and other care regimens

The patient's medications and their relationships to each other

Symptoms/changes that necessitate calling the hospice nurse

Other instructions as needed, based on the patient's unique medical condition
   and other needs

9. **Specific tips for quality and reimbursement**

   Document any variances to expected outcomes. There are many models of
   hospice programs. Those that are home health agency–based must work
   within the framework of the Medicare home care program. For example,
   sometimes a hospice patient reaches a stable period in the illness and has no
   further skilled needs or the patient is no longer homebound per Medicare
   home health care criteria. When this occurs, one option is to discharge the
   patient from Medicare home health agency reimbursement and maintain the
   patient on grant funds or other available resources. If the patient's status deteriorates and again meets the Medicare criteria, a new start of care is initiated on the HCFA form 485. Usually hospices continue volunteer support,
   nursing, and other services indicated during these periods of no reimbursement.

   The Medicare hospice benefit does not require that the patient be homebound or have identified skilled needs. Though it is a needed and viable
   program, the Medicare hospice benefit may not be indicated for all Medicare-
   eligible beneficiaries. For further information on this benefit, please refer to
   HCFA Hospice Manual 21.

   Should the patient's status deteriorate and increased personal care be
   needed, obtain a telephone order for the increased service, noting frequency
   and estimating the duration.

   Obtain a telephone order for all medication and treatment changes of the
   medical regimen, and document these in the clinical record.

   Unless the patient is in a hospice insurance program, some insurers will
   not pay for a skilled nurse visit that is made at death if the patient is dead
   when the nurse arrives at the home. From a Medicare home care perspective,
   the visit at the time of death may be covered when the orders and clinical
   record document assessment of the patient's status or signs of death/life or
   state law allows pronouncement of death by a nurse.

   Document patient deterioration

   Document dehydration, dehydrating

   Document patient change or instability

   Document pain, other symptoms not controlled

   Document status after acute episode of _____ (specify)

   Document positive urine, sputum, etc. culture; patient started on
      _____ (specify ordered antibiotic therapy)

   Document patient impacted; impaction removed manually per physician's
      orders

   Document RN in frequent communication with physician regarding
      _____ (specify)

Document febrile at _____, pulse change at _____, irr., irr.

Document change noted in _____

Document bony prominences red, opening

Document RN contacted physician regarding _____ (specify)

Document marked SOB

Document alteration in mental status

Document medications being adjusted, regulated, or monitored

Document unable to perform own ADLs, personal care

Document all interdisciplinary team meetings and communications in the POC and in the progress notes of the clinical record

All hospice team members should have input into the POC and document their interventions and goals

Document changes to the plan of care, such as medications, services, frequency, communication, and concurrence of other team members

Document coordination of services or consultation of the other members of the IDT

Document communications and care coordination with other care providers, such as skilled nursing facility or nursing home staff, inpatient team members, hired caregivers, and others

Catheter care

Documentation should include the size and type of catheter, the frequency of change, and other physician orders

Document color, appearance of urine, and urine C&S results in your clinical documentation

Document the continuing need for personal care services of the home health aide

Implement new or changed POC, teach or communicate to the patient or family, and document in the clinical record

Document specific teaching needs, teaching accomplished, and the behavioral outcomes of that teaching

Document your catheter supplies, including type and size

Document the following:

Constipation and resulting pressure on the bladder

A urinary infection, catheter position change, or the need for a different size or kind of catheter

Bladder spasms that can occur after catheter change

Increased sediment, sometimes indicating need for bladder irrigation

Catheter draining, but leaking apparent also and other catheter problems based on their unique history

Feeding-tube care

Document the gastrostomy site wound, and indicate color, any drainage, amount, and the specific care rendered

Communicate any POC changes

Document the reason for the tube feeding and the type of tube chosen

Document progress in wound healing or deterioration in wound status in the clinical documentation

Document the supplies needed on the form 485, or other POC, and obtain physician orders for all supplies or equipment

Obtain a telephone order for any additional visits not projected on the original POC and state why (e.g., RN to visit × 1 to reinsert tube). Better yet, obtain prn orders for tube dislodgment (e.g., prn × 3), patient complaint, or other tube problem needing evaluation.

Document any learning barriers

Document the specific care and teaching accomplished and the behavioral and objective outcomes of that teaching

Document patient's level of independence in care

Document that the nutritional solutions are the patient's sole source of nutrition, when appropriate. Medicare and many other insurers will pay only if it is the *sole* source of nutrition (e.g., Ensure)

Document any problems with the skin site surrounding the tube and care provided

Document the specific type and size of tube. Specify the insertion date and site, the ordered feeding schedule, and teaching needs identified and accomplished.

Document need for disease-specific nutrition products when standard formula is unsuccessful

Ostomy care

Document up with assistance only

Document any changes, including specific care provided

Document physician changed medications to _____ (specify)

Document new onset (any problem)

Document pain not controlled effectively

Document increased gas pain and discomfort

Document the specific type of ostomy, the type and size of the ordered appliances, and frequency of changes needed

Document the patient's skin condition and the specific skin care regimen ordered and provided

Document the patient's level of self-care and progress toward predetermined, patient-centered goals

There are usually many nursing needs of the patient with a new colostomy or the patient with a new caregiver who must be taught the established care regimens. These include the following:

Observation and assessment skills

Ostomy care, including healing, complications, and body image

Wound care (hands-on teaching and wound assessment/reassessment)

Teaching the safe care regimens to caregivers

Document in the clinical notes the clear progression and symptomatology and interventions that demonstrate the overall management of the patient with _____ (specify)

Document when/if the patient has respiratory changes, shortness of breath, exacerbation of conditions, dysphagia, changes in pain, and/or other symptoms and that they are identified and resolved

Remember that the clinical documentation is key to measuring compliance for quality and reimbursement purposes. Care coordination, timely verbal and initial physician orders, and assessment and addressing of spiritual and psychosocial needs should be ongoing and documented in the patient's clinical record

The documentation should support that all hospice care supports comfort and dignity while meeting patient/family needs

The documentation should include ongoing assessment and management of pain and other symptoms and the anticipation and prevention of secondary symptoms such as constipation

It is important to note that all team members, including nurses and social workers, should assess, identify, and "hear" spiritual needs that the patient and family want to be addressed. These spiritual issues are key to the provision of quality hospice care and cannot be addressed effectively and promptly by the spiritual counselor only

Document clearly symptoms, clinical changes, and assessment findings related to pain and patient care

Document patient changes, symptoms, and clinical information identified from visits and team conferences that support hospice care and a limited life expectancy

Clearly support in the documentation the rationale that supports/explains the progression of the illness from the chronic to terminal stages

Document mentation, behavioral, and/or cognitive changes

Document dysphagia, weight loss, increased shortness of breath, dyspnea, infection, sepsis, new or changed medications, etc.

Document any skin changes (e.g., inflamed, painful, weeping skin site[s])

Document when the patient is actively dying, deteriorating, or progressing toward death

Remember that the "litmus test" of care coordination rests on the quality of the clinical documentation by all team members. Review one of your patient's clinical records and ask yourself the following: "If I was unable to give a verbal report/update on this patient, would a peer be able to pick up and provide the same level of care and know (from the documentation) the current orders, medications, and other details that contribute to effective hospice care?"

This patient population usually has many clinical changes that should be documented. These include weight loss and multiple and changed medication regimens with varying routes. Side effects to the drug regimen should be observed, noted, documented, and reported

10. **Resources for hospice care and practice**

Catheter care

Available free from the Agency for Health Care Policy and Research (AHCPR) are these four resources: *Clinical Practice Guideline: Urinary Incontinence in Adults; Quick Reference Guide for Clinicians: Urinary Incontinence in Adults; Urinary Incontinence in Adults: A Patient's Guide;* and *Caregiver Guide: Helping People with Incontinence.* To receive these publications, call the AHCPR at 1-800-358-9295.

Feeding-tube care and ostomy care

For resources or support for patients, there are two organizations that your patients can contact: The United Ostomy Association at 1-800-826-0826 or 1-800-826-0826 or the National Foundation for Ileitis and Colitis at 1-800-343-3637.

WOUND AND PRESSURE ULCER CARE

1. General considerations

Pressure ulcers, malignant cutaneous wounds, and other draining or leaking skin sites are commonly seen in patients in the home setting and are cared for sensitively and skillfully by the hospice team. The enterostomal therapist may be consulted. The enterostomal therapist plays an important role in providing this special patient population with quality care.

2. Needs for visit

Physician order for hospice care, specific to the hospice program's admission criteria and policies
Standard precautions supplies
Vital signs equipment for baseline assessment
Dressing supplies
Other supplies or equipment, based on physician orders

3. Safety considerations

Infection control/standard precautions
Night-light
Extra caution on slippery surfaces
Removal of scatter rugs
Tub rail, grab bars for bathroom safety
Supportive and nonskid shoes
Handrail on stairs
Fall precautions/protocol
The phone number of whom to call with a care problem
The need to report changes in skin integrity
Protective skin measures
Smoke detector and fire evacuation plan
Assistance with ambulation
Others, based on the patient's unique condition and environment

4. Potential diagnoses and codes

Amputation, infected right or left BKA, AKA	997.62
Amputation, transmetatarsal (right or left) (surgical)	84.12
Anal rectal abscess	566
Arterial graft, S/P (surgical)	39.58
Arterial insufficiency	447.1
Arterial occlusive disease	444.22
Bullous pemphigoid	694.5
Catheter (Foley indwelling)	57.94
Cellulitis of the arm	682.3
Cellulitis of the trunk	682.2
Cellulitis RLE, LLE	682.6
Chronic ischemic heart disease	414.9

Congestive heart failure (CHF)	428.0
Coronary artery disease	414.0
CVA	436
Debridement (surgical)	86.22
Decubitus ulcer (pressure ulcer)	707.0
Diabetes mellitus, with complications (NIDDM)	250.90
Diabetes mellitus, with complications (IDDM)	250.91
Diabetic neuropathy	250.60 and 357.2
Diabetic retinopathy	250.50 and 362.01
Excoriation of skin	919.8
Femoral-popliteal bypass (right or left) (surgical)	39.29
Foot abscess	682.7
Foot wound, open	707.1
Gangrene, toe	785.4
Heel ulcer, right or left	707.0
Hypertension	401.9
I and D stitch abscess	86.04 and 998.5
Infection, postoperative	998.5
Leg injury	959.7
Open wound, lower leg (right or left)	707.1
Open wound, upper leg (right or left)	707.1
Osteomyelitis, acute	730.00
Osteomyelitis, foot	730.07
Osteomyelitis, lower leg (right or left)	730.06
Peripheral vascular disease	443.9
Peritonitis	567.9
Pressure ulcer	707.0
Protein-caloric malnutrition	263.9
Quadriplegia	344.0
Septicemia	038.9
Skin eruption	782.1
Skin, excoriation of	919.8
Skin graft	86.89
Staph infection	041.10
Stasis ulcer	454.2
Stitch abscess, excision	998.5 and 86.22
Surgical wound, open	998.3
Thrombophlebitis	451.9
Ulcer, heel with cellulitis	682.7
Ulcer, right or left heel	707.1
Urinary incontinence	788.30
Varicose leg ulcer	454.9
Vascular insufficiency	459.9
Vascular shunt bypass	32.29
Venous insufficiency	459.81
Venous ulcer	454.0
Wound evisceration	998.3
Wound, open lower leg (right or left)	707.1

5. **Associated nursing diagnoses**
   Activity intolerance
   Activity intolerance, risk for
   Anxiety
   Body image disturbance
   Body temperature, altered, risk for
   Cardiac output, decreased
   Caregiver role strain
   Caregiver role strain, risk for
   Constipation
   Coping, ineffective individual
   Denial, ineffective
   Family processes, altered
   Fatigue
   Fear
   Fluid volume deficit, risk for
   Fluid volume excess
   Home maintenance management
   Infection, risk for
   Injury, risk for
   Knowledge deficit (self-care management)
   Management of therapeutic regimen (individuals), ineffective
   Mobility, impaired physical
   Noncompliance (self-care regimen)
   Nutrition, altered: less than body requirements
   Pain
   Pain, chronic
   Self-care deficit, bathing/hygiene
   Self-care deficit, dressing/grooming
   Self-care deficit, feeding
   Self-care deficit, toileting
   Sensory/perceptual alterations (specify) (visual, auditory, kinesthetic, gustatory, tactile, olfactory)
   Sexuality patterns, altered
   Skin integrity, impaired
   Sleep pattern disturbance
   Social interaction, impaired
   Spiritual distress (distress of the human spirit)
   Spiritual well-being, potential for enhanced
   Tissue integrity, impaired
   Tissue perfusion, altered (specify type) (renal, cerebral, cardiopulmonary, gastrointestinal, peripheral)

6. **Skills and services identified**

   - *Hospice nursing*

     a. *Comfort and symptom control*
        Skilled observation and systems assessment of patient with a
        _____ (specify site or type) wound
        Skilled observation and all systems assessment of patient with a pressure ulcer

Presentation of hospice philosophy and services

Explain patient rights and responsibilities

Assess patient, family, and caregiver wishes and expectations regarding care

Assess patient, family, and caregiver resources available for care

Provision of volunteer support to patient and family

Teach family or caregiver physical care of patient

RN to provide and teach effective oral care and comfort measures

Skilled observation and assessment of wound q visit

Assess pain and other symptoms, including site, duration, characteristics, and relief measures

RN to assess patient's pain q visit to identify need for change, addition, or other plan or dose adjustment

Assessment of healing process and site for sign of infection

Comprehensive risk assessment of patient with a wound

Pack wound with _____, cover with _____ (per physician orders)

Culture wound prn

Teach patient or caregiver wound packing and irrigation techniques

Soak foot in _____ (per physician orders)

Pain assessment and effectiveness of pain management every visit

Cover wound with _____ (specify orders)

Wrap site

Assess wound on left extremity for signs and symptoms of infection

Measure vital signs q visit

RN to contact enterosotomal therapist for assessment of wound and recommendation of plan

RN to provide aseptic wound care to site (specify supplies, frequency, and specific wound orders)

RN to evaluate patient's pain and to implement pain control/relief program

Teach patient and caregiver regarding wound infection control measures

Observe for signs and symptoms of infection

Assess healing process

Change packing q _____ (specify)

Teach family or caregiver wound procedure and care regimen(s)

Pack wound with _____ (specify)

Apply wet to dry dressing of _____ (specify)

Soak site with _____ (specify)

Assess peripheral circulation

Instruct patient in dressing change

Assess wound drainage and amount

Cover with sterile 4 × 4

Remove dressing using normal saline solution

Repack wound with _____ (specify)

Pain assessment and management q visit

Assess wound for symptoms of infection, decreased circulation, or other problems

Elevate leg whenever sitting

TEDs or Ace™ wrap whenever up

Wash site gently with _____ (specify)

RN to consult with enterostomal therapist nurse for evaluation and POC and to report findings and recommendations to physician

Measure the site(s) for baseline and progress, including length, width, and depth

RN to teach infection control measures of wound care

Observation and skilled assessment of other areas for possible breakdown, including heels, hips, elbows, ankles, and other pressure-prone areas

RN to monitor for infection, necrosis, and increased exudate or other problems and to report to physician

Comfort measures of backrub and hand or other therapeutic massage

Assess pain, and evaluate the pain management's effectiveness

Teach care of bedridden patient

Measure vital signs, including pain, q visit

Assess cardiovascular, pulmonary, and respiratory statuses

Teach caregivers symptom control and relief measures

Oxygen on at _____ liters per _____ (specify physician orders)

Identify and monitor pain, symptoms, and relief measures

Teach caregiver care of weak, terminally ill patient

Observation, assessment, and supportive care to patient and family

Teach patient/family use of standardized form/tool to use between hospice team members' visits (and for care coordination between team members)

Supportive care and scopolamine patches per physician orders

Observation, assessment, and supportive care to patient and family

Teach patient/family principles of effective pain management

Effective management of pain and prevention of secondary symptoms

Observation and assessment, communication with physician related to signs and symptoms of continuing decompensation, increased symptoms, pain, discomfort, shortness of breath, and measures to alleviate and control

Pain assessment and management q visit, including source of pain (e.g., neuropathy, phantom pain, claudication, infection, other problems such as cardiac or arthritis pain)

Interventions of symptoms directed toward comfort and palliation

Teach patient and family about realistic expectations of disease process

Teach care of dying and signs/symptoms of impending death

Presence and support

Other interventions, based on patient/family needs

b. *Safety and mobility considerations*

Provide caregiver/family with home safety information and instruction related to _____ and documented in the clinical record

Teach family about safety of patient in home

Teach patient and family about energy conservation techniques

Other interventions, based on patient/family needs

   c. *Emotional/spiritual considerations*

Psychosocial assessment of patient and family regarding disease and prognosis

RN to provide emotional support to patient and family

Assess mental status and sleep disturbance changes

Observation and assessment of mental status changes/complaints of depression in new hospice patient with large draining wound

Observation of patient for neuropsychiatric complications of illness, including confusion, depression, and anxiety

RN to provide support and intervention/referral for depression

Teach patient/family about depression and signs/symptoms of exacerbation that require more intervention

Assess for and manage plans for psychosocial and/or spiritual pain (e.g., all pain, anxiety, interpersonal or other distress)

Psychosocial aspects of pain control (e.g., depression) assessed and acknowledged with team support/intervention

Ongoing acknowledgment of spirituality and related concerns of patient/family

Other interventions, based on patient/family needs

   d. *Skin care*

Pressure ulcer care as indicated

Assess skin integrity

Observation and evaluation of wound and surrounding skin

Evaluate patient's need for equipment, including supplies to decrease pressure, alternating pressure mattress, gel foam seat cushion, and heel and elbow protectors

Teach family to perform dressings between RN visits

RN to teach patient regarding care of irradiated skin sites

Teach patient, family, or caregiver about proper body alignment and positioning in bed to prevent skin tears from shearing skin

Observe and apply skilled assessment of areas for possible breakdown, including heels, hips, elbows, ankles, and other pressure-prone areas

Teach caregiver about skin care needs, including the need for frequent position changes, appropriate pressure pads and mattresses, and the prevention of breakdown

Other interventions, based on patient/family needs

   e. *Elimination considerations*

Assess bowel regimen, and implement program as needed

Check for impaction and remove in bedbound patient per physician orders

Condom catheter or indwelling catheter as indicated

Assess amount and frequency of urinary output

RN to evaluate the patient's bowel patterns and need for stool softeners, laxatives, and dietary adjustments and to develop bowel management plan

RN to teach daily catheter care

Teaching and ongoing assessment for the prevention and early identification of constipation and its correction/resolution

Initiate bowel management program per hospice physician

Teach patient, family, and aide the importance of observing and noting bowel movements between scheduled nursing visits

Obtain patient history related to norms for bowel movements to date (e.g., "all my life I go only every other day")

Implement bowel assessment management program

Bowel management program of stool softeners, laxative of choice, Fleet's Enemas prn, and other methods per patient wishes and physician orders

Other interventions, based on patient/family needs

f. *Hydration/nutrition*

Teach patient/family role of adequate nutrition in wound healing. Promote intake of high biological value proteins

Assess nutrition/hydration status

Diet counseling for patient with anorexia

Nutrition/hydration supported by offering patient's choice of favorite or desired foods or liquids

Nutrition/hydration maintained by offering patient high-protein diet and foods of choice as tolerated

Teach patient and family to expect decreased nutritional and fluid intake as disease progresses

Teach feeding-tube care to family

Other interventions, based on patient/family needs

g. *Therapeutic/medication regimens*

Assess the patient's response to therapeutic treatments and interventions, and report to the physician any changes or unfavorable responses

Teach about new antibiotic regimen

Teach about medication and medication management

RN to instruct in pain control measures and medications

Teach and observe regarding side effects of palliative chemotherapy, including constipation, anemia, and fatigue

Venipuncture q _____ (specify ordered frequency) for monitoring platelet count

Medication assessment and management

Teach new medication and effects

Assess for electrolyte imbalance

Teach patient and caregiver use of PCA pump

RN to instruct in pain control measures and medications

Nonpharmacological interventions of progressive muscle relaxation imagery, positive visualization, music, massage and touch, and humor therapy of patient's choice implemented

Teaching of patient/family, including medications and the management program, including strength, type, actions, times, and compliance tips

Encourage family/caregivers to give the patient medications on the schedule and around-the-clock

Medications changed using equianalgesic conversion tables/physician orders (e.g., from oral morphine to an equianalgesic dose of transdermal fentanyl)

Nonpharmacological or other interventions of relaxation, hot/cold
therapy, biofeedback, distraction, guided imagery, humor, music
therapy, acupuncture, TENS technology, hypnosis, massage, or others
as patient/family wishes
Other interventions, based on patient/family needs

h. *Other considerations*
Assess disease process progression
Other interventions, based on patient/family needs
RN to assess the patient's response to treatments and interventions and
to report to physician any changes, unfavorable responses, or reac-
tions

- *Home health aide or certified nursing assistant*
Effective and safe personal care
Safe ADL assistance and support
Respite care and active listening skills
Observation and reporting
Meal preparation
Homemaker services
Comfort care
Other duties

- *Hospice social worker*
Psychosocial assessment of patient and family/caregiver, including adjust-
ment to illness and its implications
Identification of optimal coping strategies
Financial assessment and counseling regarding food acquisition, ability to
prepare, and costs of needed medications or wound care supplies
Intervention/support related to terminal illness and loss
Emotional/spiritual support
Depression/fear assessed
Facilitate communication among patient, family, and hospice team
Identification of caregiver role strain necessitating respite/relief measures/
support
Referral/linkage to community services and resources as indicated
Grief counseling and intervention/support related to illness/loss
Patient/caregiver counseling and support
For patients who live alone with no support system (e.g., able, available,
willing caregiver[s]): obtain resources to enable patient to remain in
home
Identification of illness-related psychiatric condition necessitating care

- *Volunteer(s)*
Support, friendship, companionship, and presence
Comfort and dignity maintained/provided for patient and family
Errands and transportation
Advocacy and respite
Other services, based on interdisciplinary team recommendations and
patient/caregiver needs

- *Spiritual counselor*
  Spiritual assessment and care
  Counseling, intervention, and support related to that dimension of life
    related to life's meaning (consistent with patient's beliefs)
  Support, listening, and presence
  Participation in sacred or spiritual rituals or practices
  Other supportive care, based on patient's/family's needs and belief systems

- *Dietitian/nutritional counseling*
  Supportive counseling with patient/family indicating that patient will have
    a decreased appetite and usually at some point may not eat/drink
  Assessment and recommendations for swallowing difficulties
  Teaching and support of family members and caregivers
  Support and care with food and nourishment as desired by patient
  Encourage oral nutritional supplements for increased caloric and protein
    intake
  Encourage adequate fluids
  Evaluation/management of nutritional deficits and needs
  Food, dietary recommendations incorporate patient choice and wishes

- *Occupational therapist*
  Evaluation of ADLs and functional mobility
  Assess for need for adaptive equipment and assistive devices
  Safety assessment of patient's environment and ADLs
  Assessment for energy conservation training
  Assessment of upper extremity function, retraining motor skills, and/or
    splinting for contracture(s)

- *Physical therapist*
  Evaluation
  Assessment of patient's environment for safety
  Instruct in transfer training or bed mobility exercises and positioning to
    facilitate healing
  Pain assessment/reduction factors
  Strengthening exercises/program
  Assessment of gait safety and home safety measures
  Instruct/supervise caregiver and volunteers on home exercise program for
    conditioning and strength
  Assistive, adaptive devices and evaluation of equipment and teaching
  Progressive mobility
  Assist with selection of pressure-relieving devices

- *Speech-language pathologist*
  Evaluation for speech/swallowing problems
  Food texture recommendations
  Alternate functional communication

- *Bereavement counselor*
  Assessment of the needs of the bereaved family and friends
  Support and intervention, based on assessment and ongoing findings
  Presence and counseling

Supportive visits, follow-up, and other interventions (e.g., mailings, calls)

Other services related to bereavement work and support

- *Pharmacist*

    Evaluation of hospice patient with constipation on cathartics, stool soften-
    ers, and other medications for possible food/drug and drug/drug interac-
    tions

    Medication monitoring regarding therapeutic levels and dosages

    Pain consult and input into interdisciplinary plan of care related to pain
    control, palliation, and symptom management

    Assessment of medication regimen and plan for safety and compliance

- *Music, massage, art, or other therapies or services*

    Evaluation and intervention based on patient's and caregiver's unique
    wishes and needs that support care, comfort, and death in the setting of
    the patient's choice

    Pet therapy (including patient's pet, if available) and therapeutic interven-
    tion

    Assessment plan to engage patient and support comfort, quality, enjoyment,
    and dignity

7. **Outcomes for care**

- *Hospice nursing*

    Patient and caregiver verbalize satisfaction with care

    Educational tools/plans incorporated in daily care, and patient and care-
    giver verbalize understanding of safe, needed care

    Patient will decide on care, interventions, and evaluation

    Caregiver effective in care management and knows whom to call for
    questions/concerns

    Patient will express satisfaction with hospice support received and will ex-
    perience increased comfort

    Patient will be made comfortable at home through death in accordance
    with the patient's wishes

    Effective pain control and symptom control verbalized by patient

    Patient verbalizes understanding of and adheres to care and medication
    regimens

    Patient and caregiver supported through patient's death

    Comfort maintained through course of care

    Patient and family receive hospice support and care, and family members
    and friends are able to spend quality time with the patient

    Caregiver able and verbalizes comfort with role and lists when to call
    hospice team members

    Patient supported through and receives the maximum benefit from pallia-
    tive chemotherapy and radiation with minimal complications

    Patient and caregiver list adverse reactions, potential complications, and
    signs/symptoms of infection (e.g., sputum change, chest congestion)

    Comfort maintained through death with dignity

    Pain effectively managed, and patient verbalizes comfort

    Patient is protected from injury, has stable respiratory status, and is compli-
    ant with medication, safety, and care regimens

Comfort and individualized intervention of patient with immobility/
bedbound status (e.g., skin, urinary, musculature, vascular)

Spiritual and psychosocial needs met (specify) as defined by patient and
caregiver throughout course of care

Patient and caregiver will demonstrate _____% behavioral compliance
with instructions related to medications, diet, and skin care

Infection-free wound healing by _____ (specify date)

Patient states pain is _____ on 0-10 scale by next visit

Patient and caregiver demonstrate appropriate back-up or "rescue" therapies
for breakthrough pain or other symptoms (e.g., dyspnea)

Patient and caregiver correctly demonstrate/provide incisional or other
wound care

Optimal circulation and nutrition for patient to support healing

Adherence to POC by patient and caregivers and ability to demonstrate
safe and supportive care

Behavioral compliance with home care regimen

Patient and caregiver compliant with comprehensive wound care program,
including pressure reduction, pain management, nutritional support, and
positioning regimen

Wound site healing and infection free by _____ (specify date)

Wound closure occurring in patient with burns as demonstrated by measurements that show a decrease in wound size (specify)

Patient and caregiver will demonstrate _____% behavioral compliance
with instructions related to medications, diet, and wound/skin care

Optimal nutrition/hydration needs maintained/addressed as evidenced by
patient's weight maintained/decreased by/increased by _____ lbs

Patient will be maintained in home stating/demonstrating adherence
to POC

Adherence to multiple medication regimen

Lab values (specify) will be improved/WNL for patient

Caregiver and patient able to self-manage care, ADLs, diet, safety, medications, and exercise regimens

Medications regulated as demonstrated by stable blood levels

Caregiver and patient verbalize symptoms that necessitate calling the physician and intervention/follow-up

Supportive and skillful care to patient with draining wound

Comfort through death with support and care of hospice team

Mental distress, depression, and fear of dying addressed throughout care by
hospice team

Patient and family able to care for and support patient

Patient and caregiver can verbalize symptoms, changes, or accelerations
that necessitate call to physician

Patient and family demonstrate compliance to medication and other therapeutic interventions

Patient demonstrates stabilization and increased or enhanced coping skills
related to functioning and depression

Pain and symptoms managed/controlled in setting of patient/family choice
(e.g., patient/family report ability to eat, sleep, speak with pacing)

Planned and effective bowel program, as evidenced by regular bowel
movements and patient/family report of comfort

Death with dignity and pain/symptoms controlled in setting of patient/
family choice

Optimal comfort, support, and dignity provided throughout illness

Death with maximum comfort through effective symptom control with specialized hospice support

Patient and caregiver able to list adverse drug reactions/problems with
medication regimen and whom to call for follow-up and resolution

Patient's/family's privacy, independence, and choices supported with
respect and maintained through death

Enhancement and support of quality of life

Effective symptom relief and control (e.g., a peaceful and comfortable
death at home, depression controlled, some enjoyment of life)

Maximizing the patient's quality of life (e.g., alert and pain free or as
patient wishes)

Pharmacological and nonpharmacological interventions such as localized
heat application, biofeedback, massage, positioning, relaxation methods,
and music

Patient cared for and family supported through death with physical, psychosocial, spiritual, and other concerns/needs acknowledged/addressed

Patient- and family-centered hospice care provided based on the patient's/
family's unique situation and needs

Infection control and palliation through death in setting of patient's choice

Grief/bereavement expression and support provided

Patient is pain free by next _____ visit

Caregiver demonstrates ability to manage pain, where applicable

Patient maintains comfort and dignity throughout illness

Other outcomes/goals, based on the patient condition with input from the
hospice team and patient and family

- *Home health aide or certified nursing assistant*

Effective hygiene, personal care, and comfort

ADL assistance

Safe environment maintained

Respite and advocacy

- *Hospice social worker*

Problem identified and addressed, with patient/caregiver linked with appropriate support services and plan of care successfully implemented

Patient and caregiver cope adaptively with illness and death

Adaptive adjustment to changed body and body image

Psychosocial support and counseling offered to patient/caregivers experiencing loss and grief

Caregiver system assessed, and development of stable caregiver plan facilitated

- *Volunteer(s)*

Comfort, companionship, and friendship extended to patient/family

Support provided as defined by the needs of the patient/caregiver

Patient and family supported by team with care, comfort, and companionship

- *Spiritual counseling*

  Spiritual support offered and provided as defined by needs of patient/
  caregiver

  Provision of spiritual support and care based on the assessed and ongoing
  needs of the patient and family

  Spiritual support offered, and patient and family needs met

  Patient and family express relief of symptoms of spiritual suffering

  Support, listening, and presence

  Participation in sacred or spiritual rituals or practice

- *Dietitian/nutritional counseling*

  Patient and family verbalize comprehension of changing nutritional
  needs

  Family and caregiver integrate dietary recommendations into nutrition
  teaching (where appropriate)

  Patient and caregiver know whom to call for nutrition- and hydration-
  related questions/concerns

  Nutrition/hydration per patient's choices

  Caregiver integrates recommendations into daily meal planning

- *Occupational therapist*

  Patient and caregiver demonstrate maximum independence with ADLs,
  adaptive techniques, and assistive devices

  Patient and caregiver demonstrate maximum safety in ADLs and functional
  mobility

  Patient and caregiver demonstrate effective use of energy conservation

  Verbalization/demonstration of improved functional activity level and enhanced quality of life

  Patient and caregiver demonstrate effective use of diaphragmatic breathing
  to reduce shortness of breath and relaxation techniques to help in pain/
  symptom management

  Patient and caregiver demonstrate correct use of exercise and splints for
  maximum upper extremity function and joint position

- *Physical therapist*

  Prevention of complications

  Home exercise and upper extremity program taught to caregiver

  Optimal strength, mobility, and function maintained/achieved

  Compliance with home exercise program by _____ (specify
  date)

- *Speech-language pathologist*

  Communication method implemented, and patient able to be understood as
  self-reported or reported by family/caregivers

  Safe swallowing and functional communication

  Recommended lists of food/textures for safety and patient choice

- *Bereavement counselor*

  Support services related to grief provided to patient and family

  Well-being and resolution process of grief initiated and followed through
  bereavement services

- *Pharmacist*

    Regimen for bowel regimen successful as self-reported by patient and in update at team meeting

    Multiple drug regimen reviewed for food/drug and drug/drug interactions in patient on multiple medications

    Stability and safety in complex medication regimen with maximum benefit to patient

    Effective pain and symptom control and symptom management as reported by patient/caregiver

- *Music, massage, art, or other therapies or services*

    Therapeutic massage/touch effective for patient as self-reported or observed by caregivers/family

    Improved muscle tone, relaxation, and/or sleep

    Patient comfortable and relaxed (e.g., sleeping) after massage

    Music therapy intervention based on assessment to decrease pain perception and provide emotional expression and support

    Maintenance of comfort and physical, psychosocial, and spiritual health

    Patient has pet's presence as desired—in all care sites, when possible

    Holistic health maintained and comfort achieved through _____ (specify modality)

8. **Patient, family, and caregiver educational needs**

    Educational needs are the care regimens that contribute to safe and effective care at home between the hospice team's visits. These include the following:

    The basic tenets of hospice and the availability of support 24 hours a day, 7 days a week

    Home safety assessment and counseling

    The patient's medication regimen

    Anticipated disease progression

    Safe and proper body mechanics to promote patient comfort and prevent caregiver safety problems

    Other teaching specific to the patient's and family's unique needs

    Support groups available to patient's family, such as the hospice program's "Caregiver Support Group" meetings for family members and friends of the patient

    All aspects of the specific care related to wound care, including effective hand-washing techniques, safe disposal of soiled dressings, and other infection control measures

    The importance of optimal nutrition and, when possible, exercise to speed the healing process

    Medication instruction, including schedule, route, functions, and possible side effects

    Other aspects of care, based on patient's unique medical condition and needs

9. **Specific tips for quality and reimbursement**

    Document any variances to expected outcomes. There are many models of hospice programs. Those that are home health agency–based must work within the framework of the Medicare home care program. For example, sometimes a hospice patient reaches a stable period in the illness and has no further skilled needs or the patient is no longer homebound per Medicare home health care criteria. When this occurs, one option is to discharge the patient from Medicare home health agency reimbursement and maintain the patient on grant funds or other available resources. If the patient's status deteriorates and again meets the Medicare criteria, a new start of care is initiated on the HCFA form 485. Usually hospices continue volunteer support, nursing, and other services indicated during these periods of no reimbursement.

The Medicare hospice benefit does not require that the patient be homebound or have identified skilled needs. Though it is a needed and viable program, the Medicare hospice benefit may not be indicated for all Medicare-eligible beneficiaries. For further information on this benefit, please refer to HCFA Hospice Manual 21.

Should the patient's status deteriorate and increased personal care be needed, obtain a telephone order for the increased service, noting frequency and estimating the duration.

Obtain a telephone order for all medication and treatment changes of the medical regimen, and document these in the clinical record.

Unless the patient is in a hospice insurance program, some insurers will not pay for a skilled nurse visit that is made at death if the patient is dead when the nurse arrives at the home. From a Medicare home care perspective, the visit at the time of death may be covered when the orders and clinical record document assessment of the patient's status or signs of death/life or state law allows pronouncement of death by a nurse.

Document patient deterioration

Document dehydration, dehydrating

Document patient change or instability

Document pain, other symptoms not controlled

Document status after acute episode of _____ (specify)

Document positive urine, sputum, etc. culture; patient started on _____ (specify ordered antibiotic therapy)

Document patient impacted; impaction removed manually

Document RN in frequent communication with physician regarding _____ (specify)

Document febrile at _____, pulse change at _____, irr., irr.

Document change noted in _____

Document bony prominences red, opening

Document RN contacted physician regarding _____ (specify)

Document marked SOB

Document alteration in mental status

Document medications being adjusted, regulated, or monitored

Document unable to manage ADLs, personal care

Document all interdisciplinary team meetings and communication in the POC and in the progress notes of the clinical record

All hospice team members involved should have input into the POC and document their interventions and goals

Document all teaching accomplished with family or caregiver

Document progress toward goals, when identified

Document description of decubitus (pressure) ulcer

Document infected area

Document any discharge and odor and amount

Document draining wound

Document homebound status

Document up only with assistance

Document can only transfer safely

Document length, width, depth of wound

Document any changes, including specific care provided

Document medication(s) changed or medication(s) being regulated

Document RN contacted physician regarding _____ (specify)

Document febrile, temperature _____ (specify)

Document unable to perform ADLs or personal care

Document any change in the patient's status or POC

Take photograph of wound(s) to substantiate document at onset of q3 weeks, have patient sign release, take one photograph for the clinical record

Specify any learning barriers, such as arthritic hands, poor eyesight, and language barriers

Document the specific teaching accomplished and the behavioral outcomes of that teaching

Document clearly the status of the decubitus (pressure) ulcer and the clinical progress toward healing and patient-centered goal achievement

Wound care is an area in which managed-care companies and other payors are attempting to decrease allowed numbers of visits. It is the professional nurse's responsibility to remember that it is not just the dressing change that occurs. When a nurse makes a home visit, an assessment of the wound healing or deterioration and teaching occur. There should also be observation and assessment of the wound and the surrounding skin. These skills usually require the skills of a nurse. All these components contribute to safe, effective wound care.

Document progress toward wound healing

Document patient or wound deterioration

Document any change that impacts the provision of safe care

Document wound draining, amount, and site

Document any medication change(s)

Document progress or deterioration in wound healing, and take measurements at least once a week

The way to help third-party payors understand these components is to clearly record the care you provided on each skilled visit. The specifics related to the wound size, drainage, odor, involvement of tissues/structures, and your skilled assessment of the healing or potential for healing will be helpful to those having to make a payment decision about the services provided.

Wound dressing or care orders should always include the specific orders such as aseptic or clean technique, wound location, frequency of change, and any special supplies needed to safely and effectively follow the POC.

Document coordination of services or consultation of the other members of the IDT

Document communications and care coordination with other care providers, such as skilled nursing facility or nursing home staff, inpatient team members, and hired caregivers

Document in the clinical notes the clear progression and symptomatology and interventions that demonstrate the overall management of the patient with _____ (specify)

Document when/if the patient has respiratory changes, shortness of breath, exacerbation of conditions, dysphagia, changes in pain, and/or other symptoms and that they are identified and resolved

Remember that the clinical documentation is key to measuring compliance for quality and reimbursement purposes. Care coordination, timely verbal and initial physician orders, and assessment and addressing of spiritual and psychosocial needs should be ongoing and documented in the patient's clinical record

The documentation should support that all hospice care supports comfort and dignity while meeting patient/family needs

The documentation should include ongoing assessment and management of pain and other symptoms and the anticipation and prevention of secondary symptoms such as constipation

It is important to note that all team members, including nurses and social workers, should assess, identify, and "hear" spiritual needs that the patient/family want to be addressed. These spiritual issues are key to the provision of quality hospice care and cannot be addressed effectively and promptly by the spiritual counselor only

Document clearly symptoms, clinical changes, and assessment findings related to pain and patient care

Document patient changes, symptoms, and clinical information identified from visits and team conferences that support hospice care and a limited life expectancy

Clearly support in the documentation the rationale that supports/explains the progression of the illness from the chronic to terminal stages

Document mentation, behavioral, and/or cognitive changes

Document dysphagia, weight loss, increased shortness of breath, dyspnea, infection, sepsis, new or changed medications, etc.

Document changes to the plan of care, such as medications, services, frequency, communication, and concurrence of other team members

Your assessments, observations, and clinical findings are information that assists in painting a picture to support coverage and documentation requirements for hospice care

Document any hospitalizations and changed clinical findings

Document patient changes, symptoms, psychosocial issues impacting the care, and information gathered at the patient/family visits and during team meetings

The documentation should reflect ongoing effects of the terminal condition, the patient's/family's difficulty with care or coping, and the continued desire for hospice care

Document any skin changes (e.g., inflamed, painful, weeping skin site[s])

Document when the patient is actively dying, deteriorating, or progressing toward death

Remember that the "litmus test" of care coordination rests on the quality of the clinical documentation by all team members. Review one of your patient's clinical records and ask yourself the following: "If I was unable to give a verbal report/update on this patient, would a peer be able to pick

up and provide the same level of care and know (from the documentation) the current orders, medications, and other details that contribute to
effective hospice care?"

This patient population usually has many clinical changes that should be
documented. These include weight loss and multiple and changed medication regimens with varying routes. Side effects to the drug regimen should
be observed, noted, documented, and reported

10. Resources for hospice care and practice

The Agency for Health Care Policy and Research has *Pressure Ulcers: Pre-
diction and Prevention, Pressure Ulcers: Treatment, Treating Pressure Sores:
Consumer Guide,* and *Preventing Pressure Ulcers: Patient Guide,* which can
be ordered by calling 1-800-358-9295. The Wound Care Institute, Inc. offers
Wound Care Information, a newsletter on computer disk. For more information or to order, send a fax request to 1-305-944-6260 or via e-mail at tama-
ra;cawoundcare.org (no period at the end).

Another resource is *Wound Caring: A Guide to Wound Management Protocol Development,* by Johnson & Johnson (J & J) Medical, Inc. For a copy
of this booklet or other wound-related resources, contact your local representative, or call 1-800-433-5170.

PART FIVE

HOSPICE CARE OF CHILDREN
Special Patients and Families

OUTLINE FOR CARE GUIDELINES

1. **General Considerations**

2. **Needs for Visit**

3. **Safety Considerations**

4. **Potential Diagnoses and Codes**

5. **Associated Nursing Diagnoses**

6. **Skills and Services Identified**
   - Hospice Nursing
     a. Comfort and Symptom Control
     b. Safety and Mobility Considerations
     c. Emotional/Spiritual Considerations
     d. Skin Care
     e. Elimination Considerations
     f. Hydration/Nutrition
     g. Therapeutic/Medication Regimens
     h. Other Considerations
   - Home Health Aide or Certified Nursing Assistant
   - Hospice Social Worker
   - Volunteer(s)
   - Spiritual Counselor
   - Dietitian/Nutritional Counseling
   - Occupational Therapist
   - Physical Therapist
   - Speech-Language Pathologist
   - Bereavement Counselor
   - Pharmacist (for some diagnoses)
   - Music, Massage, Art, or Other Therapies or Services

7. **Outcomes for Care**

8. **Patient, Family, and Caregiver Educational Needs**

9. **Specific Tips for Quality and Reimbursement**

10. **Resources for Hospice Care and Practice**

BOX 5-1

CHILDREN'S HOSPICE INTERNATIONAL
Standards of Hospice Care for Children

Access to Care
Principle
Children with life-threatening, terminal illnesses and their families have special needs. Hospice services for children and their families offer developmentally appropriate palliative and supportive care to any child with a life-threatening condition in any appropriate setting. Children are admitted to hospice services without regard for diagnosis, gender, race, creed, handicap, age, or ability to pay.

Standards
A.C.1. Hospice care services are accessible to children and their families in a setting that is desired and/or appropriate for their needs.

A.C.2. The hospice team is available to provide continuity of care to children and their families in the home and/or in an institutional setting.

A.C.3. The hospice program has eligibility admission criteria for the children and families they serve. Care plans are developed that take into consideration the child's prognosis, and the child and family's needs and desires for hospice services. Admission to the hospice care service does not preclude the child and family from treatment choices or hopeful, supportive therapies.

A.C.4. The hospice program provides information to the community and referral sources about the services that are offered, who qualifies, and how services may be obtained and reimbursed.

Child and Family as a Unit of Care
Principle
Hospice programs provide family-centered care to enhance the quality of life for the child and family as defined by each child-and-family unit. It includes the child and family in the decision making process about services and treatment choices to the fullest degree that is possible and desired.

Standards
C.F.U.1. The unit of care is the child and family. Hospice provides family-centered care. The family is defined as the relatives and/or other significant persons who provide physical, psychological, social, and/or spiritual support for the child.

C.F.U.2. The hospice program recognizes the unique, personal values and beliefs of all children and families. The hospice respects and maintains, as possible, the wishes and dignity of every child and his or her family.

C.F.U.3. The hospice program encourages that children and their families participate in decisions regarding care, including discontinuation of hospice care at any time, and maintains documentation related to consent, advance directives, treatments, and alternative choices of care.

C.F.U.4. The hospice program provides care that considers each child's growth, development, and stage of family life cycle. Children's interests and needs are solicited and considered but are not limited to those related to their illness and disability.

Continued

BOX 5-1

CHILDREN'S HOSPICE INTERNATIONAL
Standards of Hospice Care for Children—cont'd

C.F.U.5. The hospice team seeks to assist each child and family to enjoy life as they are able and to continue in their customary life-style, functioning, and roles as much as possible, especially helping the child to live as normal a life as is possible.

Policies and Procedures
Principle
The hospice program offers services that are accountable to and appropriate for the children and families it serves.

Standards
P.P.1. The hospice program establishes and maintains accurate and adequate policies and procedures to ensure that the hospice is accountable to children, their families, and the communities they serve.

P.P.2. The hospice agency is in compliance with all local, state, and federal laws and regulations that govern the appropriate delivery of hospice care services.

P.P.3. The hospice program provides a clear and accessible grievance procedure to families, outlining how to voice complaints or concerns about services and care without jeopardizing services.

Interdisciplinary Team Services
Principle
Seriously ill children with life-threatening conditions and/or facing terminal stages of an illness and their families have a variety of needs that require a collaborative and cooperative effort from practitioners of many disciplines, working together as an interdisciplinary team of qualified professionals and volunteers.

Standards
I.T.1. The hospice program provides care to the child and family by utilizing a core interdisciplinary team, which may include the child, the family and/or significant others, physicians, nurses, social workers, clergy, and volunteers.

I.T.2. Representatives of other appropriate disciplines are involved in the team as needed (i.e., physical therapy, occupational therapy, speech therapy, nutritional consultation, art therapy, music therapy). The team might also include psychologists, child life specialists, teachers, recreation therapists, play therapists, home health aides, nursing assistants, and other specialists or services as needed.

I.T.3. The hospice core team meets on a regular basis, and an integrated plan of care is developed, implemented, and maintained for every child and family.

I.T.4. The hospice staff professionals are qualified in their particular discipline by training, experience, certification, and/or licensure. Complete orientation, training, and continuing education are provided to each hospice staff member.

I.T.5. The hospice has an active volunteer program. All volunteers are carefully and appropriately selected, trained, supervised, and evaluated, at least annually, by hospice professionals.

BOX 5-1

CHILDREN'S HOSPICE INTERNATIONAL
Standards of Hospice Care for Children—cont'd

I.T.6. All hospice personnel receive educational, psychological, and emotional support appropriate to their situational needs and desires.

I.T.7. The hospice core interdisciplinary team meets at least every 2 weeks or sooner if needed to review and update all plans of care.

Continuity of Care
Principle
Hospice is an integrated system of home and inpatient care. Hospice provides a consistent continuum of care in all settings from admission to the final bereavement services.

Standards
C.C.1. Hospice services are available to children and their families on a consistent basis: 7 days a week and 24 hours a day in institutions or at home.

C.C.2. Appropriate hospice team members are available to children and their families on an on-call basis when the office is closed.

C.C.3. The hospice program has a communication system that assures confidentiality and privacy and can be used to update team members about each child and family's status so that needs can be addressed as soon as possible.

C.C.4. All children and families receive a timely and comprehensive assessment of their physical, psychosocial, emotional, spiritual, and financial needs.

C.C.5. The hospice team, with the family, develops an integrated, written, interdisciplinary plan of care for each child and family. The plan addresses the unique and individual needs of the child and family, including assessment, identified present and potential problems, interventions, and the type and level of services to be provided.

C.C.6. The hospice team addresses and documents the concerns, needs, and desires of the child and family in developing and implementing the plan of care. This document is updated as indicated by the changing status of the child or family.

C.C.7. The hospice agency maintains appropriate documents and clinical records. The clinical record includes properly executed consents for medical/hospice treatment. Confidentiality of hospice records is maintained.

Pain and Symptom Management
Principle
Children should be as symptom free as possible, and pain and/or other symptoms of their illness should be managed to achieve the greatest possible level of comfort.

Standards
P.S.M.1. The hospice team assists the children in achieving comfort through the most effective treatments available.

P.S.M.2. Palliative therapies are discussed with children and their families and provided to children to ensure the most effective and adequate pain and symptom management.

Continued

BOX 5-1

CHILDREN'S HOSPICE INTERNATIONAL
Standards of Hospice Care for Children—cont'd

P.S.M.3. Alternative methods of pain and symptom management are discussed and incorporated into the care of the child as appropriate.

Bereavement Program
Principle
Families of children who die may continue to need appropriate professional and supportive services for a period following the death.

Standards
B.P.1. The hospice program has a structured and active bereavement program. Bereavement services are provided to the surviving family members and/or significant others. Special attention may need to be given to siblings who may not be able to articulate their needs for support.

B.P.2. The level and type of services provided are determined by the family member(s) and appropriate hospice team members.

B.P.3. Bereavement services are available and provided for at least 13 months following the death of the child, extending throughout the second year if possible.

Utilization Review/Quality Improvement
Principle
The hospice program should monitor and ensure the appropriate allocation and utilization of resources and the effectiveness of services.

Standards
U.R.1. The hospice program has a written continuous quality improvement and utilization review program. The program includes criteria to assess the overall functioning components of the hospice program and the effectiveness of its services.

U.R.2. The continuous quality improvement and utilization review program is an ongoing process and implemented on a regular basis, with results of the evaluation reported to appropriate individuals and/or committees for action.

U.R.3. The hospice program provides a written evaluation tool for all recipients of services to document their satisfaction or dissatisfaction with the services received. A written plan outlining how evaluation information will be used to improve services is available to all consumers.

ACQUIRED IMMUNE DEFICIENCY SYNDROME (AIDS) (CARE OF THE CHILD WITH)

1. General considerations

Children with HIV and AIDS are susceptible to numerous infections, including encephalopathy with associated developmental delays, cardiomyopathy, diarrhea, and thrush. The hospice team and the child and family work together to meet these children's myriad needs for care, love, infection control, and symptom relief.

Please refer to "Care of the Medically Fragile Child," "Care of the Child with Cancer," or "Infusion Care" should these sections also pertain to your patient.

2. Needs for visit

Physician order for hospice care, specific to the hospice program's admission criteria and policies

Standard precautions supplies

Vital signs equipment for baseline assessment

Other supplies or equipment, based on physician orders

3. Safety considerations

Infection control/standard precautions

Night-light

Medication safety and storage

Infant/child safety considerations (e.g., car seat, electrical outlet protection, sleeping position)

Municipal water source/safety

Pet care (e.g., infection control)

Symptoms that necessitate immediate reporting/assistance

Safety related to home medical equipment

Smoke detector and fire evacuation plan

Others, based on patient's unique condition and environment

4. Potential diagnoses and codes

AIDS (general)	042
Anemia	042 and 285.9
Bacterial infections, recurrent	042
Candidiasis	042 and 112.9
Candidiasis, esophageal	042 and 112.84
Candidiasis, oral	042 and 112.0
Candidiasis, vaginal	042 and 112.1
Cardiomyopathy	042 and 425.4
Cervical cancer	042 and 180.9
Chorioretinitis	042 and 363.20
Cytomegalovirus	042 and 078.5
Cytomegalovirus retinitis	078.5, 363.20, and 042
Developmental delays, neurological	042
Diarrhea	042 and 008.69

Encephalitis	042 and 323.0
Encephalopathy, AIDS	042 and 348.3
Endocarditis	042 and 424.90
Esophagitis	042 and 530.1
Failure to thrive	042 and 783.4
Herpes simplex	042 and 054.79
Herpes zoster	042 and 053.79
Histoplasmosis	042 and 115.99
HTLV III	042
Kaposi's sarcoma	042 and 176.9
Lymphocytic interstitial pneumonia	042 and 516.8
Meningitis	042 and 047.8
Mycobacterium avium intracellulare	042 and 031.0
Neurological developmental delays	042 and 315.9
Neuropathy, peripheral	042 and 357.4
Neutropenia	042 and 288.0
Peripheral neuropathy	042 and 359.4
Pneumocystis carinii pneumonia	042 and 136.3
Pneumonia (bacterial)	042 and 482.9
Pneumonia (NOS)	042 and 486
Pneumonia (viral)	042 and 480.9
Polymyositis	042 and 710.4
Polyradiculopathy	042 and 357.4
Protein-caloric malnutrition	042 and 263.9
Quadriplegia	042 and 344.00
Retinal detachment	042 and 361.9
Retinal hemorrhage	042 and 362.81
Seizures	042 and 780.3
Sepsis	042 and 038.9
Shigella	042 and 004.9
Shigella, dysentery	042 and 004.9
Thrombocytopenia	042 and 289.5
Toxoplasmosis	042 and 130.9
Tuberculosis (pulmonary)	042 and 011.9
Wasting syndrome	042 and 799.4

5. **Associated nursing diagnoses**
   Activity intolerance
   Activity intolerance, risk for
   Airway clearance, ineffective
   Anxiety
   Body image disturbance
   Body temperature, altered, risk for
   Bowel incontinence
   Cardiac output, decreased
   Caregiver role strain
   Caregiver role strain, risk for
   Coping, ineffective family: compromised
   Coping, ineffective family: disabling
   Coping, ineffective individual
   Family processes, altered

Fatigue

Fear

Fluid volume deficit, risk for

Gas exchange, impaired

Grieving, anticipatory

Growth and development, altered

Infection, risk for

Injury, risk for

Knowledge deficit (related to managing disease)

Nutrition, altered: less than body requirements

Oral mucous membrane, altered

Pain

Pain, chronic

Powerlessness

Protection, altered

Self-care deficit, bathing/hygiene

Self-care deficit, dressing/grooming

Self-care deficit, feeding

Self-care deficit, toileting

Sensory/perceptual alterations (specify) (visual, auditory, kinesthetic, gustatory, tactile, olfactory)

Sexual dysfunction

Sexuality patterns, altered

Skin integrity, impaired

Skin integrity, impaired, risk for

Social interaction, impaired

Social isolation

Spiritual distress (distress of the human spirit)

Swallowing, impaired

Thought processes, altered

Tissue integrity, impaired

Tissue perfusion, altered (specify type) (renal, cerebral, cardiopulmonary, gastrointestinal, peripheral)

Urinary elimination, altered

6. **Skills and services identified**

- *Hospice nursing*

  a. *Comfort and symptom control*

     Complete initial assessment of the child with an impaired immune response and multiple system infections

     Presentation of hospice philosophy and services

     Explain patient rights and responsibilities to parents

     Assess child, family, and caregiver wishes and expectations regarding care

     Assess child, family, and caregiver resources available for care

     Teach family or caregiver physical care of child

     Provision of volunteer support to child and family

     Assess pain and other symptoms, including site, duration, characteristics, and relief measures

     RN to provide and teach effective oral care and comfort measures

RN assessment of pulmonary status, including dyspnea, changed or abnormal breath sounds, retractions, respiratory rate, flaring, and other symptoms of respiratory compromise

RN to observe and assess all systems and symptoms every visit

RN to report changes or new symptoms to physician

RN to assess and monitor child's use of and response to aerosol therapy medication

RN to assess child for candidal diaper rash or oral thrush

RN to evaluate caregiving ability, particularly if parents or other caregivers are HIV+

RN to monitor child's blood pressure and other vital signs

Instruct child, parents, and caregivers in all aspects of effective handwashing techniques and proper care of bodily fluids and excretions

RN to instruct parents and caregivers to call physician for symptoms of fever, increased irritability, vomiting, diarrhea, suspected ear or other infection, decreased appetite, new cough, or any new symptom or complaint

RN to instruct parents regarding the need to isolate HIV+ child from anyone with known infections, such as other children at school who have chicken pox, measles, or other communicable infections that are life threatening for the child with AIDS

RN to instruct parents or caregivers regarding signs and symptoms that necessitate calling RN or physician

RN to provide support to child with new tumor necessitating surgery, chemotherapy, or radiation

RN to address sexuality concerns with young adolescent with AIDS and the importance of safe sexual expression, including the use of condoms, abstinence, or other techniques

Teach child/family about realistic expectations of disease process

Teach care of dying and signs/symptoms of impending death

Presence and support

Other interventions, based on child/family needs

b. *Safety and mobility considerations*

Provide child with home safety information and instruction related to _____ and documented in the clinical record

Instruct on pet care and avoidance of cross contamination, and check with physician about certain types of pets

RN to teach child and parents safe use of oxygen therapy

RN to instruct child and family about safety and standard precautions in the home

RN to teach parents and caregivers about all aspects of child's needed care for safe and effective management at home

Other interventions, based on child/family needs

c. *Emotional/spiritual considerations*

Psychosocial assessment of child and family regarding disease and prognosis

RN to provide emotional support to child and caregivers with chronic/terminal illness and associated implications, especially if parent is HIV+

Assess grief, denial, and guilt of parents and caregivers
Other interventions, based on child/family needs

d. *Skin care*
RN to teach parents and caregivers all aspects of wound care, including safe disposal of dressing supplies
Other interventions, based on child/family needs

e. *Elimination considerations*
Assess bowel regimen, and implement program as needed
RN to closely monitor parenteral feeding catheter site for infection and other problems
Other interventions, based on child/family needs

f. *Hydration/nutrition*
RN to weigh child q visit and review intake diary
RN to instruct parents or caregivers regarding prescribed diet
RN to monitor for adverse effects of medication, particularly steroids
RN to teach parents and caregivers about the importance of optimal hydration and nutrition
Other interventions, based on child/family needs

g. *Therapeutic/medication regimens*
RN to teach parents and caregivers about new medications
RN to instruct parents or caregivers on all aspects of medications, including schedule, functions, and side effects
RN to assess the child's unique response to treatments and interventions and to report to the physician changes, unfavorable responses, or reactions
Other interventions, based on child/family needs

h. *Other considerations*
Assess disease process progression
Other interventions, based on child/family needs

• ***Home health aide or certified nursing assistant***
Effective and safe personal care
Safe ADL assistance and support
Respite care
Active listening skills
Meal preparation
Observation and reporting
Homemaker services
Assist with diversional therapy (e.g., playing games)
Comfort care
Other duties

• ***Hospice social worker***
Psychosocial assessment (age appropriate) of patient and family/caregiver, including adjustment to long-term illness and its implications
Identification of optimal coping strategies
Financial assessment and counseling regarding food acquisition, ability to prepare, and costs of needed medications

Intervention/support related to terminal illness and loss
Emotional/spiritual support
Depression/fear assessed and addressed
Facilitate communication among patient, family, and hospice team
Referral/linkage to community services and resources as indicated
Grief counseling and intervention/support related to illness/loss
Patient/caregiver counseling and support
Identification of illness-related psychiatric condition necessitating care

- *Volunteer(s)*
Support, friendship, companionship, and presence
Comfort and dignity maintained/provided for patient and family
Errands and transportation
Other services, based on interdisciplinary team recommendations and
    patient/caregiver needs

- *Spiritual counselor*
Spiritual assessment and care
Counseling, intervention, and support related to that dimension of life
    related to life's meaning (consistent with child's beliefs)
Support, listening, and presence
Participation in sacred or spiritual rituals or practices
Other supportive care, based on patient's/family's needs and belief sys-
    tems

- *Dietitian/nutritional counseling*
Supportive counseling with patient/family indicating that patient will have
    a decreased appetite and usually at some point may not eat/drink
Assessment and recommendations for swallowing difficulties
Teaching and support of family members and caregivers
Support and care with food and nourishment as desired by patient
Evaluation/management of nutritional deficits and needs
Food and dietary recommendations incorporate child's choices and wishes

- *Occupational therapist*
Evaluation of ADLs and functional mobility
Assess for need for adaptive equipment and assistive devices
Safety assessment of patient's environment and ADLs
Assessment for energy conservation training
Assessment of upper extremity function, retraining motor skills

- *Physical therapist*
Evaluation
Assessment of patient's environment for safety
Safe transfer training or bed mobility exercises
Pain assessment/reduction factors
Strengthening exercises/program
Assessment of gait safety and home safety measures
Instruct/supervise caregiver and volunteers on home exercise program for
    conditioning and strength
Assistive, adaptive devices and evaluation of equipment and teaching

- *Speech-language pathologist*
  Evaluation for speech/swallowing problems
  Food texture recommendations
  Alternate functional communication

- *Bereavement counselor*
  Assessment of the needs of the bereaved family and friends
  Support and intervention, based on assessment and ongoing findings
  Presence and counseling
  Supportive visits, follow-up, and other interventions (e.g., mailings, calls)
  Other services related to bereavement work and support

- *Pharmacist*
  Evaluation of hospice patient with constipation on cathartics, stool softeners, and other medications for possible food/drug and drug/drug interactions
  Medication monitoring regarding therapeutic levels and dosages
  Pain consult and input into interdisciplinary plan of care related to pain control, palliation, and symptom management
  Assessment of medication regimen and plan for safety and compliance

- *Music, massage, art, or other therapies or services*
  Evaluation and intervention based on patient's and caregiver's unique wishes and needs that support care, comfort, and death in the setting of the patient's choice
  Assessment plan to engage patient and support comfort, quality, enjoyment, and dignity

7. **Outcomes for care**

- *Hospice nursing*
  Comfort through death for child and family with support and care of hospice team
  Parent able to care for and support child with hospice assistance
  Parent can verbalize symptoms, changes, or questions that necessitate call to hospice
  Parent demonstrates compliance to medication and other care and therapeutic interventions
  Pain and symptoms managed/controlled in setting of family choice
  Death with dignity and pain/symptoms controlled in setting of family choice
  Optimal comfort, support, and dignity provided to child throughout illness
  Death with maximum comfort through effective symptom control with specialized hospice support
  Parent able to list adverse drug reactions/problems with medication regimen and whom to call for follow-up and resolution
  Enhancement and support of child's/family's quality of life
  Effective symptom relief and control (e.g., a peaceful and comfortable death at home, pain and other symptoms controlled, and some enjoyment of life and play)

Pharmacological and nonpharmacological interventions used effectively for comfort and supportive care through illness

Child/family cared for and family supported through death with physical, psychosocial, developmental, spiritual, and other concerns/needs acknowledged/addressed

Infection control and palliation through illness in setting of child/family choice

Grief/bereavement expression and support provided to family

Patient is pain free by next _____ visit

Parent and caregiver demonstrate ability to manage pain and other symptoms, where applicable

Parent and caregiver demonstrate appropriate backup or "rescue" therapies for breakthrough pain or other symptoms (e.g., dyspnea)

Parent and child verbalize satisfaction with care

Support growth and developmental tasks of childhood

Successful pain and symptom management as verbalized by patient/caregiver

Patient will demonstrate adequate breathing patterns as evidenced by a lack of respiratory distress symptoms

Patient will be comfortable through illness

Patient and caregiver will demonstrate _____% compliance with instructions related to care

Patient and caregiver demonstrate and practice effective hand washing and other infection-control measures (specify, e.g., disposal of waste, cleaning linens, other aspects of care at home)

Adherence to POC by patient and caregivers and able to demonstrate safe and supportive care of child

Nutritional needs maintained/addressed as evidenced by patient's weight maintained/increased by _____ lbs.

Patient's pulmonary status will be maintained/improved

Child and parent integrate information and care regarding implications of disease and terminal nature

Lab values (specify) will be improved/WNL for child

Catheter will remain patent and infection free

Caregiver adheres to/demonstrates compliance with multiple medication regimens (e.g., times, storage, refrigeration)

Child's educational play, and support needs met as verbalized by caregiver and adherence to plan

Palliative and symptomatic interventions to ensure optimal level of functioning in child

- ***Home health aide or certified nursing assistant***
  Effective hygiene, personal care, and comfort
  ADL assistance
  Safe environment maintained
  Comfort and life enjoyment, including play and activities of choices

- ***Hospice social worker***
  Problem identification and addressed with child/caregiver and linked with appropriate support services and plan of care successfully implemented
  Patient/caregiver copes adaptively with illness and death

Adaptive adjustment to changed body and body image

Psychosocial support and counseling offered/initiated to patient/caregivers experiencing loss and grief

- *Volunteer(s)*

  Comfort, companionship, and friendship extended to patient/family

  Support provided as defined by the needs of the patient/caregiver

  Patient and family supported by team with care, comfort, and companionship

- *Spiritual counselor*

  Spiritual support offered and provided as defined by needs of patient/caregiver

  Provision of spiritual support and care based on the assessed and ongoing needs of the patient and family

  Spiritual support offered, and patient and family needs met

  Patient and family express relief of symptoms of spiritual suffering

- *Dietitian/nutritional counseling*

  Family and caregiver integrate recommendations into nutrition teaching (where appropriate)

  Patient and parent know whom to call for nutrition- and hydration-related questions/concerns

  Nutrition/hydration per patient's choices

  Caregiver integrating recommendations into daily meal planning (age dependent)

  Parent and caregiver verbalize comprehension of changing nutritional needs

- *Occupational therapist*

  Patient and caregiver demonstrate maximum independence with ADLs, adaptive techniques, and assistive devices

  Patient and caregiver demonstrate maximum safety in ADLs and functional mobility

  Patient and caregiver demonstrate effective use of energy conservation

  Verbalization/demonstration of improved functional activity level and enhanced quality of life

  Patient and caregiver demonstrate effective use of diaphragmatic breathing to reduce shortness of breath and relaxation techniques to help in pain/symptom management

- *Physical therapist*

  Prevention of complications

  Home exercise and upper extremity program taught to parent/caregiver

  Optimal strength, mobility, and function maintained/achieved

  Compliance with home exercise program by _____ (specify date)

- *Speech-language pathologist*

  Communication method implemented, and patient able to be understood as self-reported or reported by family/caregivers

  Safe swallowing and functional communication

  Recommended lists of foods/textures for safety and choice

- *Bereavement counselor*
  Support services related to grief provided to patient and family
  Well-being and resolution process of grief initiated and followed through
    bereavement services

- *Pharmacist*
  Regimen for bowel regimen successful as self-reported by patient and in
    update at team meeting
  Multiple drug regimen reviewed for food/drug and drug/drug interactions in
    patient on multiple medications
  Stability and safety in complex medication regimen, with maximum benefit
    to patient
  Effective pain and symptom control and symptom management as reported
    by patient/caregiver

- *Music, massage, art, or other therapies or services*
  Therapeutic massage/touch effective for child as self-reported or observed
    by caregivers/family
  Improved muscle tone, relaxation, and/or sleep
  Patient comfortable and relaxed (e.g., sleeping) after massage
  Music therapy intervention based on assessment to decrease pain percep-
    tion, provide emotional expression and support
  Maintenance of comfort, physical, psychosocial, and spiritual health
  Holistic health maintained and comfort achieved through _____
    (specify modality)

8. **Patient, family, and caregiver educational needs**
   Educational needs are the care regimens that contribute to safe and effective
   care at home between the hospice team's visits. These include the following:
   The basic tenets of hospice and the availability of support 24 hours a day, 7
     days a week
   Home safety assessment and counseling
   Anticipated disease progression
   The patient's medication regimen
   Safe and proper body mechanics to promote comfort and avoid caregiver
     safety problems
   Other teaching specific to the child's and family's unique needs
   Symptom management
   Importance of adequate hydration and nutrition
   Standard precaution protocols
   Home safety concerns, issues, and teaching
   The avoidance and prevention of infection, when possible
   The importance of medical follow-up
   Support groups and resources in the community available to the parent and
     child
   Other identified information needed, based on the child's and family's unique
     medical and other needs

9. **Specific tips for quality and reimbursement**
   Document any variances to expected outcomes. The care provided is directed
   toward symptom and infection control and treatment. These children and ado-

lescents are usually so ill that there are many skills the professional nurse and other team members must provide.

Document the coordination occurring among team members based on the POC. The interdisciplinary conference notes should be reflected in the clinical record. Refer to these meetings or communications on any form used by third-party payors (e.g., your program's update form).

In addition:

Write the specific care and teaching instructions provided

Document your progress toward goals

Document any exacerbation of symptoms that necessitated another visit, and be sure there is a physician order for care

Document all POC changes

Document all interactions/communications with the physician

Document the skills used in the provision of professional nursing care practice when caring for the child (e.g., teaching, training, observation, assessment, catheters, IV site care)

Many times these children are closely case managed to identify problems early on; communicate information about the child's and family's statuses and course of care necessitating intervention

Discuss other measurable changes and information that communicate the status of the child and the need for skilled home care services

Document changes to the plan of care, such as medications, services, frequency, communication, and concurrence of other team members

Document coordination of services or consultation of the other members of the IDT

Document communications and care coordination with other care providers, such as inpatient team members and hired caregivers

Document in the clinical notes the clear progression and symptomatology and interventions that demonstrate the overall management of the child with _____ (specify)

Document when/if the patient has respiratory changes, shortness of breath, exacerbation of conditions, changes in pain, and/or other symptoms and that they are identified and resolved

Remember that the clinical documentation is key to measuring compliance for quality and reimbursement purposes. Care coordination, timely verbal and initial physician orders, and assessment and addressing of spiritual and psychosocial needs should be ongoing and documented in the patient's clinical record

The documentation should support that all hospice care supports comfort and dignity while meeting child/family needs

The documentation should include ongoing assessment and management of pain and other symptoms and the anticipation and prevention of secondary symptoms such as constipation

It is important to note that all team members, including nurses and social workers, should assess, identify, and "hear" spiritual needs that the patient/family want to be addressed. These spiritual issues are key to the provision of high-quality hospice care and cannot be addressed effectively and promptly by the spiritual counselor only

Document clearly symptoms, clinical changes, and assessment findings related to pain and patient care

Document weight loss, increased shortness of breath, dyspnea, infection, sepsis, new or changed medications, etc.

Document any skin changes (e.g., inflamed, painful, weeping skin site[s])

Remember that the "litmus test" of care coordination rests on the quality of the clinical documentation by all team members. Review one of your patient's clinical records and ask yourself the following: "If I was unable to give a verbal report/update on this child/family's course of care, would a peer be able to pick up and provide the same level of care and know (from the documentation) the current orders, medications, and other details that contribute to effective hospice care?"

This patient population usually has many clinical changes that should be documented. These include weight loss and multiple and changed medication regimens with varying routes. Side effects to the drug regimen should be observed, noted, documented, and reported

Your assessments, observations, and clinical findings are information that assists in painting a picture to support coverage and documentation requirements for hospice care

Document any hospitalizations and changed clinical findings

Document patient changes, symptoms, psychosocial issues impacting the care, and information gathered at the child/family visits and during team meetings

Document all care provided and outcomes of that care

Document the child's/parent's responses to care, changes, and communications with the physician and other hospice team members

Document the course of care, including why the infant/child was admitted for care, the plan, and support provided

10. **Resources for hospice care and practice**

The Centers for Disease Control and Prevention (CDC)

National AIDS Hotline: 1-800-342-2437 or 1-800-342-AIDS

The National AIDS Information Clearinghouse: 1-800-458-5231

The AIDS Pediatric Clinical Trials Information Service: 1-800-TRIALS-A (1-800-874-2572)

The National Hemophiliac Foundation: 1-212-431-8541

The CDC National AIDS Clearinghouse offers *Adolescents and HIV Disease* and *HIV and Your Child: Consumer Guide.* For more information, call 1-800-458-5231.

A helpful drug resource is the *Pharmacological Treatment of AIDS.* Kirk Ryan, Pharm.D., the author, can be reached by sending an e-mail message to kirkryan@creative.net

Guidelines for the Use of Antiretroviral Agents in Pediatric HIV Infection is available free from the Department of Health and Human Services (HHS) by calling 1-800-458-5231 or 1-800-448-0440.

The Candlelighters Childhood Cancer Foundation offers many services for parents and children, including resources, services, advocacy, and support. Call 1-301-657-8401 or 1-800-366-2223 (CCCF) for information.

CANCER (CARE OF THE CHILD WITH)

1. **General considerations**

   The news that a child's prognosis is terminal is devastating. Brain tumors, leukemias, and solid tumors, such as Wilms', are some of the cancers seen in pediatric hospice. It is said that cancer is the leading cause of death from disease in children who are 3 to 15 years old and the second cause of death from all causes, surpassed only by death from injuries.

   Cancer care in children utilizes all facets of nursing skills. Death at any age is sad, but the suffering and death of children magnify the emotional turmoil. Parents know their child best, and in this role they are the teachers for care providers. Parental control should be maintained as much as possible. The child, the siblings, and the parents become the unit of care for comfort, support, and intervention.

   Please refer to "AIDS (Care of the Child With)," "Care of the Medically Fragile Child," and "Infusion Care" should these sections also pertain to your patient.

2. **Needs for visit**

   Physician order for hospice care, specific to the hospice program's admission
        criteria and policies
   Standard precautions supplies
   Vital signs equipment for baseline assessment
   Other supplies or equipment, based on physician orders

3. **Safety considerations**

   Infection control/standard precautions
   Night-light
   Medication safety and storage
   Child safety considerations (e.g., car seat, electrical outlet protection, sleeping
        position)
   Symptoms that necessitate immediate reporting/assistance
   Safety related to home medical equipment
   Smoke detector and fire evacuation plan
   Others, based on the patient's unique condition and environment

4. **Potential diagnoses and codes**

Acute lymphocytic leukemia	204.00
Acute myelogenous leukemia	205.00
Aplastic anemia	284.9
Astrocytoma	191.9
Bone marrow transplant	41.00
Chronic leukemia	208.10
Chronic myelogenous leukemia	205.10
Ewing's tumor	170.9
Glioblastoma	191.9
Leukopenia	288.00
Metastases, general	199.1

Neuroblastoma	194.0
Wilms' tumor	189.0

5. **Associated nursing diagnoses**
   Activity intolerance
   Activity intolerance, risk for
   Adjustment, impaired
   Anxiety
   Aspiration, risk for
   Body image disturbance
   Body temperature, altered, risk for
   Breathing pattern, ineffective
   Cardiac output, decreased
   Caregiver role strain
   Caregiver role strain, risk for
   Constipation
   Coping, family: potential for growth
   Coping, ineffective family: compromised
   Coping, ineffective family: disabling
   Decisional conflict (specify) (e.g., treatment regimen options)
   Denial, ineffective
   Diarrhea
   Family processes, altered
   Fatigue
   Fear
   Fluid volume deficit, risk for
   Grieving, anticipatory
   Growth and development, altered
   Infection, risk for
   Injury, risk for
   Knowledge deficit (diagnoses and treatment)
   Mobility, impaired physical
   Nutrition, altered: less than body requirements
   Oral mucous membrane, altered
   Pain
   Pain, chronic
   Parental role conflict
   Parenting, altered
   Protection, altered
   Role performance, altered
   Self-care deficit, bathing/hygiene
   Self-care deficit, dressing/grooming
   Self-care deficit, feeding
   Self-care deficit, toileting
   Sensory/perceptual alterations (specify) (visual, auditory, kinesthetic, gusta-
      tory, tactile, olfactory)
   Sexuality patterns, altered
   Skin integrity, impaired, risk for
   Sleep pattern disturbance
   Social interaction, impaired

Spiritual distress (distress of the human spirit)
Swallowing, impaired
Tissue integrity, impaired
Tissue perfusion, altered (specify type) (renal, cerebral, cardiopulmonary, gastrointestinal, peripheral)
Urinary elimination, altered

6. **Skills and services identified**

   • *Hospice nursing*

   a. *Comfort and symptom control*
   Admission of infant/child to hospice with _____ (specify)
   Presentation of hospice philosophy and services
   Explain patient rights and responsibilities to parents
   Assess parent and caregiver wishes and expectations regarding care
   Assess parent, family, and caregiver resources available for care
   Teach parent or caregiver physical care of child
   Provision of volunteer support to child and family
   Assess pain and other symptoms, including site, duration, characteristics, and relief measures
   RN to provide and teach effective oral care and comfort measures
   Anticipate and encourage child and family input into care regimen(s)
   Teach caregivers observational aspects of care, including fever, bleeding, bruising, and other signs unique to the disease or treatment
   RN to monitor for seizure activity and perform neurological checks q visit
   Teach the importance of effective hand washing and other infection-control measures, including the prevention and avoidance of infection when possible
   RN to instruct caregiver to call physician for symptoms of fever, irritability, vomiting, diarrhea, suspected ear or other infection, decreased appetite, cough, or other complaint
   Ongoing assessment and observation of cardiovascular, pulmonary, and respiratory statuses
   Teach new pain and symptom control measures to parent
   Identify and monitor pain, symptoms, and relief measures
   Observation, assessment, and supportive care to child and family
   Teach child/family use of standardized form/tool for pain to use between hospice team members' visits (and for care coordination between team members and child/family)
   Teach parent principles of effective pain management
   Effective management of pain and prevention of secondary symptoms
   Interventions of symptoms directed toward comfort and palliation
   Observation and assessment and communication with physician related to signs, new symptoms, increasing irritability, thrush, others
   Pain assessment and management q visit, including source of pain
   Teach parent/family about realistic expectations of disease process
   Teach care of dying and signs/symptoms of impending death
   Presence and support
   Other interventions, based on child/family needs

b. *Safety and mobility considerations*

Parent and caregiver provided with home safety information and instruction

Teach parent regarding home safety and infection control measures

Other interventions, based on child/family needs

c. *Emotional/spiritual considerations*

Psychosocial assessment of child and family regarding disease and prognosis

RN to provide emotional support to child and family

Assess child's and parent's coping skills

RN to provide emotional support to child and family with chronic or terminal illness and associated implications

Assess for and manage plans for psychosocial and/or spiritual pain (e.g., fear, anxiety, interpersonal and other distress)

Observation of child for neuropsychiatric complications of illness, including pain, irritability, and depression

Psychosocial aspects of pain control (e.g., depression) assessed and acknowledged with team support/intervention

Ongoing acknowledgment of spirituality and related concerns of child/family and their belief systems

Other interventions, based on child/family needs

d. *Skin care*

RN to teach parents and caregivers all aspects of skin care

Other interventions, based on child/family needs

e. *Elimination considerations*

Assess bowel regimen, and implement program as needed

Other interventions, based on child/family needs

f. *Hydration/nutrition*

Teach the importance of optimal nutrition and hydration

Assessment and referral for child with thrush and painful swallowing

Nutrition/hydration supported by offering foods/beverages of child's choice, when possible

Other interventions, based on child/family needs

g. *Therapeutic/medication regimens*

Symptom control for side effects of radiation or chemotherapy

RN to assess the child's unique response to treatments and interventions and to report to the physician changes, unfavorable responses, or reactions

Teach new medications and effects

Teach parent about medications and the management program, including strength, type, actions, times, and compliance tips

Encourage parent to give the child medications on the schedule and around the clock

Nonpharmacological or other interventions of relaxation, guided imagery, humor, music therapy, art therapy, bubble blowing, magic presentations and wands, and massage for comfort during painful interventions

Other interventions, based on child/family needs

h. *Other considerations*
Assess disease process progression
Other interventions, based on child/family needs

- **Home health aide or certified nursing assistant**
Effective and safe personal care
Safe ADL assistance and support
Respite care and active listening
Observation and reporting
Meal preparation
Assist with diversional therapy (e.g., playing games)
Homemaker services
Comfort care
Other duties

- **Hospice social worker**
Psychosocial assessment of patient and parent/caregiver, including adjustment to long-term illness and its implications
Identification of optimal coping strategies
Financial assessment and counseling regarding food acquisition, ability to prepare food, and costs of needed medications
Intervention/support related to terminal illness and loss
Emotional/spiritual support
Depression/fear assessed and addressed
Facilitate communication among patient, family, and hospice team
Referral/linkage to community services and resources as indicated
Grief counseling and intervention/support related to illness/loss
Patient and caregiver counseling and support
Illness-related psychiatric condition necessitating care

- **Volunteer(s)**
Support, friendship, companionship, presence, fun, and play (based on child's illness/age)
Comfort and dignity maintained/provided for patient and family
Errands and transportation
Other services, based on interdisciplinary team recommendations and patient/caregiver needs

- **Spiritual counselor**
Spiritual assessment and care
Counseling, intervention, and support related to that dimension of life related to life's meaning (consistent with patient's beliefs)
Support, listening, and presence
Participation in sacred or spiritual rituals or practices
Other supportive care, based on patient's/family's needs and belief systems

- **Dietitian/nutritional counseling**
Supportive counseling with patient/parent indicating that patient will have a decreased appetite and usually at some point may not eat/drink
Assessment and recommendations for swallowing difficulties
Teaching and support of family members and caregivers
Support and care with food and nourishment as desired by patient
Evaluation/management of nutritional deficits and needs

Food and dietary recommendations incorporate patient's choice and wishes

Allow child to eat whatever and whenever desired, with small, frequent feedings

Tube feeding, as necessary

Teach child to manage own tube feedings, "special care," when possible

- *Occupational therapist*
  Evaluation
  Energy conservation techniques
  Adaptive, assistive, and safety supports/devices and training
  ADL training
  Teach compensatory techniques

- *Physical therapist*
  Evaluation
  Assessment of patient's environment for safety
  Safe transfer training or bed mobility exercises
  Pain assessment/reduction factors
  Strengthening exercises/program
  Assessment of gait safety and home safety measures
  Instruct/supervise caregiver and volunteers on home exercise program for conditioning and strength
  Assistive, adaptive devices and evaluation of equipment and teaching

- *Speech-language pathologist*
  Evaluation for speech/swallowing problems
  Food texture recommendations
  Alternate functional communication

- *Bereavement counselor*
  Assessment of the needs of the bereaved family and friends
  Support and intervention, based on assessment and ongoing findings
  Presence and counseling
  Supportive visits, follow-up, and other interventions (e.g., mailings, calls)
  Other services related to bereavement work and support

- *Pharmacist*
  Evaluation of hospice patient with constipation on cathartics, stool softeners, and other medications for possible food/drug and drug/drug interactions
  Medication monitoring regarding therapeutic levels and dosages
  Pain consult and input into interdisciplinary plan of care related to pain control, palliation, and symptom management
  Assessment of medication regimen and plan for safety and compliance

- *Music, massage, art, or other therapies or services*
  Evaluation and intervention based on patient's and caregiver's unique wishes and needs that support care, comfort, and death in the setting of the patient's choice
  Assessment plan to engage patient and support comfort, quality, enjoyment, and dignity (e.g., play)

7. **Outcomes for care**

- *Hospice nursing*

    Comfort through death for child and family with support and care of hospice team

    Parent able to care for and support child with hospice support

    Parent can verbalize changes or symptoms that necessitate call to hospice

    Parent demonstrates compliance to medication and other care and therapeutic interventions

    Pain and symptoms managed/controlled in setting of family choice

    Death with dignity and pain/symptoms controlled in setting of family choice

    Optimal comfort, support, and dignity provided throughout illness

    Death with maximum comfort through effective symptom control with specialized hospice support

    Parent able to list adverse drug reactions/problems with medication regimen and whom to call for follow-up and resolution

    Enhancement and support of child's/family's quality of life

    Effective symptom relief and control (e.g., a peaceful and comfortable death at home, pain and other symptoms controlled, some enjoyment of life and play)

    Pharmacological and nonpharmacological interventions used effectively for comfort and supportive care through illness

    Child/family cared for and family supported through death with physical, psychosocial, developmental, spiritual, and other concerns/needs acknowledged/addressed

    Infection control and palliation through illness in setting of patient's choice

    Grief/bereavement expression and support provided to family

    Patient is pain free by next _____ visit

    Parent and caregiver demonstrate ability to manage pain and other symptoms, where applicable

    Observation and assessment of child's behavior, including expressions, usual activity level, and changes noted, to assist in pain identification and management

    Patient and parent verbalize satisfaction with care

    Educational tools/plans incorporated in daily care, and child and caregiver verbalize understanding of safe, needed care

    Patient and parent decide on care, interventions, and evaluation

    Caregiver effective in care management and knows whom to call for questions/concerns

    Parent and caregiver will express satisfaction with hospice support received and will experience increased comfort

    Child will be made comfortable at home through death in accordance with the family/parent wishes

    Effective pain control and symptom control communicated by child

    Parent and caregiver verbalize understanding of and adhere to care and medication regimens

    Child and family supported through patient's death

    Comfort maintained through course of care

The patient and family receive support and care, and family members and friends are able to spend quality time with the patient

Child and caregivers supported through and receive the maximum benefit from surgery, chemotherapy, and/or radiation

Patient and caregiver list adverse reactions, potential complications, and signs/symptoms of infection (e.g., sputum change, chest congestion)

Comfort maintained through death with dignity

Patient protected from injury and compliant with medication, safety, and care regimens

Comfort and individualized intervention of child with cancer

Spiritual and psychosocial needs met (specify) as defined by child/parent/caregiver throughout course of care

Patient states pain is _____ on 0-10 scale by next visit

Patient/caregiver demonstrates appropriate backup or "rescue" therapies for breakthrough pain or other symptoms (e.g., dyspnea)

Other outcomes/goals, based on the patient condition with input from the hospice team and patient and family

- *Home health aide or certified nursing assistant*
  Effective hygiene, personal care, and comfort
  ADL assistance
  Safe environment maintained

- *Hospice social worker*
  Problems identified and addressed, with patient/parent linked with appropriate support services and plan of care successfully implemented
  Patient and parent cope adaptively with illness and death
  Adaptive adjustment to changed body and body image
  Psychosocial support and counseling offered to patient/caregivers experiencing loss and grief

- *Volunteer(s)*
  Comfort, companionship, respite, and friendship extended to child/family
  Support provided as defined by the needs of the patient/caregiver
  Patient and family supported by team with care, comfort, and companionship

- *Spiritual counseling*
  Spiritual support offered and provided as defined by needs of patient/caregiver
  Provision of spiritual support and care as based on the assessed and ongoing needs of the patient and family
  Spiritual support offered, and patient and family needs met
  Patient and family express relief of symptoms of spiritual suffering

- *Dietitian/nutritional counseling*
  Family and caregiver integrate recommendations into nutrition teaching (where appropriate)
  Parent and caregiver know whom to call for nutrition- and hydration-related questions/concerns
  Nutrition/hydration per child's choices

Parent integrating recommendations into daily meal planning

Parent and caregiver verbalize comprehension of changing nutritional needs

- *Occupational therapist*

  Maximize independence in ADLs for patient/caregiver

  Optimal function maintained/attained

  Patient and caregiver demonstrate ADL program for maximum safety

  Patient and caregiver demonstrate maximum independence with ADL, adaptive techniques, and assistive devices

  Patient and caregiver demonstrate maximum safety in ADL and functional mobility

  Patient and caregiver demonstrate effective use of energy conservation

  Verbalization/demonstration of improved functional activity level and enhanced quality of life

  Patient and caregiver demonstrate effective use of diaphragmatic breathing to reduce shortness of breath and relaxation techniques to help in pain/symptom management

- *Physical therapist*

  Prevention of complications

  Home exercise and upper extremity program taught to parent or other team member (e.g., HHA)

  Optimal strength, mobility, and function maintained/achieved

  Compliance with home exercise program by _____ (specify date)

- *Speech-language pathologist*

  Communication method implemented, and child able to be understood as self-reported or reported by family/caregivers

  Safe swallowing and functional communication

  Recommended lists of foods/textures for safety and patient choice

- *Bereavement counselor*

  Support services related to grief provided to patient and family

  Well-being and resolution process of grief initiated and followed through bereavement services

- *Pharmacist*

  Regimen for bowel regimen successful as self-reported by patient and in update at team meeting

  Multiple drug regimen reviewed for food/drug and drug/drug interactions in patient on multiple medications

  Stability and safety in complex medication regimen, with maximum benefit to patient

  Effective pain and symptom control and symptom management as reported by patient/caregiver

- *Music, massage, art, or other therapies or services*

  Therapeutic massage/touch effective for patient as self-reported or observed by caregivers/family

  Improved muscle tone, relaxation, and/or sleep

  Patient comfortable and relaxed (e.g., sleeping, playing) after massage

Music therapy intervention based on assessment to decrease pain perception and provide emotional expression and support

Maintenance of comfort and physical, psychosocial, and spiritual health

Holistic health maintained and comfort achieved through _____
(specify modality)

8. **Patient, family, and caregiver educational needs**

Educational needs are the care regimens that contribute to safe and effective care at home between the hospice team's visits.

These include the following:

The basic tenets of hospice and the availability of support 24 hours a day, 7 days a week

Home safety assessment and counseling

The patient's medication regimen

Anticipated disease progression

Safe and proper body mechanics to promote patient comfort and avoid caregiver safety problems

Other teaching specific to the patient's and family's unique needs

Support groups available to patient's family, such as the hospice program's "Caregiver Support Group" meetings for family members and friends

The medication regimen, including schedule, route, functions, and side effects

Signs and symptoms that necessitate calling the physician or RN

The importance of round-the-clock medications for pain control

Pain and other symptom control measures

Information about the disease process

Other support services for the patient, parents, and caregivers

9. **Specific tips for quality and reimbursement**

Document coordination of services or consultation of the other members of the IDT

Document all care provided and outcomes of that care

Document the child's/parent's responses to care, changes, and communications with the physician and other hospice team members

Document the course of care, including why the infant/child was admitted for care, the plan, and support provided

Document in the clinical notes the clear progression, symptomatology, interventions, and overall management of the child with _____
(specify)

Document when/if the patient has respiratory changes, shortness of breath, exacerbation of conditions, changes in pain, and/or other symptoms and that they are identified and resolved

Remember that the clinical documentation is key to measuring compliance for quality and reimbursement purposes. Care coordination, timely verbal and initial physician orders, and assessment and addressing of spiritual and psychosocial needs should be ongoing and documented in the patient's clinical record

The documentation should support that all hospice care supports comfort and dignity while meeting child's/family's needs

The documentation should include ongoing assessment and management of pain and other symptoms and the anticipation and prevention of secondary symptoms such as constipation

It is important to note that all team members, including nurses and social workers, should assess, identify, and "hear" spiritual needs that the patient/family want to be addressed. These spiritual issues are key to the provision of quality hospice care and cannot be addressed effectively and promptly by the spiritual counselor only

Document clearly symptoms, clinical changes, and assessment findings related to pain and patient care

Document weight loss, increased shortness of breath, dyspnea, infection, sepsis, new or changed medications, etc.

Document any skin changes (e.g., inflamed, painful, weeping skin site[s])

Remember that the "litmus test" of care coordination rests on the quality of the clinical documentation by all team members. Review one of your patient's clinical records and ask yourself the following: "If I was unable to give a verbal report/update on this child's/family's course of care, would a peer be able to pick up and provide the same level of care and know (from the documentation) the current orders, medications, and other details that contribute to effective hospice care?"

This patient population usually has many clinical changes that should be documented. These include weight loss, multiple and changed medication regimens with varying routes. Side effects to the drug regimen should be observed, noted, documented, and reported

Your assessments, observations, and clinical findings are information that assists in painting a picture to support coverage and documentation requirements for hospice care

Document any hospitalizations and changed clinical findings

Document patient changes, symptoms, psychosocial issues impacting the care, and information gathered at the child/family visits and during team meetings

Document communications and care coordination with other care providers, such as inpatient team members and hired caregivers

Document changes to the plan of care, such as medications, services, frequency, communication, and concurrence of other team members

10. **Resources for hospice care and practice**
    The American Brain Tumor Association offers helpful resources for children and parents about the varying types of tumors and other information. *When Your Child Is Ready To Return to School* addresses homework and important safety details should the patient/child wish to continue school and learning, depending on the pathology and course of care and illness. Another is *Alex's Journey,* which is the story of a child with a brain tumor. Information and these free resources can be obtained by calling 1-708-827-9910 or the patient number, which is 1-800-886-2282.

    Radiotherapy Days, a 20-page, four-color paperback for children ages 8 to 12, is useful to caregivers who need to explain radiotherapy to children. To order, send $5.00 per copy to Mount Sinai Medical Center, Radiotherapy Days, Department of Pediatric Hematology/Oncology, Box 1208,

One Gustave L. Levy Place, New York, NY 10029. Make check payable to MSMC.

The Make-A-Wish Foundation fulfills special wishes for children with a life-threatening illness and their families. 1-800-722-WISH (9474).

The Wisconsin Pain Initiative offers *Children's Cancer Pain Can Be Relieved* by calling 1-608-262-0978. *Acute Pain Management in Infants, Children, and Adolescents: Operative and Medical Procedures* is available free through the Agency for Health Care Policy and Research at 1-800-358-9295.

Friends Network, PO Box 4545, Santa Barbara, CA 93140, offers *Funletter Update,* a national activities letter for children and families living with cancer. Call for an issue by calling (805) 565-7031.

The Candlelighters Childhood Cancer Foundation offers many services for parents and children, including resources, services, advocacy, and support. Call 1-301-657-8401 or 1-800-366-2223 (CCCF) for information.

CARE OF THE MEDICALLY FRAGILE CHILD

1. **General considerations**

   The news that a child's prognosis is terminal is devastating. Congenital anomalies, accidents, or progressive disease include some of the problems or diagnoses when an infant or child is referred and admitted to hospice. The child, the siblings, and the parents become the unit of care for comfort, support, and intervention.

   Please refer to "Care of the Child with AIDS," "Care of the Child with Cancer," or "Infusion Care" should these sections also pertain to your patient.

2. **Needs for visit**

   Physician order for hospice care, specific to the hospice program's admission criteria and policies

   Standard precautions supplies

   Vital signs equipment for baseline assessment

   Other supplies or equipment, based on physician orders

3. **Safety considerations**

   Infection control/standard precautions

   Night-light

   Infant/child safety considerations (e.g., car seat, electrical outlet protection, sleeping position, immunizations)

   Phone number of whom to call with a problem

   Medication access and storage

   Oxygen safety

   Equipment safety (if there is home medical equipment/technology)

   Symptoms and problems that necessitate emergency call to 911

   If ventilator, TPN, or infusion patient—adequate electricity, refrigerator, clean storage area, and access to a telephone

   Smoke detector and fire evacuation plan

   Others, based on the patient's unique condition and environment

4. **Potential diagnoses and codes**

AIDS	042
Apnea	786.09
Apnea (newborn)	770.8
Asthma	493.90
Bacteriuria	791.9
Biliuria	791.4
Bone marrow transplant (surgical)	41.00
Brain injury, traumatic	854.00
Bronchial pulmonary dysplasia	770.7
Bronchiolitis	466.19
Cardiac dysrhythmia	427.89
Cerebral palsy	343.9
Child maltreatment syndrome	995.50
Cholelithiasis	574.20

Chronic renal failure	585.0
Cleft lip	749.10
Cleft palate	749.00
Cystic fibrosis	277.00
Dehydration	276.5
Diabetes mellitus, with complic.	250.91
Diarrhea	787.91
Down's syndrome	758.0
Encephalitis	323.9
Failure to thrive	783.4
Fetal/neonatal jaundice	774.6
Immaturity, extreme	765.00
Jaundice	782.4
Liver transplant (surgical)	50.59
Meningitis, bacterial	320.9
Meningitis, viral	047.9
Metabolism disorder	277.9
Muscular dystrophy	359.1
Nasogastric tube	96.07
Newborn feeding problems	779.3
Normal delivery	650
Normal development, lack of	783.4
Pancreatitis	577.0
Pneumonia	486.0
Preterm infant	765.0
Pulmonary insufficiency, newborn	770.8
Reactive airway disease	493.90
Rectal prolapse	569.1
Respiratory problem, postbirth	770.8
Respiratory syncytial virus	079.6
Seizure disorder	780.3
Sickle cell anemia	282.60
Sickle cell crisis	282.62
Sickle cell trait	282.5
Spina bifida	741.90
Spinal cord injury	952.9
Tracheal stenosis	519.1
Tracheomalacia	519.1
Tracheostomy, attention to	V55.0
Wasting syndrome	799.4

5. **Associated nursing diagnoses**
   Airway clearance, ineffective
   Anxiety
   Aspiration, risk for
   Body temperature, altered, risk for
   Breathing pattern, ineffective
   Cardiac output, decreased
   Caregiver role strain, risk for

Communication, impaired verbal
Coping, family: potential for growth
Coping, ineffective family: compromised
Coping, ineffective family: disabling
Coping, ineffective individual
Decisional conflict (care and treatment)
Family processes, altered
Fatigue
Fear
Fluid volume deficit, risk for
Fluid volume excess
Gas exchange, impaired
Growth and development, altered
Infant behavior, disorganized
Infant behavior, disorganized: risk for
Infant feeding pattern, ineffective
Infection, risk for
Injury, risk for
Knowledge deficit (specify)
Knowledge deficit (care, health maintenance, and disease process)
Pain
Pain, chronic
Parent/infant/child attachment, altered: risk for
Parental role conflict
Parenting, altered
Parenting, altered, risk for
Protection, altered
Self-care deficit (specify)
Sleep pattern response
Spiritual distress (distress of the human spirit)
Urinary elimination, altered
Ventilation, inability to sustain spontaneous

6. **Skills and services identified**

  • *Hospice nursing*

    a. *Comfort and symptom control*
      Admission of infant/child to hospice with _____ (specify)
      Comprehensive skilled assessment of all systems of infant/child with
        _____ (specify) admitted
      Presentation of hospice philosophy and services
      Explain to parents patient rights and responsibilities
      Assess child, family, and caregiver wishes and expectations regarding
        care
      Assess child, family, and caregiver resources available for care
      Teach family or caregiver physical care of child
      Provision of volunteer support to child and family
      Assess pain and other symptoms, including site, duration, characteristics, and relief measures

RN to provide and teach effective oral care and comfort measures

Support play, growth and development, and health maintenance through length of care

Establish an environment of mutual trust and respect to enhance learning

Communicate only brief amounts of complex information related to the infant's care at any given time

Assess respiratory rate and depth and lung sounds for improvement or deterioration

Teach parent management of cardiorespiratory monitor

Teach parent oxygen administration and safety considerations with infant at risk for hypoxemia and history of bradycardia and apnea

Ongoing assessment and observation of cardiovascular, pulmonary, and respiratory statuses

Teach new pain and symptom control measures to parents

Identify and monitor pain, symptoms, and relief measures

Observation, assessment, and supportive care to child and family

Teach child/family use of standardized form/tool for pain to use between hospice team members' visits (and for care coordination between team members and child/family)

Teach parent principles of effective pain management

Effective management of pain and prevention of secondary symptoms

Interventions of symptoms directed toward comfort and palliation

Observation and assessment and communication with physician related to signs, new symptoms, increasing irritability, thrush, others

Pain assessment and management q visit, including source of pain (e.g., neuropathy, infection, muscles, thrush/swallowing, dental disease, otitis)

Teach parent/family about realistic expectations of disease process

Teach care of dying, signs/symptoms of impending death

Presence and support

Other interventions, based on child/family needs

b. *Safety and mobility considerations*

Child and parent provided with home safety information and instruction related to _____ and documented in the clinical record

Teach parent about home safety and infection-control measures

Encourage family members to refrain from smoking or allowing others to smoke in the home

Schedule frequent rest periods with activities to promote optimal oxygenation

Parent provided with home safety information and instruction

Other interventions, based on child/family needs

c. *Emotional/spiritual considerations*

Psychosocial assessment of patient and family regarding disease and prognosis

RN to provide emotional support to child and family

Observation of child for neuropsychiatric complications of illness, including pain, irritability, and depression

Assess for and manage plans for psychosocial and/or spiritual pain (e.g., fear, anxiety, interpersonal and other distress)

Psychosocial aspects of pain control (e.g., depression) assessed and acknowledged with team support/intervention

Ongoing acknowledgment of spirituality and related concerns of child/family and their belief systems

Other interventions, based on child/family needs

d. *Skin care*

RN to teach parents and caregivers all aspects of skin care

Other interventions, based on child/family needs

e. *Elimination considerations*

Assess bowel regimen, and implement program as needed

Other interventions, based on child/family needs

f. *Hydration/nutrition*

Monitor length, weight, head circumference, and review of food diary for infant with failure to thrive

Reinforce feeding techniques and intake and output diary

Teach the importance of optimal nutrition and hydration

Assessment and referral for child with thrush and painful swallowing

Nutrition/hydration supported by offering foods/beverages of child's choice, when possible

Other interventions, based on child/family needs

g. *Therapeutic/medication regimens*

Administer prescribed medications as ordered, including aerosol treatments, and monitor for adverse effects

Instruct regarding medication administration and side effects

RN to assess the child's unique response to treatments and interventions and to report to the physician changes, unfavorable responses, or reactions

Teach new medications and effects

Teach parent about medications and the management program, including strength, type, actions, times, and compliance tips

Encourage parent to give the patient medications on the schedule and around the clock

Nonpharmacological interventions of relaxation, guided imagery, humor, music therapy, art therapy, bubble blowing, magic presentations and wands, and massage for comfort and during painful interventions

Other interventions, based on patient/family needs

h. *Other considerations*

Assess disease process progression

Other interventions, based on patient/family needs

- **Home health aide or certified nursing assistant**

Effective and safe personal care

Safe ADL assistance and support

Respite care

Observation and reporting
Meal preparation
Assist with diversional therapy (e.g., playing games)
Homemaker services
Comfort care
Other duties

- *Hospice social worker*
  Psychosocial assessment of patient and family/caregiver, including adjustment to long-term illness and its implications
  Identification of optimal coping strategies
  Financial assessment and counseling regarding food acquisition, ability to prepare food, and costs of needed medications
  Intervention/support related to terminal illness and loss
  Emotional/spiritual support
  Depression/fear assessed and addressed
  Facilitate communication among patient, family, and hospice team
  Referral/linkage to community services and resources as indicated
  Grief counseling and intervention/support related to illness/loss
  Patient/caregiver counseling and support
  Identification of illness-related psychiatric condition necessitating care

- *Volunteer(s)*
  Comfort, dignity, and respite maintained/provided for patient and family
  Errands and transportation
  Other services, based on interdisciplinary team recommendations and patient/caregiver needs

- *Spiritual counselor*
  Spiritual assessment and care
  Counseling, intervention, and support related to that dimension of life related to life's meaning (consistent with patient's beliefs)
  Support, listening, and presence
  Participation in sacred or spiritual rituals or practices
  Other supportive care, based on patient/family needs and belief systems

- *Dietitian/nutritional counseling*
  Supportive counseling with parent/family indicating that child will have a decreased appetite and usually at some point may not eat/drink
  Assessment and recommendations for swallowing difficulties
  Teaching and support of family members and caregivers
  Support and care with food and nourishment as desired by patient
  Evaluation/management of nutritional deficits and needs
  Food and dietary recommendations incorporate patient choice and wishes

- *Occupational therapist*
  Evaluation of ADLs and functional mobility
  Assess for need for adaptive equipment and assistive devices
  Safety assessment of patient's environment and ADLs
  Assessment for energy conservation training
  Assessment of upper extremity function, retraining motor skills and/or splinting for contracture(s)

- *Physical therapist*
  Evaluation
  Assessment of environment for safety
  Safe transfer training or bed mobility exercises
  Pain assessment/reduction factors
  Strengthening exercises/program
  Assessment of gait safety and home safety measures
  Instruct/supervise parents and volunteers on home exercise program for conditioning and strength
  Assistive, adaptive devices and evaluation of equipment and teaching

- *Speech-language pathologist*
  Evaluation for speech/swallowing problems
  Food texture recommendations
  Alternate functional communication

- *Bereavement counselor*
  Assessment of the needs of the bereaved family and friends
  Support and intervention, based on assessment and ongoing findings
  Presence and counseling
  Supportive visits and follow-up, other interventions (e.g., mailings, calls)
  Other services related to bereavement work and support

- *Pharmacist*
  Evaluation of hospice patient with constipation on cathartics, stool softeners, and other medications for possible food/drug, drug/drug interactions
  Medication monitoring regarding therapeutic levels and dosages
  Pain consult and input into interdisciplinary plan of care related to pain control, palliation, and symptom management
  Assessment of medication regimen and plan for safety and compliance

- *Music, massage, art, or other therapies or services*
  Evaluation and intervention based on child's/parent's unique wishes and needs that support care, comfort, and death in the setting of the patient's choice
  Assessment plan to engage child and support comfort, quality, enjoyment, dignity, and quality of life

7. **Outcomes for care**

  - *Hospice nursing*
    Comfort through death for child and family with support and care of hospice team
    Parent able to care for and support child with hospice support
    Parent can verbalize symptoms, changes, or symptoms that necessitate call to hospice
    Parent demonstrates compliance with medication regimen and other care and therapeutic interventions
    Pain and symptoms managed/controlled in setting of family choice
    Death with dignity and pain/symptoms controlled in setting of family choice
    Optimal comfort, support, and dignity provided throughout illness

Death with maximum comfort through effective symptom control with specialized hospice support

Parent able to list adverse drug reactions/problems with medication regimen and whom to call for follow-up and resolution

Enhancement and support of child's/family's quality of life

Effective symptom relief and control (e.g., a peaceful and comfortable death at home, pain and other symptoms controlled, some enjoyment of life and play)

Pharmacological and nonpharmacological interventions used effectively for comfort and supportive care through illness

Child/family cared for and family supported through death with physical, psychosocial, developmental, spiritual, and other concerns/needs acknowledged/addressed

Infection control and palliation through illness in setting of choice

Grief/bereavement expression and support provided to family

Child/adolescent is pain free by next _____ visit

Parent and caregiver demonstrate ability to manage pain and other symptoms, where applicable

Observation and assessment of child's behavior, including expressions, usual activity level, and changes noted, to assist in pain identification and management

Parent and child verbalize satisfaction with care

Educational tools/plans related to care of infant with _____ incorporated into care routines (e.g., rest, fluids)

Safe and infection-free delivery of total parenteral nutrition at home

Child remains at home without or with minimal complications

Infant or child is pain free and comfortable

Child will demonstrate an adequate breathing pattern as evidenced by lack of respiratory distress (e.g., no retractions, not using accessory muscles, appears comfortable)

Child will maintain a patent airway and mobilization of secretions by use of respiratory treatments, oral medications, and effective cough

Child will maintain sufficient fluid intake to prevent dehydration (_____ cc in 24 hours)

Parent and caregiver will identify factors/triggers that seem to cause exacerbations

Prevention of multiple hospital admissions for infusion therapy with case management and phone intervention program by _____ (specify date)

Parent and caregiver will meet the developmental and play needs of child

Parent and caregiver demonstrate the ability to perform taught/learned health-related behaviors

Parent can list medications, their schedule, use, and side effects

Parent experiences decreased worry

Family bonding evidenced by loving relationship with infant

Parent effective in child's health maintenance and knows whom to call for questions/concerns

Patient and caregiver demonstrate appropriate backup or "rescue" therapies for breakthrough pain or other symptoms (e.g., dyspnea)

- *Home health aide or certified nursing assistant*
  Effective hygiene, personal care, and comfort
  ADL assistance
  Safe environment maintained

- *Hospice social worker*
  Problems identified and addressed, with patient/caregiver linked with appropriate support services and plan of care successfully implemented
  Patient and caregiver cope adaptively with illness and death
  Adaptive adjustment to changed body and body image
  Psychosocial support and counseling offered/initiated to patient/caregivers experiencing loss and grief

- *Volunteer(s)*
  Comfort, companionship, and friendship extended to patient/family
  Support provided as defined by the needs of the patient/caregiver
  Patient and family supported by team with care, comfort, and companionship

- *Spiritual counseling*
  Spiritual support offered and provided as defined by needs of patient/caregiver
  Provision of spiritual support and care as based on the assessed and ongoing needs of the patient and family
  Parent and caregiver verbalize comprehension of changing nutritional needs

- *Dietitian/nutritional counseling*
  Family and caregiver integrate recommendations into nutrition teaching (where appropriate)
  Parent and caregiver know whom to call for nutrition- and hydration-related questions/concerns
  Nutrition/hydration per patient's choices
  Caregiver integrates recommendations into daily meal planning

- *Occupational therapist*
  Patient and caregiver demonstrate maximum independence with ADL, adaptive techniques, and assistive devices
  Patient and caregiver demonstrate maximum safety in ADL and functional mobility
  Patient and caregiver demonstrate effective use of energy conservation
  Verbalization/demonstration of improved functional activity level and enhanced quality of life
  Patient and caregiver demonstrate effective use of diaphragmatic breathing to reduce shortness of breath and relaxation techniques to help in pain/symptom management
  Patient and caregiver demonstrate correct use of exercise and splints for maximum upper extremity function and joint position devices to increase functioning

- *Physical therapist*
  Prevention of complications
  Home exercise and upper extremity program taught to parent
  Optimal strength, mobility, and function maintained/achieved

Compliance with home exercise program by _____ (specify
date)

- *Speech-language pathologist*
  Communication method implemented and child able to be understood as
  self-reported or reported by family/caregivers
  Safe swallowing and functional communication
  Recommended lists of foods/textures for safety and child choice

- *Bereavement counselor*
  Support services related to grief provided to patient and family
  Well-being and resolution process of grief initiated and followed through
  bereavement services

- *Pharmacist*
  Bowel regimen successful as self-reported by patient and in update at team
  meeting
  Multiple drug regimen reviewed for food/drug and drug/drug interactions in
  patient on multiple medications
  Stability and safety in complex medication regimen, with maximum benefit
  to patient
  Effective pain and symptom control and symptom management as reported
  by patient/parent

- *Music, massage, art, or other therapies or services*
  Therapeutic massage/touch effective for patient as self-reported or observed
  by caregivers/family
  Improved muscle tone, relaxation, and/or sleep
  Patient comfortable and relaxed (e.g., sleeping, playing) after massage
  Music therapy intervention based on assessment to decrease pain percep-
  tion and provide emotional expression and support
  Maintenance of comfort and physical, psychosocial, and spiritual health
  Holistic health maintained and comfort achieved through _____
  (specify modality)

8. **Patient, family, and caregiver educational needs**
   Educational needs are the care regimens that contribute to safe and effective
   care at home between the hospice team's visits. These include the following:
   The basic tenets of hospice and the availability of support 24 hours a day, 7
   days a week
   Home safety assessment and counseling
   Anticipated disease progression
   The patient's medication regimen
   Safe and proper body mechanics to promote patient comfort and prevent
   caregiver safety problems
   Other teaching specific to the patient's and family's unique needs
   Support groups available to patient's family, such as the hospice program's
   "Caregiver Support Group" meetings for family members and friends of
   the patient
   Health maintenance and growth and development information
   The importance of immunizations
   Signs and symptoms that necessitate calling the physician

Potential complications of new technologies (e.g., TPN)

Home medical equipment vendor's name and number should be readily accessible in the home care clinical record should there be a problem

Other information, based on the child's unique condition

9. **Specific tips for quality and reimbursement**

Document all care provided and outcomes of that care

Document the child's/parent's responses to care, changes, and communications with the physician and other hospice team members

Document the course of care including why the infant/child was admitted for care, the plan, and support provided

Document in the clinical notes the clear progression and symptomatology, interventions, and overall management of the child with _____ (specify)

Document when/if the patient has respiratory changes, shortness of breath, exacerbation of conditions, changes in pain, and/or other symptoms and that they are identified and resolved

Remember that the clinical documentation is key to measuring compliance for quality and reimbursement purposes. Care coordination, timely verbal and initial physician orders, and assessment and addressing of spiritual and psychosocial needs should be ongoing and documented in the patient's clinical record

Document changes to the plan of care such as medications, services, frequency, communication, and concurrence of other team members

Document coordination of services or consultation of the other members of the IDT

Document communications and care coordination with other care providers such as inpatient team members and hired caregivers

The documentation should support that all hospice care supports comfort and dignity while meeting child/family needs

The documentation should include ongoing assessment and management of pain and other symptoms and the anticipation and prevention of secondary symptoms such as constipation

It is important to note that all team members, including nurses and social workers, should assess, identify, and "hear" spiritual needs that the patient/family want to be addressed. These spiritual issues are key to the provision of quality hospice care and cannot be addressed effectively and promptly by the spiritual counselor only

Document clearly symptoms, clinical changes, and assessment findings related to pain and patient care

Document weight loss, increased shortness of breath, dyspnea, infection, sepsis, new or changed medications, etc.

Document any skin changes (e.g., inflamed, painful, weeping skin site[s])

Remember that the "litmus test" of care coordination rests on the quality of the clinical documentation by all team members. Review one of your patient's clinical records and ask yourself the following: "If I was unable to give a verbal report/update on this child/family's course of care, would a peer be able to pick up and provide the same level of care and know (from the documentation) the current orders, medications, and other details that contribute to effective hospice care?"

This patient population usually has many clinical changes that should be documented. These include weight loss and multiple and changed medication regimens with varying routes. Side effects to the drug regimen should be observed, noted, documented, and reported

Your assessments, observations, and clinical findings are information that assists in painting a picture to support coverage and documentation requirements for hospice care

Document any hospitalizations and changed clinical findings

Document patient changes, symptoms, psychosocial issues impacting the care, and information gathered at the child/family visits and during team meetings

10. **Resources for hospice care and practice**

The American Sudden Infant Death Syndrome Institute offers a pamphlet entitled *Coping with Infant Loss Grief and Bereavement* that can be obtained by calling 1-800-232-SIDS or 1-404-843-1030.

The National Easter Seal Society offers brochures about many childhood problems and can be reached at 1-800-221-6827. The National Information Center for Children and Youth With Disabilities offers information; call 1-800-695-0285.

The Agency for Health Care Policy and Research (AHCPR) offers a *Quick Reference Guide for Clinicians: Acute Pain Management in Infants, Children, and Adolescents: Operative and Medical Procedures,* which presents pain assessment tools and pain assessment and management information. This resource can be obtained free by calling 1-800-358-9295.

The American Psychiatric Association offers a free 18-page pamphlet entitled *Childhood Disorders,* which addresses information about autism, signs of depression, attention deficit disorder, development disorders, and other conditions. This resource can be obtained by calling 1-800-368-5777 or writing to American Psychiatric Association, Division of Public Affairs, Department SG, 1400 K Street, N.W., Washington, D.C. 20005.

The Candlelighters Childhood Cancer Foundation offers many services for parents and children, including resources, services, advocacy, and support. Call 1-301-657-8401 or 1-800-366-2223 (CCCF) for information.

PART SIX

PLANNING AND IMPLEMENTING NUTRITIONAL CARE

A. **Anorexia or cachexia: Whose problem?**
B. **Treating the family when the patient cannot or will not eat**
   Helpful phrases in discouraging the "He must eat or he will die" syndrome
   include the following:
   - "When his illness is this far along, he doesn't use very much energy"
   - "Just give him a little of what he wants"
   - "His system is so sick, he can't digest much anyway"
   - "Giving him only fluids will be fine"
   - "It's okay if he doesn't meet his needs; he can't use food appropriately
     anyway"
   - "Pushing him to eat will only make him more uncomfortable"
   - "He's sick. Feed him if he wants food or will take it, but don't force him"
     "He'll still be sick even if he eats"
   - "His illness controls his appetite. Don't trouble him with eating, but let him
     sit with you during meals and enjoy your company"
C. **Treating the patient who can and wants to eat**
   The following are some simple suggestions for treating the patient who can
   and wants to eat:
   1. Feed the patient when hungry, changing mealtimes if needed. Note the
      patient's best meals, and make these the largest ones.
   2. Serve a small portion of the patient's favorite foods on a small plate
   3. Gently encourage, but do not nag, the patient to eat; remove uneaten food
      without undue comment
   4. Cold foods are generally preferred to hot foods. Reassure parents of a
      dying child that they do not have to serve a hot, nutritious meal daily for
      the child; encourage them not to feel guilty if the child wants nothing or
      wants only a fast-food hamburger or fries
   5. Set an attractive table and plate, using a plate garnish or table flower if
      enjoyed by the patient. In an institutional setting, serve the patient's food
      on trays set with embroidered tray cloths and pretty china or stoneware
      rather than traditional paper underliners and dishes. Allow the patient's
      personal china and utensils from home to be used if feasible
   6. Make mealtimes sociable and enjoyable; vary the place of eating, and
      remove bedpans from the room
   7. Children can be encouraged to drink by playing games; it is fun for a
      child to drink fluids in out-of-the-ordinary ways, such as through a
      syringe, in small medicine cups, and by eating juice bars or popsicles.
      Remove toys from the bed, turn off the television, and bring in friends for
      a meal. Children will enjoy a sack lunch on occasion, and they enjoy
      eating foods that have been cut into interesting shapes or made to re-
      semble favorite characters
   8. Suggest that the patient rest before eating; most children and adults feel
      more like eating when they are relaxed
   9. Encourage high-calorie foods day or night, including eggnog, milkshake,
      custard, pudding, peanut butter, cream soups, cheese, fizzy drinks, pie,
      sherbet, and cheesecake. In an institutional setting, consider serving foods
      from a hot trolley instead of or in addition to allowing patients to choose
      their meals in advance. Consider soup and soft sandwiches for midday
      meals. Try to supply as much variety in food selection as possible, includ-
      ing regional favorites

10. Provide lipped dishes for patients who have arm and hand weakness; use rubber grips on ordinary cutlery for those with a weak grip
11. In an institutional setting, have a dining room available, with a homelike atmosphere, where patients and families can eat together. Allow the family to eat with the patient in the patient's room if desired. Have staff available to feed patients who are unable to feed themselves. Do not hurry patients to eat
12. Liberalize diets as much as possible; rarely are diabetic or low-sodium diets essential, but if they are, consider low–simple-sugar foods and no regular salt packets instead of a more restricted diet.

D. **Dietary treatment for common symptoms in terminal illness**

Belching

- Allow the patient to make the final choice of foods to eat or avoid, but consider testing the patient's tolerance to gas-producing foods such as the following: beer, carbonated beverages, alcohol, dairy products (if lactose intolerant), nuts, beans, onions, peas, corn, cucumbers, radishes, cabbage, broccoli, brussels sprouts, spinach, cauliflower, high-fat foods, yeast, and mushrooms
- Encourage the patient to eat solids at mealtimes and drink liquids between meals instead of with solid foods
- Advise the patient against eating quickly and reclining immediately after eating; encourage the patient to relax before, during, and after meals
- Advise the patient to avoid overeating, sucking through straws, and chewing gum and to keep the mouth closed when chewing and swallowing

Constipation

- Encourage the patient to eat foods high in fiber (bran; whole grains; fruits, especially pineapples, prunes, and raisins; vegetables; nuts; and legumes) if adequate fluid intake can be maintained. Avoid high-fiber foods if dehydration, severe constipation, or obstruction is anticipated.
- Increase fluid intake as tolerated; encourage fruit juices, prune juice, and cider. If liked by the patient, a recipe (1-2 ounces with the evening meal of a mixture of 2 cups applesauce, 2 cups unprocessed bran, and 1 cup 100% prune juice) is effective and may reduce laxative use
- Discontinue calcium and iron supplementation if used; limit cheese, rich desserts, and other foods if the patient is constipated

Diarrhea

- Let the patient make the final choice of foods to eat or avoid, but suggest omission of the following foods if they cause diarrhea: milk, ice cream, whole-grain breads and cereals, nuts, beans, peas, greens, fruits with seeds and skins, fresh pineapple, raisins, cider, prune juice, raw vegetables, gas-forming vegetables, alcohol, and caffeine-containing beverages
- Encourage the patient to eat bananas, applesauce, peeled apple, tapioca, rice, peanut butter, refined grains, crackers, pasta, cream of wheat, oatmeal, and cooked vegetables
- Encourage the patient to avoid liquids with a meal and instead to drink liquids an hour after a meal
- Encourage the patient to relax before, during, and after a meal
- Enteral and/or parenteral nutritional support in the AIDS patient may be appropriate if the patient has a lengthy life expectancy and the cause of the diarrhea is known and treatable; whether administered by tube feeding or

orally, the diet should be high in calories and protein and low in fiber, lactose, and fat

- If dehydration is a problem, encourage high-potassium foods

Hypercalcemia

- Allow the hypercalcemic patient to eat foods high in calcium (such as dairy products, if desired), but encourage the patient to avoid calcium and vitamin D supplementation; restriction of high-calcium foods is rarely helpful
- Encourage the patient to drink lots of fluids, particularly carbonated beverages containing phosphoric acid if the patient enjoys them

Mental disorders

- Encourage the patient to avoid alcohol and caffeine-containing foods, such as coffee, tea, and chocolate, if they contribute to anxiety, sleep deprivation, or depression.
- If the patient is *drowsy or apathetic,* suggest that the family feed the patient. Encourage them to prepare the patient's favorite foods, usually in soft form to be served with a spoon or bite-size so the patient might self-feed. Help the family protect the patient and others from the patient by shutting off the stove or removing its knobs, removing matches, and locking doors to cabinets or closets that contain poisons, alcohol, or medications. Put away electrical appliances such as mixers, food processors, can openers, and waffle irons; unplug microwave ovens
- If the patient is *agitated or confused,* caution the family about the dangers of hand-feeding the patient. Suggest feeding with a spoon and not allowing the patient to handle feeding utensils, plates, glass, etc. Encourage the family to tell the patient what time of day it is, what meal is served, and what foods are served. Remind the patient that the foods served are favorites. Make mealtimes enjoyable by reminiscing about pleasant events in the patient's life. Consider the pros and cons of waking the patient if asleep at mealtimes
- If the patient is *stuporous or comatose,* counsel the family that semistarvation and dehydration are not painful to the patient; explore with them the pros and cons of enteral and parenteral nutritional support if they request information

Mouth problems

- If the patient says that foods taste *bitter,* encourage poultry, fish, dairy products, eggs, milk, and cheese; bitter-tasting foods usually include red meat, sour juices, coffee, tea, tomatoes, and chocolate. Suggest cooking foods in glass or porcelain instead of metal containers, and avoid serving foods on metal or with metallic utensils. Encourage sweet fruit drinks, carbonated beverages, and popsicles and seasonings, herbs, and spices to enhance flavors.
- If the patient says that foods taste *old,* try adding sugar; sour and salty tastes often taste "old."
- If the patient says that foods taste *too sweet,* suggest drinking sour juices and cooking with lemon juice, vinegar, spices, herbs, and mint; add pickles to appropriate foods
- If the patient says that foods have *no taste,* suggest marinating appropriate foods, serving highly seasoned foods, adding sugar, and serving foods at room temperature

- If the patient has *difficulty swallowing,* suggest small, frequent meals of soft foods (puréed if needed); advise against foods that might irritate the mouth and esophagus, such as acidic juices or fruits, spicy foods, very hot or cold foods, alcohol, and carbonated beverages
- If the patient has *mouth sores,* suggest blenderized and cold foods; gravies, cream soups, eggnog, milkshake, cream pies, cheesecake, macaroni and cheese, and casseroles are well-liked. Suggest the patient avoid alcohol and acidic, spicy, rough, hot, and highly salted foods
- If the patient has a *dry mouth,* suggest frequent sips of water, juice, ice chips, popsicles, ice cream, fruitades or smoothies, or slushy-frozen baby foods mixed with fruit juice. Sucking on hard candy may stimulate saliva. Solid foods should be moist, pureed as needed, and not too tart or too hot or cold if mouth sores are present

Nausea and vomiting
- Encourage the patient to avoid eating if nauseated or if nausea is anticipated.
- Suggest small meals of cool nonodorous foods. Many patients find it helpful to avoid fatty, greasy, or fried foods; avoid mixing hot and cold foods at the same meal; avoid high-bulk meals; and avoid nausea-precipitating foods, such as overly sweet foods, alcohol, spicy foods, and tobacco with meals
- Encourage the patient to eat slowly and not overeat. Relaxing before and after meals, avoiding physical activity, and lying flat for 2 hours after eating may also help
- Suggest that the patient not prepare own food

Obstruction (gastrointestinal)
- If oral intake is not contraindicated, encourage the patient to eat small meals that are low in fiber, low in residue, and blenderized or strained. Many patients prefer to eat their favorite foods, enjoy large meals, and then vomit frequently. A gastric tube, open to straight or intermittent drain, may alleviate the need for regular vomiting
- With "squashed stomach syndrome," encourage the patient to eat small, frequent meals and avoid nausea-producing foods, odorous foods, gas-producing foods, and high-fat or fried foods. Limit fluid with meals; patients should take fluids an hour before and after meals.

E. **Aggressive nutrition support through tube feedings and parenteral feedings:** Potential benefits of enteral and parenteral feedings in terminally ill patients
- Correcting fluid and electrolyte imbalance may result in the following:
  1. Increased mental alertness
  2. Decreased nausea
  3. Stabilized cardiac arrhythmias
- Added calories and other nutrients may prolong life, giving the patient and family more time to get their psychosocial and material affairs in order
- Aggressive nutritional support may result in the following:
  1. Enhancement of the patient's and family's confidence that "everything is being done" to decrease cachexia and help the patient live as long as possible
  2. Increased emotional support to the patient and family by reducing their fear of abandonment

3. Improvement of the patient's overall sense of well-being; cosmetic benefits may improve self-esteem
4. Improvement of patient and family interrelationships

Potential physical burdens of enteral nutritional support in terminally ill patients

- Nasogastric tubes are irritating to most patients, outright painful to many, and almost always painful upon insertion
- Nasogastric feedings cause uncomfortable distension, nausea, diarrhea, dehydration, and hyperosmolality in many patients
- A gastrostomy or jejunostomy tube requires surgery, although it might result in increased comfort when compared with nasogastric tubes
- Vomiting, aspiration, and subsequent pneumonia sometimes occur in terminally ill patients fed via nasogastric tubes or gastric tubes. These problems are most common when the patient is recumbent and noncommunicative and has reduced oral and hypopharyngeal sensation, dysphagia, reduced competence of upper and lower esophageal sphincters, reduced esophageal peristalsis, delayed gastric emptying, and reflux exacerbated by a supine position
- Excess stomal leakage and wound dehiscence with enterostomy feedings occur, especially if the abdominal tumor is large and exerts pressure on the tube in the stomach or jejunum

Potential physical burdens of parenteral nutritional support in terminally ill patients

- Intravenous fluids can be distressful and painful, especially in patients with scarred and collapsed veins
- Patients' activities are usually restricted with parenteral feedings because they are tethered to the infusion apparatus
- Sepsis may occur in malnourished patients receiving total parenteral nutrition (TPN) and is an unnecessary and uncomfortable complication
- Fluid overload, ascites, peripheral edema, pulmonary edema, and pressure symptoms from edematous masses can occur with TPN and intravenous (IV) solutions
- The cost of TPN can be excessive for family and palliative care programs
- TPN might exacerbate the patient's disease
- Thrombosis is a potential result of the use of TPN and IV solutions in terminally ill patients
- Lung puncture is an unnecessary risk of TPN in terminally ill patients
- Increased urine flow with TPN and IV fluids may result in the need for catheterization in patients too weak to void large volumes
- Increased gastrointestinal secretions may require nasogastric suctioning
- Increased pulmonary secretions may require suctioning
- Death rattle, with accumulating pharyngeal secretions, is more likely to occur with increased fluid

Modified from Gallagher-Allred CR: *Nutritional care of the terminally ill,* Rockville, Md, 1989, Aspen.

Patient Profile

Name: _____   Referring MD.: _____

Caregiver: _____   Hospice nurse: _____

Age: _____   Date of intake: _____

Diagnosis: _____   Date of death: _____

Additional medical information: (medical history and condition on admission)

Medications: (admission and updates; D/C meds by marking through medication name with colored marker)

Date: Medication:

_____

_____

_____

Weekly team update: (prognosis, medical-nursing conditions, family concerns, etc.)

Date: Update:

_____

_____

_____

_____

Nutritional Assessment

Nutritional status (admission):   excellent ☐

                                         adequate for ADL ☐

                                         poor ☐

PO intake (admission):   good ☐   fair ☐   poor ☐

Nutritional problems:

Date identified	Date resolved	Problem

Patient/family views on PO intake, tube feeding, parenteral feeding:

Nutritional action needed: ☐ none by RD; nurse can handle

                                    ☐ RD to phone patient/family

                                    ☐ RD to visit patient/family

Figure 6-1 Patient summary and nutritional screening form. (Modified from Gallagher-Allred CR: *Nutritional care of the terminally ill,* Rockville, Md., 1989, Aspen.)

PART SEVEN

PAIN

Assessment and Management Resources

PAIN ASSESSMENT FORM

PAIN ASSESSMENT

GENERAL INFORMATION

Primary pain site _____   Date of pain onset ___ / ___ / ___
                          (Indicate on body illustration as Site A)

Brief pain history (patient's viewpoint)_____

Describe cause of pain _____

Describe how pain feels to patient _____

Pain relief methods tried (check all that apply):   ☐ Medication   ☐ Deep Relaxation
   ☐ Heat   ☐ Cold   ☐ Massage   ☐ Meditation   ☐ Music   ☐ Visual Imagery
   Other (specify): _____

Pain is relieved by (describe) _____

Pain is worsened by (describe circumstances or activities) _____

Times when pain is worse: ☐ Early morning (pre-dawn)   ☐ Morning   ☐ Afternoon   ☐ Evening   ☐ Night

Activities pain prevents patient from doing _____

Patient desires pain relief: ☐ Yes   ☐ No (if no, explain) _____

Associated symptoms (if any)_____

Comments: _____

PAIN LOCATION/TYPE/FREQUENCY/INTENSITY

Indicate on the body illustrations below any pain locations other than the primary site already marked. (Label additional sites B, C, D.) Code pain type, frequency and intensity as applicable. Children may use the facial expressions to assist in determining pain intensity.

TYPE	SITE A	SITE B	SITE C	SITE D
Code: I = Internal; A = Acute; E = External; C = Chronic				

FREQUENCY				
Code: O = Occasional; F = Frequent; C = Constant				

INTENSITY

Scale:
0   1   2   3   4   5   6   7   8   9   10
No Pain   Moderate Pain   Worst Pain

	SITE A	SITE B	SITE C	SITE D
At Present				
1 Hour After Medication				
3 Hours After Medication				
Worst It Gets				
Best It Gets				

PAIN MEDICATION

Medication	Time Used		Strength	Frequency	Results/Side Effects Experienced
	☐ Past	☐ Present			
	☐ Past	☐ Present			
	☐ Past	☐ Present			
	☐ Past	☐ Present			
	☐ Past	☐ Present			
	☐ Past	☐ Present			

Signature and Title of Assessor _____   Date ___ / ___ / ___

PATIENT NAME—Last, First, Middle Initial   ID#

Form 3459P   © 1995 Briggs Corporation, Des Moines, IA 50306
To order, phone 1-800-247-2343   PRINTED IN U.S.A.   **PAIN ASSESSMENT**

(Reprinted with permission of Briggs Health Care Products, Des Moines, Iowa.)

INITIAL PAIN ASSESSMENT TOOL

Date_____

Patient's Name_____Age_____Room_____

Diagnosis_____Physician_____

Nurse_____

I. LOCATION: Patient or nurse mark drawing.

II. INTENSITY: Patient rates the pain. Scale used _____

Present:_____
Worst pain gets:_____
Best pain gets:_____
Acceptable level of pain:_____

III. QUALITY: (Use patient's own words, e.g. prick, ache, burn, throb, pull, sharp) _____

IV. ONSET, DURATION VARIATIONS, RHYTHMS:_____

V. MANNER OF EXPRESSING PAIN:_____

VI. WHAT RELIEVES THE PAIN?_____

VII. WHAT CAUSES OR INCREASES THE PAIN?_____

VIII. EFFECTS OF PAIN: (Note decreased function, decreased quality of life.)
Accompanying symptoms (e.g. nausea)_____
Sleep_____
Appetite_____
Physical activity_____
Relationship with others (e.g. irritability)_____
Emotions (e.g. anger, suicidal, crying)_____
Concentration_____
Other_____

IX. OTHER COMMENTS:_____

X. PLAN:_____

(From McCaffery, Beebe A: *Pain: clinical manual for nursing practice,* St Louis, 1989, Mosby, p 21. May be duplicated for use in clinical practice.)

PAIN INTENSITY SCALES

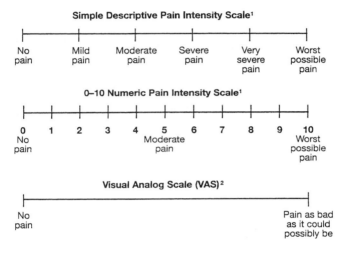

Simple Descriptive Pain Intensity Scale[1]

No pain | Mild pain | Moderate pain | Severe pain | Very severe pain | Worst possible pain

0–10 Numeric Pain Intensity Scale[1]

0 No pain | 1 | 2 | 3 | 4 | 5 Moderate pain | 6 | 7 | 8 | 9 | 10 Worst possible pain

Visual Analog Scale (VAS)[2]

No pain | Pain as bad as it could possibly be

[1] If used as a graphic rating scale, a 10-cm baseline is recommended.
[2] A 10-cm baseline is recommended for VAS scales.

(From Cancer Pain Management Guideline Panel: *Management of cancer pain. Clinical Practice Guideline,* AHCPR Publication No. 94-0592, Rockville, Md, 1994, Agency for Health Care Policy and Research, Public Health Service, U.S. Department of Health and Human Services, p 23.)

FACES PAIN RATING SCALE

Explain to child that each face is for a person who feels happy because there is no pain (hurt) or sad because there is some or a lot of pain. FACE 0 is very happy because there is no hurt. FACE 1 hurts just a little bit. FACE 2 hurts a little more. FACE 3 hurts even more. FACE 4 hurts a whole lot, but FACE 5 hurts as much as you can imagine, although you don't have to be crying to feel this bad. Ask child to choose face that best describes own pain. Record the number under chosen face on pain assessment record.

(From Wong DL: *Wong and Whaley's clinical manual of pediatric nursing,* ed 4, St Louis, 1996, Mosby, p 316.)

PAIN FLOW SHEET

Patient _____   Date _____

*Pain rating scale used _____

Purpose: To evaluate the safety and effectiveness of the analgesic(s).

Analgesic(s) prescribed: _____

Time	Pain rating	Analgesic	R	P	BP	Level of arousal	Other†	Plan & comments

*Pain rating: A number of different scales may be used. Indicate which scale is used and use the same one each time. For example, 0-10 (0 = no pain, 10 = worst pain).

†Possibilities for other columns: bowel function, activities, nausea and vomiting, other pain relief measures. Identify the side effects of greatest concern to patient, family, physician, nurses.

(From McCaffery, Beebe A: *Pain: clinical manual for nursing practice,* St Louis, 1989, Mosby, p 27. May be duplicated for use in clinical practice.)

NURSE'S POWER AND RESPONSIBILITY IN RELATION TO MEDICATION FOR PAIN RELIEF

Nurse Is Expected To:	Comments
1. Determine whether the analgesic is to be given and, if so, when.	1. Many analgesics are on PRN basis (PRN means use clinical judgment). Assess and apply knowledge. Based on this assessment, a PRN analgesic order may be given around the clock (ATC), on a regular basis (e.g., q3h).
2. Choose the appropriate analgesic(s) when more than one is ordered.	2. More than one analgesic is often available. Which one does the nurse give? Two at the same time? Avoid one? This decision is based on pharmacological knowledge along with skills in assessment and evaluation.
3. Be alert to the possibility of certain side effects as a result of the analgesic.	3. Nurse plays key role in identifying life-threatening side effects (e.g., respiratory depression). Identifies constipation, which can seriously influence patient's comfort as much as pain itself.
4. Evaluate effectiveness of analgesic at regular frequent intervals following each administration, but especially the initial dose.	4. This is a vital step in ensuring effective pain control. Assessment and evaluation are continuous processes. A flow sheet is recommended.
5. Report promptly and accurately to the physician when a change is needed.	5. Every new prescription of analgesic for the individual patient is merely a guess that must be evaluated. Too small a dosage should be changed as quickly as too large a dosage.
6. Make suggestions for specific changes (e.g., drug, route, dosage, and interval).	6. The nurse has unique blend of knowledge: pharmacological information and direct observation of patient. The result is that nurse is in ideal position to make an educated guess about what may work better for the individual patient.
7. Advise the patient about the use of analgesics, both prescription and nonprescription.	7. Nurse has a key educational role about dosage, side effects, addressing misconceptions, preventive schedule, and how to talk with physician or nurse about questions or problems with drug.

IMMEDIATE HELP FOR PHARMACOLOGICAL CONTROL OF PAIN

Patient in home care setting unexpectedly unable to take oral analgesics

Time involved: Reading time, 4 minutes; implementation time, about 10 minutes.

Situation: Patient of any age being cared for at home with moderate to severe pain controlled with oral analgesics is now unexpectedly unable to swallow or has uncontrolled nausea and vomiting. His next dose of analgesics is due in 1 hour, and he cannot take it orally, even in liquid form. Moderate to severe pain will occur unless analgesics can be administered by another route, but no provision has been made for this (e.g., there are no drugs or equipment for IM, SC, IV, or rectal administration). It would take 2 hours or longer to obtain such drugs or equipment. How can the oral analgesics he has been taking be used to provide pain relief now?

Possible solution: Take all oral forms of analgesics due in the next oral dose, dissolve them in warm water, and administer rectally.

Expected outcome: Pain relief will be satisfactory, but perhaps not ideal. Pain may increase somewhat, but moderate to severe pain will not occur.

HOW TO USE ORAL ANALGESICS RECTALLY IN AN EMERGENCY

- Obtain the physician's approval for changing the route of administration.
- Instruct the patient or family via telephone or do this yourself if you are in the home at the time:
  1. Assemble all the oral analgesics to be given at the next dose, including narcotics and nonnarcotics.
  2. Review the ingredients and formulations.

  Caution: The only known exception to the following instructions concerns sustained-release formulations. Be especially alert to sustained-release morphine (MS Contin, Roxanol SR). If sustained-release morphine is included, administer only a portion of the dose due because dissolving the tablets will convert morphine to immediate-release morphine with a duration of approximately 4 hours. Thus if sustained-release morphine doses are given every 8 hours, each dose would be divided in half and given every 4 hours.

  Although there is no research to support this practice, many home care nurses report that satisfactory analgesia can be obtained from any of the oral analgesics by converting them to the rectal route as explained here. Some medications are more irritating than others, but hopefully this is only a temporary measure. Oral analgesics given rectally with successful pain relief include tablets of oxycodone plus acetaminophen, hydromor-

Modified from McCaffery, Beebe A: *Pain: clinical manual for nursing practice,* St Louis, 1989, Mosby, p 45.

phone, liquid or tablets of morphine, methadone, and several of the NSAIDs.

3. Place the tablets in a small but strong container (e.g., cup), and crush them with the bowl of a small spoon.

4. Measure a teaspoon (5 ml), or more if necessary, of very hot tap water. Pour over the crushed tablets. Mix or crush further until fairly well dissolved. Let it sit while you find the equipment needed to insert it into the rectum. It should be about body temperature when it is inserted. Warm again if it gets cold or hardens.

5. Several types of equipment may be improvised for rectal insertion of the liquid. An ideal arrangement is a syringe with a short length of small-lumen rubber catheter attached. If this is not available, any of the following will suffice if the patient is placed in a position where gravity can assist (e.g., bending over or lying on his side):

   a. Any equipment used to administer enemas. The main problem is likely to be that the tubing is so long that some of the medication is lost by adhering to the sides of the tubing. Using more water to dissolve the tablets may help.

   b. Douche equipment, with some modification of the usual tip for insertion. Again, long tubing may be a problem.

   c. Baster (pointed tube with bulb attached, often used for basting turkey) or rubber ear syringe (not used much anymore, but it has a small rubber tip and a bulb). With either of these, immediately before insertion into the rectum, suction up the liquid, point the open end upward, and squeeze out as much air as possible without losing the liquid. Maintain that amount of bulb compression until the tube is inserted in the rectum. Then compress completely and withdraw.

   d. Any clean, small-lumen rubber tubing attached to a funnel.

   e. If all else fails, a plastic straw may be attached to a funnel shaped of aluminum foil or wax paper.

6. Lubricate the end of the tubing prior to insertion. A water-soluble lubricant (e.g., K-Y Jelly) is best, but if it is not available, use a small amount of any lubricant such as Vaseline, butter, or cooking oil.

7. Slowly insert the tube about 1½ inches into the rectum.

8. After the liquid has been inserted, position the patient on his left side for better absorption.

9. Get a pain rating from the patient at the time the medication is given rectally and then at half-hour intervals. If pain is not relieved or has increased after 1 hour, give another dose rectally. If there is no relief after 1 hour, consider giving 50% to 100% of the previous rectal dose. If there is some relief but not enough, consider giving an additional 25% of the previous dose.

QUICK ALTERNATIVES TO LIQUID FORM OF RECTAL ADMINISTRATION

1. Except for sustained-release tablets, the tablets or capsules themselves may simply be inserted about 1½ inches into the rectum. If lubricant is necessary, moisten with water or use a water-soluble lubricant such as K-Y Jelly. Absorp-

tion takes longer, since the tablets must first dissolve, and seems less reliable than the liquid formulation. However, small tablets or those without a coating may work well.

2. If the volume is small, put the crushed tablet in an empty capsule. Simply empty any capsule for use unless the patient is allergic to whatever it contained. Again, absorption may take longer than with the liquid formulation.

IMMEDIATE HELP FOR PHARMACOLOGICAL CONTROL OF PAIN

Maximal use of nonprescription analgesics when prescription analgesics are unavailable*

Time involved: Reading time, 3 minutes; implementation time, after ingredients are obtained, 5 minutes.

Situation: Unexpected moderate to severe pain of known cause (e.g., dislocated shoulder or broken bone from accidental fall) occurring in a healthy adult patient. A physician is contacted, but it will be 2 hours or longer before the patient can be seen by the physician. Also, due to time, location, and other factors, it is not possible to obtain any prescription analgesic. Using nonprescription analgesics available from a general store, what can be done to obtain maximal analgesia on a one-time-only basis?

Possible solution: Consider a combination of the following, if available, and obtain the physician's consent.

Expected outcome: Significant pain relief, but it may not be sufficient.

Maximal Pain Relief with Nonprescription Drugs

1. Acetaminophen 1000 mg in liquid form, if possible, or tablets (three regular tablets or two "extra strength" tablets)
2. Ibuprofen 800 mg (four tablets of 200 mg each)
3. Antacid (1 teaspoon of a concentrated liquid, if possible)
4. Caffeine 100 to 200 mg (a strong cup of brewed coffee, or one to two "keep awake" nonprescription tablets)
5. Carbonated beverage (e.g., 7-Up) or one with caffeine (e.g., Pepsi)
6. Alcohol (e.g., wine, gin). Many social drinks combine a carbonated beverage with alcohol (e.g., gin and tonic). A social drink may be relaxing or distracting

Caution: Use of the above should be restricted to emergencies or "one time only." Consult a physician and determine the patient's previous response to each ingredient. Drugs that have produced unwanted side effects should be eliminated.

Rationale: No research supports the safety or effectiveness of the above combination. Separate research studies suggest that these ingredients would be an effective combination and are pharmacologically compatible (i.e., they may be given together). Regarding each item, the rationale is as follows:

1. Acetaminophen relieves pain in a manner different from other nonnarcotics. It is well tolerated (i.e., side effects are unlikely). Combinations of acetaminophen and aspirin have been approved for sale as nonprescription analgesics. Patients on NSAIDs are allowed to take acetaminophen

---

*Or, when the physician won't return your call, when the physician has refused to prescribe anything, when the pharmacy loses the prescription, or in other frustrating situations.
Modified from McCaffery, Beebe A: *Pain: clinical manual for nursing practice,* St Louis, 1989, Mosby, p 46.

2. Ibuprofen is an NSAID somewhat similar to aspirin but better tolerated (e.g., fewer GI upsets). The maximal recommended single dose of ibuprofen when it is prescribed by a physician is 800 mg. (The nonprescription recommended dose is limited to 400 mg.) If ibuprofen is unavailable or undesirable for any reason, aspirin can be substituted in a dose of 1000 mg. Aspirin could be given along with ibuprofen and the other ingredients. Omitting it from the above list may be unnecessary, but it could increase the risk of GI upset and decrease the effectiveness of the ibuprofen (probably to a limited extent). There are no data on the combination of ibuprofen and aspirin as a single dose. They are sometimes combined in the treatment of rheumatoid arthritis. The recommendation in this instance to give either aspirin or ibuprofen, but not both, is merely a qualified guess. On a single-dose basis for analgesia only, ibuprofen may do what aspirin does but with fewer side effects. Adding aspirin to the ibuprofen may increase the risks more than the analgesia (possibly is a duplication of effort)
3. Antacids are recommended in combination with NSAIDs to prevent stomach upset. Antacids may also hasten the absorption of NSAIDs
4. Caffeine, in doses of 100 to 200 mg, has been shown to increase the effectiveness of both acetaminophen and aspirin. If patients do not ordinarily consume caffeine beverages, they are probably not tolerant to them, so the dose should be kept to the minimum of 100 mg to prevent side effects such as nervousness. If the patient is a regular user of caffeine (e.g., 4 cups or more of coffee a day), the larger dose of 200 mg may be advisable
5. Carbonation seems to result in a much faster onset of action, probably by helping to dissolve tablets and promoting absorption
6. Alcohol has some analgesic as well as tranquilizing and sedating properties. If the patient drinks alcohol enough to be familiar with his response to it, it can be given in the amount usually tolerated. However, it does increase the likelihood of GI irritation, especially along with aspirin

   Nausea or anxiety: If the patient has a history of vomiting in response to varied stimuli (a "weak stomach"), give a nonprescription antiemetic or sedative. Most over-the-counter (OTC) antiemetics are sedating. Sedation alone may decrease nausea or anxiety. An OTC product for "motion sickness" or anything for an allergy or cold may help (e.g., one that contains diphenhydramine, or Benadryl). There is some indication that diphenhydramine is analgesic or potentiates analgesia. If needed, give it along with the analgesic combination.

PART EIGHT

HOSPICE DEFINITIONS, ROLES, AND ABBREVIATIONS

KEY HOSPICE DEFINITIONS AND ROLES

Abuse According to Medicare, *abuse* describes practices that, either directly or indirectly, result in unnecessary costs to the Medicare program. An example is providing medically unnecessary services or services that do not meet professionally recognized standards.

Access The availability of health care and the ability of an individual to receive services such as hospice, including all factors related to cost, location, transportation, and ability to receive care.

Accreditation A rigorous process that examines various components of hospice operations and clinical practice. The achievement of accreditation designates that the organization has gone through the accreditation process and meets predetermined standards as measured by on-site nurses and other survey team "visitors."

A process that an organization or program undertakes to demonstrate it has met established standards or requirements (e.g., the Joint Commission for Accreditation of Healthcare Organizations [JCAHO] and the Community Health Accreditation Program [CHAP]).

Activities of daily living (ADLs) Basic, usually self-care, activities that must be done daily to care for our bodies and overall health. These activities include personal hygiene tasks such as bathing and grooming and obtaining and preparing food. Others include toileting and transferring in and out of bed. These activities are important indicators because they demonstrate the patient's functional status or health care needs.

Advance directives Effective December 1, 1991, participating hospices (and other participating organizations, such as home health agencies and hospitals) must comply with the advance directive provisions of S4206 of the Omnibus Budget Reconciliation Act (OBRA) of 1990. This means the hospice must inform adult patients in writing of state laws regarding advance directives and of their policies regarding the implementation of advance directives. The hospice must document in the individual's clinical record whether the individual has executed an advance directive and cannot impose conditions on the provision of care or otherwise discriminate against an individual based on whether that individual has executed an advance directive (since the law does not require an individual to do so). Moreover, the hospice must educate staff and the community on issues concerning advance directives. Two common forms of advance directives are a living will and a durable power of attorney for health care.

Advocacy A role assumed by a health care professional designed to maximize patient self-determination through education, support, and affirmation of patient health care decisions.

Agency for Health Care Policy and Research (AHCPR) An agency of the U.S. Department of Health and Human Services that sponsors research projects and develops clinical practice guidelines related to the delivery of health care services.

Autonomy Respect for patients as individuals who are capable of making their own choices about health care and lifestyle options.

Benchmark A systematic process to measure or quantify; a standard for comparing two similar types of products and services when trying to identify areas for improvement in an organization.

Bereavement Bereavement consists of counseling services provided to the hospice patient's family or survivors after the patient's death. An assessment is usually performed by a bereavement professional or specially trained volunteers to identify families or family members who may be at risk for bereavement problems.

Capitated risk The financial risk involved in not being able to estimate accurately the cost of services and contract appropriately for care or services to a capitated population.

Capitation A set dollar amount established to cover the cost of health care services delivered to an individual. The amount is based on the number of members in the plan, not the amount of services used.

Care plan A plan of action for care that is developed, delivered, and evaluated by a hospice interdisciplinary team. This may also be called the *plan of care,* and the format varies among organizations.

Caregiver Anyone who provides care or services to or for a patient.

Case management A system for overseeing a patient's care across health care settings or systems. In hospice, this is often a primary care model with the case manager, nurse, or therapist rendering the skilled care and supervising or collaborating with other ordered professional service providers. Communication among the services and disciplines involved in the care must be documented in the clinical record. In these care conferences, input is given to the case manager to assist the disciplinary team in achieving predetermined or desired patient outcomes. Case management incorporates the principles of managed care. Hospice nurses may also interface with the insurance company nurse who is the case manager.

Case (Care) manager One person who is responsible for the overall care of the patient and use of resources for that care. The case (or care) manager may be a nurse, social worker, or therapist.

   The primary person (registered nurse or other health care professional) responsible for developing patient care outcomes for his or her case load. A case manager is accountable for meeting outcomes within an appropriate length of stay, the effective use of resources, and preestablished standards. A case manager collaborates with the health care team and the patient to accomplish those outcomes.

Catheter Any rounded or tubular medical device that is inserted into veins, cavities, or other body passages. The purpose of a catheter is to improve or replace function. Examples include a urinary Foley catheter in the bladder from which urine drains into a collection bag, suction catheters, and intravenous catheters inserted into the vein that allow for the delivery of fluids.

Certification Organizations desiring to participate in the Medicare program must meet participation conditions for certification (the Medicare Conditions of Participation). State agencies (such as the Department of Health) certify to the Department of Health and Human Services (DHHS) that the hospice or other types of organizations satisfy, and continue to satisfy, health care quality requirements for participation in the Medicare program.

Chaplaincy services The chaplain serves a population that spans the life continuum, from birth through death. The chaplain, like the professional nurse and other hospice team members, interfaces with patients and their families and friends at some of the most difficult times of their lives. Many people who have significant health concerns struggle to come to terms with the meaning of life. The chaplain assists patients and families with this process, regardless of whether they have any formal religious beliefs. The role varies, based on the setting, the patient and family, or other needs. Responsibilities may include patient assessment and support, bereavement counseling, serving on ethics committees, hospice staff support, or performing the sacrament of the sick. The chaplain facilitates the patient's movement toward his or her own resolution of life's questions.

Patients who may benefit from chaplaincy services include those for whom the NANDA nursing diagnoses *spiritual distress (distress of the human spirit)* and *spiritual well-being (potential for enhanced)* have been identified as appropriate. Other patients may have a need for spiritual care based on their health problems. For example, the elderly patient who is temporarily homebound as a result of a recent fall and fracture and misses going to church services on Sunday morning may need a call made to her priest or minister to arrange visits to her home.

Chronic A slow or persistent illness or health problem that must be treated or monitored throughout the patient's life. Examples include diabetes, glaucoma, some cancers, and some chronic lung conditions.

Classification system A system of categorizing elements of similar groups using preestablished criteria.

Client One who receives care. Also called the *patient, customer,* or *consumer* of health care services or products. An individual, customer, consumer, or patient who receives care or services.

Clinical care All the events that encompass the diagnosis and treatment of illness and the attainment of specific patient outcomes; it is the process of the health care team member and the physician working closely with the patient and the patient's family to meet predetermined and patient self-determined clinical outcomes.

Clinical path (CP) A structured plan for care, often categorized by diagnosis or patient problem, that defines specific care interventions, team members, and other information across a time line. Clinical management tools that organize, sequence, and time the major interventions of nursing staff, physicians, rehabilitation therapists, and other health professionals for a particular case type of condition. The pathways describe a standard of practice and are, in essence, a clinical budget.

Coinsurance The amount or percentage of the cost of services that consumers may be required to pay under a cost-sharing agreement with their insurance plan or program. It may also be called a *copayment.*

Collaboration The active process of working together and valuing another's input toward reaching patient goals. The act of working together to achieve a common goal(s). In health care, collaboration is a joint effort by staff from many disciplines planning together to improve the processes, which leads to improved patient care.

Community health nursing A synthesis of nursing practice and public health practice applied to promoting and preserving the health of the population. Health promotion, health maintenance, health education and management, and the coordination and continuity of care contribute to a holistic approach to the management of the health care of individuals, families, and groups within a community.

Continuous quality improvement (CQI) An ongoing process, also called *performance improvement* (PI), that seeks to continuously improve patient care, delivery of services, staff education, and other important parts of operations or other parts of an organization. Accreditation standards demand continuous quality improvement. Home care or hospice team members may be involved in various parts of CQI/PI or be asked to serve on certain committees.

A conceptual framework for evaluating the quality of care that emphasizes an analytical approach to understanding the contributions of all components of the health care system in achieving results and constantly incorporating improvements into the system.

Cost containment Those measures or requirements established by organizations involved in the delivery of health care to control the increases in utilization or expenditures.

Critical path A tool for case management and managed care that is an abbreviated version of the physician, nursing, rehabilitation therapists, and other service processes that must occur in a timely fashion to achieve an appropriate length of stay. Those key incidents may be categorized according to tests, activities, treatment, medication, diet, discharge planning, teaching, and outcomes. This can also be referred to as a *clinical path.* (See *Clinical paths.*)

Data Products of measurement (singular form: *datum*) compiled in such a fashion that discussion can be formulated or inference can be obtained.

Dementia Changes in brain function that cause memory loss, confusion, or the loss of ability to safely function independently.

Diagnoses The identification of problems or diseases. The singular form of the term is *diagnosis.*

Diagnostic-related groups (DRGs) A code of classifying patient illnesses according to principal diagnosis and treatment requirements. Under Medicare, each DRG has its own price (weight) that a hospital is paid regardless of the actual cost of treatment.

Dietitian The role of the registered dietitian (RD) is expanding as more patients are cared for in the community setting. Hospices have professional dietitians available to make home visits and provide consultative services to promote optimal patient nutrition. Another important component of the dietitian's role is as inservice educator for the care team. The RD also explains the nutrition/hydration parts of advanced directives.

Often, after being hospitalized, patients receive instructions on nutrition with regard to their unique needs and medical condition. Some of the common reasons home care patients consult with a dietitian are for enteral/parenteral nutrition considerations, anorexia, cancer, COPD, pressure ulcers, end stage renal failure, diabetes, AIDS, and other diseases, as well as assessment and monitoring of nutritional needs. Often, the family or caregiver needs the information from the RD more than the patient does.

More innovative insurers are reimbursing for this care when organizations clearly articulate the patient's need and justify the visits as part of the comprehensive plan.

Documentation The writing of clinical notes that contains information needed for communication and legal and other reasons.

Effective management A health care management style that shares the focus of patient care with administration of the program and effectively seeks improvement through the simplification and review of all systems involved in care or service delivery.

Enteral nutrition Provision of nourishment via a tube inserted into the nose and down to the stomach or through a surgical site through the stomach. A G-tube is one way to administer enteral nutrition.

Enterostomal therapy nurse Some organizations have an enterostomal therapy (ET) nurse available as a consultant and clinical specialist. This role is particularly important in the home care and hospice settings, which have a high volume of patients with ostomy and wound problems. The clinical specialist role is also important in serving the educational needs of the clinical visiting staff and community.

Equity of care A health care system that differentiates levels of care based on assessed patient needs, not individual or group characteristics (e.g., ability to pay).

ET nurse (enterostomal therapy nurse) A nurse specialist with special education and training who cares for patients with wounds or assists other nurses and team members to care for these patients. The ET nurse may also visit patients with an ostomy, a urinary or fecal diversion from usual function, and other skin care challenges.

Evaluation visit (assessment visit) The first or initial home hospice visit to determine whether the patient meets the criteria for admission. It is often the first skilled visit, made when the nurse already has specific physician's orders and is providing a skilled service to the patient.

Extended care services Patient care services provided as an alternative to inpatient hospitalization, in a skilled nursing facility, rehabilitation facility, or subacute facility offered after an acute illness or injury.

Fee for service A health plan in which beneficiaries choose their health care provider and the health plan pays the provider charge for services. This type of plan usually includes some element of utilization review or prior approval by the plan for certain, if not all, services.

Fraud Medicare defines *fraud* as making false statements or representations of material facts in order to obtain some benefit or payment for which no entitlement would otherwise exist. These acts may be committed either for the person's own benefit or for the benefit of some other party. Examples of fraud include billing for services that were not furnished and/or supplies not provided and falsely representing the nature of the services furnished (e.g., describing a noncovered service in a misleading way that makes it appear as if a covered service were actually furnished).

Gatekeeper One who has the overall responsibility for a patient's course of care and reviews, approves, or disapproves all requests for health care services. This role has traditionally been filled by a physician but may be filled by a managed care provider, a payor, or a subcontracted utilization review group.

Goals The end point of care or the desired results for care. For example, if the goal is to provide safe mobility, everything done should support that goal. The team members work together to achieve the patient goals. The desired result of an action or series of actions an individual or organization might strive for; a goal is different from an objective in that a goal is more broad based, and objectives are more quantifiable and specific and are derived from a goal statement.

G-tube A stomach or gastrostomy tube used to place nutrients into the stomach when the patient cannot safely swallow or eat.

Health Care Financing Administration (HCFA) An agency of the U.S. government under the Department of Health and Human Services (HHS) responsible for the Medicare and Medicaid programs. This direction includes various requirements, policies, payment for services, and many other operational aspects of the programs. HCFA sets the coverage policy and payment and other guidelines and directs the activities of government contractors (e.g., carriers and fiscal intermediaries).

Health maintenance organization (HMO) A health care provider organization that offers a comprehensive health service plan to its beneficiaries through an established network of primary care physicians, specialists, clinics, and hospitals. It provides these services on a prepaid, fixed-cost basis.

Homebound A criterion for meeting Medicare home care requirements. Synonomous with the phrase *confined primarily to the home as a result of medical reasons,* the term connotes that it is a "considerable and taxing effort" for the patient to leave home (applicable only to hospices that are home health agencies).

Home care/Home health The provision of a range of health services, products, supplies, and equipment to patients in their homes. A range of health care services and products provided to a patient in his or her place of residence. Medicare home care currently reimburses skilled nursing, speech-language pathology, physical and occupational therapy, medical social work, and home health aide services.

Home health agency (HHA) An organization that provides care to patients in their homes. The agency may or may not be licensed, depending on state requirements. Medicare-certified agencies must have a survey or a special review to accept Medicare patients.

Home health aide The aide's primary supportive function is to provide personal care and ADL assistance. This role and the associated functions are very important to the patient and family. The HHA usually spends more actual time with the patient and family than does any other team member. The HHA's contribution is invaluable to both the team process and the achievement of positive patient outcomes.

Home medical equipment (HME) Walkers, wheelchairs, commodes, beds, infusion pumps, TENS units, oxygen, suction machines, and other products related to patient care are HME. Most HME is considered Medicare Part B, which has a 20% co-payment requirement for patients. Under the Medicare hospice benefit, most medical equipment and supplies are included in the care because the hospice benefit is a managed care payment program. Because Medicare has made many changes to the HME rules, you need to consult your HME representative for specific rules, indications, and coverage requirements. Some equipment requires Certificates of Medical Necessity (CMNs), which are completed by the physician. Most private insurers now provide some coverage for patients needing HME at home. The HME products and supplies needed and used by the hospice patients should be mentioned in the clinical documentation because they may help support the medical necessity and level of needed hospice care.

Hospice care Hospice care is sometimes appropriate for patients with a terminal illness. Hospice care focuses on the comfort and quality of life to assist the patient and family in making every remaining day the best that it can be. Hospice is a philosophy, and care can be provided in any setting, such as home, a skilled nursing facility, or an inpatient hospice unit. Palliative care, emotional support, and control of pain and other symptoms are some of the areas of expertise addressed by the hospice team. Through team meeting and individual visits, the physician, the spiritual counselor, the primary nurse, the hospice volunteers, the social worker, the hospice clinical specialist, and others assist the patient and family in meeting their unique needs.

After death, bereavement support services are provided to the family as a key component of continued hospice care.

Hospice nursing Hospice nursing uses knowledge gained as a professional nurse to execute skills, render judgments, and evaluate process and outcome while supporting and caring for a diverse group of patients and families. Teaching, assessment, pain management, support, presence, active listening, and evaluation skills are some of the many areas of expertise that are hallmarks of hospice nursing. For Medicare, nursing care is provided by or under the supervision of a registered nurse.

ICD-9 code A coding methodology developed to identify specific clinical diagnoses for the purpose of data collection and payment. DRGs are assigned an ICD-9 code.

Instrumental care (IADLS) The provision of assistance with instrumental activities of daily living, such as shopping, cooking, transportation, financial management, homemaking, and home maintenance.

Integrated delivery network A provider of health care services that offers a wide continuum of services to its customer population. It usually comprises one or more acute care hospitals, skilled and intermediate nursing facilities, outpatient and ambulatory surgery centers, home health care agencies, hospices, and physicians who either are employees of the group or are tightly controlled by utilization management techniques.

Intermediary (also called the *Regional Home Health Intermediary [RHHI]*)—The Medicare Part A RHHI is an organization that has entered into an agreement with the Health Care Financing Administration (HCFA) to process Medicare claims and make payment determinations or adjudications for home care and hospice organizations. Hospices are generally assigned to the RHHI based on their geographic location.

Length of stay/service (LOS) The number of hospice or home care days for each patient. Each patient's hospitalization is subject to review to determine the appropriateness of the length of stay (ALOS, average length of stay).

Managed care Care that is organized to achieve specific patient outcomes within fiscally responsible time frames (length of stay) using resources that are appropriate in amount and sequenced to the specific case type and population of the individual patient. Care is structured by case management care plans and clinical paths that are based on knowledge by case type regarding usual length of stay, critical events and their timing, anticipated outcomes, and resource utilization.

Managed care plan or organization (MCP or MCO) Any organization providing a network of patient care services, including physician and clinic or hospital care, for a set, agreed-upon payment. These plans employ a variety of cost-containment measures, discounts, and utilization review services in an effort to control or manage the risk of providing health care.

Medicaid A health program that is administered at the state level for patients who qualify. The basis for qualification is financial. Medicaid coverage varies by state. Sometimes even the name is different; for example, in California it is called *MediCal.*

Medical Social Services (MSS) Social services in hospice provide support to the patient and family and are related to the patient's medical condition. When social concerns impede the effective implementation of the POC, a social worker is appropriate. These concerns may include family, finances, grief work, housing, and caregiver issues. The social worker has an important role in assisting hospice patients and families through their unique situation and journey.

Medicare A federal program for people who are over age 65 or disabled or who have end stage renal disease (ESRD). Medicare is complex but has two main parts, Part A and Part B, that cover different services, such as inpatient hospitalization (after the Medicare beneficiary pays a deductible), home care, and hospice. Medicare is a medical insurance program, and like all insurance programs, it has exclusions, eligibility, and coverage rules.

Medicare health maintenance organization (HMO) An alternative insurance product for Medicare beneficiaries that allows commercial insurers to contract with the Health Care Financing Administration to provide similar Medicare-covered services. Providers must have a contract with such insurers to provide beneficiary care. The advantages of such a program are that beneficiaries do not have to submit paperwork for payment, do not have to pay a copayment or deductible, and may appear to have a richer benefit package. However, beneficiaries are limited in the number of providers to whom they may go for services and the number or types of services allowed.

Medicare hospice The Medicare definition of hospice is that a hospice is a public agency or private organization that is primarily engaged in providing care to terminally ill individuals, meets the conditions of participation for hospices, and has a valid provider agreement. An individual may elect to receive Medicare coverage of election periods for hospice care. For patients to be eligible for Medicare hospice care, they must be entitled to Medicare Part A and be certified as being terminally ill. An individual is considered to be terminally ill if the individual has a medical prognosis that his or her life expectancy is 6 months or less if the terminal illness runs its normal course. The patient "elects" the benefit and is the one who can "revoke" or decide to discontinue the Medicare benefit, thus reverting to traditional Medicare benefits. There are four levels of care and reimbursement through the Medicare hospice benefit: (1) routine home care, (2) continuous home care, (3) inpatient respite care, and (4) general inpatient care.

Occupational therapy (OT) OT helps the patient attain the maximum level of physical and psychosocial independence. Areas of expertise include fine motor coordination, perceptual-motor skills, sensory testing, adaptive/assistive equipment, ADLs, and specialized upper extremity/hand therapies. The kinds of problems frequently addressed by OT include CVAs, amputations, and lung processes for conservation of energy skills.

Occupational Safety and Health Administration (OSHA) All clinicians have heard much in recent years about the need for practice of universal or standard precautions. Nurses are well aware of the dangers of hepatitis B and HIV. Employees must create infection-control policies that support the use of these precautions. In addition, nurses, home health aides, and other team members must be educated about the policy. In practice, this means that hepatitis B immunizations are available when the job requires exposure to blood or other potentially infectious body fluids. The hospice must also provide protective equipment and supplies, including gloves, face masks or other protective shields, fluidproof aprons, gowns, and other needed protection. These should be provided by the organization free of charge to the hospice nurses and staff. OSHA also issues guidelines on blood or other body fluid transport, blood spill clean up, and the safe disposal of infectious waste.

Outcomes Outcomes are quantifiable or measurable goals of care to be achieved in a specific time frame (e.g., the patient, by a certain date, can name all medications and the times to take them).

Outcome, clinical The results or effects of clinical processes on patients. The results may be described by outcome criteria.

Outcomes criteria The ends to be achieved. From a knowledge of the usual course of events and the factors relevant to the patient group involved, the clinician should be able to determine the desired results for a given patient at the end of a program or service of care. Services should have been carried out in a fashion adequate to achieve the purpose of the outcome criteria.

Payor The payor or insurance company financially responsible for the services or care provided to patients. Example include Medicare or other insurance companies.

    The organization responsible for paying a health care provider for the health care products and/or services provided to a patient or beneficiary.

Performance improvement See p. 455, *CQI.*

Performance measure A quantifiable standard or measurement to determine how successful a health care provider has been in meeting established outcomes or goals of care.

Personal emergency response systems (PERSs) PERSs are a unique technology that links the frail or elderly with community resources, neighbors, or a friend at the push of a button or through voice-activated mechanisms. Although different types exist, all are telephone service dependent. PERSs may be appropriate for single patients returning home after surgery, patients who live alone or spend many hours at home alone, or patients at risk from falls. PERSs allow subscribers to signal for help at the push of a button. For the system to be effective, the emergency device must be worn at all times. Hospice nurses are in a unique position to identify this safety need in the community setting so that a referral can be initiated.

Pharmacist The role of the clinical pharmacist in hospice and home care is growing as the emphasis on quality and addressing patient needs from an interdisciplinary model continues. In practice, nurses are acutely aware of many patients who are inappropriately medicated or overmedicated.

    Traditionally, the pharmacist has been considered the provider of a product— drugs. While this is certainly true, the pharmacist can offer many other services to the home care team.

    Many patients are elderly and have multiple risk factors for therapeutic misadventures secondary to drug therapy. These patients may have multiple pathological conditions and different prescribers. They may exhibit polypharmacy (both prescription and nonprescription medications) and are at a greater risk for adverse effects from medications because of altered physiology secondary to aging and disabilities (e.g., poor eyesight, impaired hearing, arthritic fingers). Don't forget that a pharmacist can offer more than the provision of drugs; the pharmacist is the drug expert. This discipline is an excellent position to review medication regimens and screen for drug interactions (i.e., drug-drug, drug-disease, drug-food), adverse drug reactions, and incorrect doses or dosage forms and make recommendations. The pharmacist can suggest simplifying the patient's medication regimen by altering drug delivery systems or medication administration scheduling or by suggesting ways to monitor and assess the therapeutic or toxic effect of drugs. Hospice providers can always turn to a pharmacist for drug information, the provision of inservice education, or participation in case conferences and home care/hospice rounds.

Physical therapy (PT) PT services usually are based on patient need and diagnosis. In hospice the most common kinds of patient problems requiring PT include CVAs, hip fractures, surgery, acute exacerbations of osteoarthritis, and pathological fracture (care focuses on safety, pain management, and positioning). One of the primary PT skills focuses on teaching the patient and family the home exercise regimens.

Physician certification The physician is an important member of the hospice care team. Medicare requires that the physician certify that the patient is terminally ill. The timeline for signature varies, depending on state licensure, but must be obtained before billing (Balanced Budget Act of 1997).

In subsequent hospice periods the organization must obtain written certification no later than 2 calendar days after the first day of each period. The certification includes: (1) the statement that the individual's medical prognosis includes a life expectancy of 6 months or less, (2) the signatures of the physicians.

Preferred provider organization (PPO) A health services program that provides its members with services from contracted providers of care. Beneficiaries receive better cost coverage by using a contracted provider; they can use a noncontracted provider but will be responsible for a copayment or additional fee for service.

Pressure ulcer An area of redness or skin breakdown, possibly affecting surrounding tissues, usually over a bony prominence and related to immobility.

Process A series of activities or events that are related and sequenced in such a fashion as to effect a prescribed or established patient outcome.

Quality A degree of excellence. The achievement of individualized outcomes. *Quality* is defined by the organization and also by the patient/family.

Quality assessment The measurement or assessment of care provided to an individual or a group.

Quality assurance The systematic review of all activities included in the provision of services or the production of a product that meets preestablished criteria, which provides a sense of confidence that a certain level of quality has been achieved.

Quality improvement The achievement of a level of performance or quality status that has not been met before in this process.

Respiratory therapy Respiratory therapy services usually involve patients who need oxygen or have other respiratory problems or illnesses.

Sentinel event A significant or serious patient event or outcome that needs to be evaluated immediately. Sentinel events are commonly risk management issues.

Speech-language pathology (S-LP) S-LP services are a vital rehabilitation service indicated for various speech pathologies or swallowing problems. Patients who may need S-LP services have the following problems: tracheostomy, laryngectomy, and various neuromuscular diseases.

Standard A level of performance or set of conditions considered acceptable by some authority or by the individual or individuals engaged in performing or maintaining the set of conditions in question.

Structure The framework of an organization that supports and defines how the components of a process are bound together to meet or achieve a given outcome (e.g., in hospice organizations the policies, procedures, and clinical competency checklists and standards define in part how patient care will be delivered).

Time line Identifies when an event or a series of events should occur, following a preestablished and agreed-upon framework for those events to happen or specific outcomes to be achieved.

Total quality management A system of continuous quality improvement that empowers employees to review and concentrate on the systems or processes affecting group achievements and that is directed from senior management.

Variance The difference between what is expected and what actually happens. Variances are differentiated by system (internal or external), practitioner, and patient.

Volunteers Volunteers are the backbone of hospice services and provide respite and advocacy services. Some programs are solely volunteer driven, although this model is changing as reimbursement and costs make significant changes in health care generally. Volunteers are specially trained and selected for multifaceted skills that include well-honed listening skills and the ability to demonstrate empathy and provide support. Activities or duties in which volunteers may participate are as varied as hospice but may include bereavement, direct care, and transportation assistance.

KEY HOSPICE ABBREVIATIONS

The following abbreviations are those most commonly used in the practice of hospice and home care. Please refer to your hospice's own designated list of approved abbreviations for daily use in documentation.

ADLs	Activities of daily living
ADR	Adverse drug reaction
ALS	Amyotrophic lateral sclerosis (Lou Gehrig's disease)
AMI	Acute myocardial infarction
APHA	American Public Health Association
ASCVD	Arteriosclerotic cardiovascular disease
ASD	Atrial septal defect
ASHD	Arteriosclerotic heart disease
BP	Blood pressure
BPH	Benign prostatic hypertrophy
BRP	Bathroom privileges
BS	Blood sugar
CA	Cancer
CABG	Coronary artery bypass graft
CBC	Complete blood count
CDC	Centers for Disease Control and Prevention
CHAP	Community Health Accreditation Program
CHF	Congestive heart failure
CLIA	Clinical Laboratory Improvement Act
CNS	Clinical nurse specialist
COPD	Chronic obstructive pulmonary disease
COPs	(Medicare) Conditions of Participation
CPM	Continuous passive motion
CPR	Cardiopulmonary resuscitation
C/S	Cesarean section
CVA	Cerebral vascular accident
CXR	Chest x-ray
DJD	Degenerative joint disease
DM	Diabetes mellitus
DNI	Do not intubate
DNR	Do not resuscitate
DOE	Dyspnea on exertion
DRG	Diagnosis related group
DX	Diagnosis
ET	Enterostomal therapist
FBS	Fasting blood sugar
FMR	Focused medical review
FX	Fracture
HCFA	Health Care Financing Administration
HEP	Home exercise program
HHA	Home health agency or home health aide
HHC	Home health care
HHS	Health and Human Services

HME	Home medical equipment
IDDM	Insulin-dependent diabetes mellitus
IDG	Interdisciplinary group
IDT	Interdisciplinary team
IG	Inspector General
IM	Intramuscular
IV	Intravenous
JCAHO	Joint Commission on Accreditation of Healthcare Organizations
LLE	Left lower extremity
LLL	Left lower lung
LUE	Left upper extremity
MI	Myocardial infarction
MOW	Meals on Wheels
MSS	Medical social services
NHP	Nursing home placement
NIDDM	Non-insulin-dependent diabetes mellitus
NIH	National Institutes of Health
OBRA	Omnibus Budget Reconciliation Act
OIG	Office of Inspector General
ORT	Operation Restore Trust
OSHA	Occupational Safety and Health Administration
OT	Occupational therapy
PCA	Patient-controlled analgesia
PERLA	Pupils equal, react to light and accommodation
PICC (line)	Peripherally inserted central catheter
PKU	Phenylketonuria
PO	By mouth (orally)
POC	Plan of care
PRE	Progressive resistive exercises
PRN	As needed
PSDA	Patient Self-Determination Act (of 1991)
PT	Physical therapy
PVD	Peripheral vascular disease
RHHI	Regional home health intermediary
RLE	Right lower extremity
RLL	Right lower lung
ROM	Range of motion
RUE	Right upper extremity
S-LP	Speech-language pathology
SNF	Skilled nursing facility
SNV	Skilled nursing visit
SOB	Shortness of breath
S/P	Status post
SQ	Subcutaneous
SX	Symptoms
TC	Telephone call
TENS	Transcutaneous electrical nerve stimulation
TF	Tube feeding
TIA	Transient ischemic attack

TITLE XVIII	The Medicare section of the Social Security Act
Title XIX	The Medicaid section of the Social Security Act
Title XX	The Social Services section of the Social Security Act
TKR	Total knee replacement
TO	Telephone order
TPN	Total parenteral nutrition
TPR	Temperature, pulse, and respiration
TUR	Transurethral resection of prostate
TURP	Transurethral resection of prostate
TX	Treatment
UA/C&S	Urinalysis/culture and sensitivity
UE	Upper extremity
URI	Upper respiratory infection
UTI	Urinary tract infection
VO	Verbal order
WIC	Women, Infants, and Children Program
WNL	Within normal limits

PART NINE

DIRECTORY OF RESOURCES

RESOURCES

1. **Administration**
2. **Advance Directives**
3. **Aides**
4. **AIDS/HIV**
5. **Articles**
6. **Book Resources**
7. **Clinical Resources**
8. **End-of-Life Issues**
9. **Ethics**
10. **Fraud and Abuse**
11. **Government**
12. **Hospice Nursing Certification**
13. **Internet Sites**
14. **Journals**
15. **Medicare**
16. **National Organizations**
17. **Nutrition Resources**
18. **Orientation**
19. **Other Resources**
20. **Pain**
21. **Patient Resources**
22. **Pediatric**
23. **Physician Resources**
24. **Spiritual**
25. **Volunteers**

ADMINISTRATION

Kilburn L: *Hospice operations manual: hospice for the next century.* To order, call 800-646-6460, or write to the following address for further information: NHO Store, 200 State Road, South Deerfield, MA 01373.

Marrelli T: *The nurse manager's survival guide: practical answers to everyday problems,* ed 2, St Louis, 1997, Mosby. Call 800-993-6397 or 941-697-2900 for more information.

Medical guidelines for determining prognosis in selected non-cancer diseases, ed 2, Arlington, Va, 1996, National Hospice Organization (NHO). This book can be obtained by writing to NHO at the following address: 200 State Road, South Deerfield, MA 01373.

NHO Standards and Accreditation Committee: *Standards of a hospice program of care,* Arlington, Va, 1998, National Hospice Organization. Write to the following address for further information: 1901 North Moore Street, Suite 901, Arlington VA 22209 (703-243-5900).

ADVANCE DIRECTIVES (SEE ALSO "END-OF-LIFE ISSUES")

The American Bar Association Commission on Legal Problems of the Elderly
1800 M Street, NW
Washington, DC 20036

American Health Decisions
319 E. 46th Street #9V
New York, NY 10017
212-268-8900

Hastings Center
Institute of Society, Ethics, and the Life Sciences
255 Elm Road
Briarcliff Manor, NY 10510
914-478-0500

Pacific Center for Health Policy and Ethics
444 Law Center
University of Southern California
Los Angeles, CA 90089
213-740-2541

U.S. Department of Health and Human Services
Office of Public Affairs
Health Care Financing Administration
6325 Security Boulevard
Baltimore, MD 21207
202-245-6977

AIDES (HOSPICE AIDE, HOME HEALTH AIDE, CERTIFIED NURSING ASSISTANT [CNA])

Home Health Aide Digest. For subscriptions, write to 404 Parkwood Ave, Kalamazoo, MI 49001 (800-340-3356; fax 616-344-8274).

Marrelli T, Whittier S: *Home health aide: guidelines for care,* Englewood, Fla, 1996, Marrelli and Associates. For more information, call 800-993-6397 or 941-697-2900.

Marrelli T, Friend L: *Home health aide: guidelines for care instructor manual,* Englewood, Fla, 1997, Marrelli and Associates. For more information, call 800-993-6397 or 941-697-2900.

AIDS/HIV

Carr D, editor: *Pain in HIV/AIDS,* Washington, DC, 1994, France-USA Pain Society. Available from Roxane Pain Institute (800-335-9100).

Eberle S, Kubota M: *A primary care guide to HIV disease,* Santa Rosa, Calif, 1997, Sonoma County Academic Foundation for Excellence in Medicine.

Flaskerud JH, Ungvarski PJ: *HIV/AIDS: a guide to nursing care,* ed 3, Philadelphia, 1995, WB Saunders.

Ross Labs offers a free videotape entitled *Taking charge: managing the symptoms of HIV.* This videotape addresses interventions for pain and fatigue in patients with AIDS. Ask your local Ross representative for the tape, or call 800-227-5767 if you do not know who the representative in your area is. Ask for Tape #H358V.

ARTICLES

American Occupational Therapy Association: Occupational therapy and hospice: a position paper, *Am J Occup Ther* 40:839, 1986.

Cody C: Hospice update: documentation in non-cancer diseases, *Home Care Nurse News* 2(10):5, 1995.

Marrelli T: Hospice update: accreditation, *Home Care Nurse News* 3(3):5, 1996.

Marrelli T, Hilliard L: Documentation and effective patient care planning, *Home Care Provider* 1(4):198, 1996.

BOOK RESOURCES

Anderson MD et al: *Medical care of the dying,* Victoria, BC, Canada, 1993, Victoria Hospice Society.

Aspen Reference Group: *Palliative care patient and family counseling manual,* Gaithersburg, Md, 1996, Aspen.

Byock I: *Dying well: the prospect for growth at the end of life,* New York, 1997, Riverhead Books. Available from NHO Store, 200 State Road, South Deerfield, MA 01373-0200 (800-646-6460).

Callanan M, Kelley P: *Final gifts,* New York, 1993, Bantam.

Connor SR: *Hospice: practice, pitfalls, promise,* Bristol, Pa, 1997, Taylor and Francis.

Doyle D, Hanks GWC, McDonald N, editors: *The Oxford textbook of palliative medicine,* New York, 1993, Oxford University Press.

Finkelman AW: *Psychiatric home care,* Frederick, Md, 1997, Aspen.

Groenwald SL, Frogge MH, Goodman M, et al: *Cancer nursing: principles and practice,* ed 4, Boston, 1997, Jones and Bartlett.

Irish DP, Lundquist KF, Nelson VJ: *Ethnic variations in dying, death, and grief,* Bristol, Pa, 1993, Hemisphere.

Jaffe M, Skidmore-Roth L: *Home health nursing care plans,* St Louis, 1996, Mosby.

Kübler-Ross E: *Death: the final stage of growth,* Englewood Cliffs, NJ, 1975, Prentice-Hall.

Larson DG: *The helper's journey: working with people facing grief, loss, and life-threatening illness,* Champaign, Ill, 1993, Research Press.

Marrelli T: *Handbook of home health standards and documentation guidelines for reimbursement,* ed 3, St Louis, 1998, Mosby. For more information, call 800-993-6397 or 941-697-2900.

Marrelli T, Whittier S: *Home health aide: guidelines for care,* Englewood, Calif, 1996, Marrelli and Associates. For more information, call 800-993-6397 or 941-697-2900.

Marrelli T, Friend L: *Home health aide: guidelines for care instructor manual,* Englewood, Calif, 1997, Marrelli and Associates. For more information, call 800-993-6397 or 941-697-2900.

McCorkle R, Grant M, Frank-Stromborg M, et al: *Cancer nursing: a comprehensive textbook,* ed 2, Philadelphia, 1996, WB Saunders.

Medical guidelines for determining prognosis in selected non-cancer diseases, ed 2, Arlington, Va, 1996, National Hospice Organization (NHO). For more information, write the NHO at 1901 North Moore Street, Suite 901, Arlington, VA 22209.

Robert D: *Profits of death: an insider exposes the death care industries,* Chandler, Ariz, 1997, Five Star Publications.

Sheehan DC, Forman WB: *Hospice and palliative care: concepts and practice,* Boston, 1996, Jones and Bartlett.

Sigrist D: *Journey's end: a guide to understanding the dying process,* Rochester, NY, 1995, Hospice of Rochester Genesee Regional Home Care. For more information, write to Hospice of Rochester Genesee Regional Home Care, 49 Stone Street, Rochester, NY 14604.

Storey P: *Primer of palliative care,* ed 2, Gainesville, Fla, 1996, American Academy of Hospice and Palliative Medicine. For more information, write the American Academy of Hospice and Palliative Medicine at P.O. Box 14288, Gainesville, FL 32604-2288, or call 352-377-8900.

CLINICAL RESOURCES

Home Care Nurse News is a monthly clinically focused newsletter for clinicians and managers practicing in home care and hospice. To review an issue, call Marrelli and Associates, Inc., at 800-993-NEWS (6297) or 941-697-2900.

Home Care of the Hospice Patient is an informational/instructional booklet for caregivers in the home. For more information, write Purdue Frederick Company, 100 Connecticut Avenue, Norwalk, CT 06850-3590. (800-733-1333)

National Hospice Organization (NHO): *NHO medical guidelines for determining prognoses in selected non-cancer diseases.* These guidelines may be obtained by calling the NHO or by writing the NHO Store, 200 State Road, South Deerfield, MA 01373-0200. (800-646-6460)

Pressure ulcer treatment. Clinical practice guideline, No. 15, Rockville, Md, 1994, U.S. Department of Health and Human Services, Public Health Service, Agency for Health Care Policy and Research. AHCPR Pub. No. 95-0653.

END-OF-LIFE ISSUES

The Center to Improve Care of the Dying (CICD), George Washington University, 1001 22nd Street, NW, Suite 820, Washington, DC 20037 (202-467-2222). Research, advocacy, and educational activities to improve the care of the dying. Press releases, Amicus brief, Supreme Court opinions, and other material are available to download from the following web site: http://www.gwu.edu/~cicd/CICD.HTM.

Choice in Dying, 200 Varick Street, Suite 1001, New York, NY 10014-4810. This organization provides copies of state-specific advance directive forms. A list of other materials, including educational videotapes and literature, is available. Call 800-989-WILL (9455) or 212-366-5540.

Commission on Aging with Dignity offers the "Five Wishes" living will free of charge. It can be obtained by writing to P.O. Box 11180, Tallahassee, FL 32302-3180 or by calling toll-free 888-5-WISHES.

DeathNET is a World Wide Web information center specializing in end-of-life issues and "right to die" materials and services. Access their website at http://www.islandnet.com/deathnet. For more information, call 800-331-3055.

Webb M: *The good death: the new American search to reshape the end of life,* New York, 1997, Bantam.

ETHICS

Alzheimer's disease: ethics and the progression of dementia, *Clin Geriatr Med* 10(2):379, 1994.

D'Olimpio J: The Hospice Ethics Committee, *CARING* 14(11):31, 1995.

Healthcare Ethics. For subscriptions, call 800-333-7373. This publication also publishes *Healthcare Ethics Literature Review.*

FRAUD AND ABUSE

The Department of Health and Human Services has a toll-free hotline to report fraud and abuse by providers in the Medicare and Medicaid programs: 800-447-8477. Their mailing address is Office of Inspector General, Department of Health and Human Services, HHS-TIPS Hot Line, P.O. Box 23489, Washington, DC 20026.

GOVERNMENT

Health Care Financing Administration (HCFA) (800-638-6833)

Medicare Hospice Benefits (free flyer)

Medicare Handbook (free; includes detailed information about Medicare programs, including hospice)

Health Care Financing Administration (HCFA) manuals are available through the following subscription services:

Government Printing Office
Superintendent of Documents (Sup Docs)
Washington, DC 20402
202-512-1800
Web site: www.fedbbs.access.gpo.gov

National Technical Information Services (NTIS)
Department of Commerce
5285 Port Royal Road
Springfield, VA 22161
1-800-553-NTIS (6847)
Web site: 222.fedworld.gov/NTISHome.html

Hospice Under Medicare is a booklet by the National Hospice Organization (NHO) and is available from NHO Store (800-646-6460).

Medicare Hospice Benefits is a free brochure (Publication No. HCFA 02154). For more information, call the Health Care Financing Administration (HCFA) at 800-638-6833.

Medicare Hospice Manual (HCFA Pub. 21) is available by calling the U.S. Department of Commerce's National Technical Information Service (NTIS) at 703-487-4630. Medicare-certified hospices will receive the manual from their designated regional home health intermediary (RHHI). (The RHHIs process and adjudicate the hospice and home care claims.)

HOSPICE NURSING CERTIFICATION

Berry P, Zeri K, Egan K: *The hospice nurse's study guide: a preparation for the CRNH candidate,* ed 2, Pittsburgh, 1997, The Hospice Nurses Association.

The National Board of Certification of Hospice Nurses (NBCHN) offers a specialty certification for RNs in hospice (CRNH). For information, call 412-361-2470.

Hospice and Palliative Nurses Association: *Standards of hospice nursing practice and professional performance,* Pittsburgh, 1995, Hospice Nurses Association. Call 412-361-2470 for information to obtain.

INTERNET SITES

AHCPR (Agency for Health Care Policy and Research)
http://www.ahcpr.gov

Alzheimer's Disease Education and Research
http://www.alzheimers.org/adear

American Academy of Hospice and Palliative Medicine
http://www.aahpm.org

Food and Drug Administration
http://www.fda.gov

Health and Human Services, Department of (DHHS)
http://www.dhhs.gov

Hospice Hands
http://hospice-care.com

House of Representatives
http://www.house.gov

Library of Congress
http://www.loc.gov

Marrelli and Associates, Inc.
http://www.marrelli.com

National Committee for Quality Assurance (HMOs)
http://www.ncqa.org

National Institutes of Health (NIH)
http://www.nih.gov

Occupational Safety and Health Administration
http://www.osha.gov

Social Security Administration
http://www.ssa.gov

White House
http://www.whitehouse.gov

JOURNALS

The Hospice Journal is available from The Haworth Press, Inc., 10 Alice Street, Binghamton, NY 13904-1580 or by calling 800-HAWORTH (429-6784).

Journal of Health Care Chaplaincy is a biannual publication available from The Haworth Press, Inc., 10 Alice Street, Binghamton, NY 13904-1580. Call 800-3-HAWORTH (342-9678) or fax 1-607-722-6362 for more information.

MEDICARE

Health Care Financing Administration (HCFA) (1-800-638-6833)

Medicare Hospice Benefits (free flyer)

Medicare Handbook (free; includes detailed information about Medicare programs, including hospice)

Health Care Financing Administration (HCFA) manuals are available through the following subscription services:

Government Printing Office
Superintendent of Documents (Sup Docs)
Washington, DC 20402
202-512-1800
Web site: http://www.fedbbs.access.gpo.gov

National Technical Information Services (NTIS)
Department of Commerce
5285 Port Royal Road
Springfield, VA 22161
800-553-NTIS (6847)
Web site: 222.fedworld.gov/NTIShome.html

Hospice Under Medicare is a booklet by the National Hospice Organization (NHO). It is available from NHO Store (800-646-6460).

Medicare Hospice Benefits is a free brochure (Publication No. HCFA 02154). Call the Health Care Financing Administration (HCFA) (800-638-6833).

Medicare Hospice Manual (HCFA Pub. 21) can be ordered by calling the U.S. Department of Commerce's National Technical Information Service (NTIS) at 703-487-4630. Medicare-certified hospices will receive the Manual from their designated regional home health intermediary (RHHI). (The RHHIs process and adjudicate the hospice and home care claims.)

NATIONAL ORGANIZATIONS

American Academy of Hospice and Palliative Medicine (Formerly called *The Academy of Hospice Physicians*) (AAHPM)
P.O. Box 14288
Gainesville, FL 32604-2288.
352-377-8900

American Federation of Home Health Agencies (AFHHA)
1320 Fenwick Lane, Suite 100
Silver Spring, MD 20910
301-588-1454
Web site: http://www.his.com/~afhha/usa.html

Home Care Association of America (HCAA)
9570 Regency Square Blvd.
Jacksonville, FL 32225
800-386-4222
Web site: http://www.hcaa-homecare.com

Home Health Services & Staffing Association
155-D South Asaph Street
Alexandria, VA 22314
703-386-9863

Hospice Association of America
228 Seventh St., SE
Washington, DC 20003
202-547-7424
Web site: http://www.nahc.org

Hospice Association of America
519 C Street, NE
Washington, DC 20002-5809
202-546-4759

Hospice Foundation of America
777 17th St., #401
Miami Beach, FL 33139
800-854-3402
2001 "S" St., Suite 300
Washington, DC 20009
202-638-5419
E-mail: hospicefdn@charitiesusa.com

Hospice and Palliative Nurses Association
Medical Center East, Suite 375
211 North Whitfield St.
Pittsburgh, PA 15206-3031
212-361-2470
Web site: http://www.roxane.com/hna

National Association for Home Care (NAHC)
228 Seventh St., SE
Washington, DC 20003
202-547-7424
Web site: http://www.hahc.org

National Association for Medical Equipment Services (NAMES)
625 Slaters Lane, Suite 2000
Alexandria, VA 22314-1171
703-836-6263

National Family Caregivers Association (NCFA)
9621 East Bexhill Drive
Kensington, MD 20895-3104
301-942-6430
Web site: http://www.nfcacares.org

National Funeral Directors Association
800-228-6332 or 414-541-2500
Learning Resource Center Catalog of
  books, videos, and audio tapes. Free
  consumer brochures include the fol-
  lowing titles: *Anatomical Gifts; Em-
  balming; Co-worker Death; Funeral
  Service and Hospice: Mutual
  Concern, Cooperation & Care;
  Parent Death; Making Funeral Ar-
  rangements; A Caring Response to
  an AIDS-Related Death; Choosing a
  Funeral Ceremony; Living With
  Dying; Living When Your Spouse
  Has Died; Grief: a Time to Heal;
  What Can We Do To Help?;* and
  Suicide.

National Hospice Organization (NHO)
1901 North Moore St., Suite 901
Arlington, VA 22209
703-243-5900
Web site: http://www.nho.org

National Prison Hospice Association
  (NPHA)
P.O. Box 941
Boulder, CO 80306-0941
303-666-9638
Web site: http://npha.org

NUTRITION RESOURCES

Gallagher-Allred CR: *Nutritional care of the terminally ill,* Gaithersburg, Md,
  1989, Aspen.
Gallagher-Allred C, Amenta MO, editors: *Nutrition and hydration in hospice
  care: needs, strategies, ethics,* New York, 1993, The Haworth Press. Published
  simultaneously in *The Hospice Journal* 9(2-3), 1993.

ORIENTATION

Marrelli T: *Handbook of home health orientation,* St Louis, 1998, Mosby. Call
  800-993-6397 or 941-697-2900 for more information.
Marrelli T, Hilliard L: *Manual of home health practice: guidance for effective
  clinical operations,* St. Louis, 1998, Mosby. Call 800-993-6397 or 941-697-
  2900 for more information.

OTHER RESOURCES

Hospice Helpline (800-658-8898), provided by the National Hospice Organization
  (NHO), offers information about hospice care in general and hospices in the
  caller's community.
Hospice Link (800-331-1620) is a nationwide toll-free service provided by the
  Hospice Education Institution to the general public and to health care professionals seeking referrals to local hospices and palliative care services or bereavement groups.

National Hospice Organization (NHO) Store offers a catalog of consumer education brochures, books, technical materials, videos, posters, and promotional items. For more information, write to NHO Store at 200 State Road, South Deerfield, MA 01373-0200 (800-646-6460; fax 800-499-6464).

NHO Standards and Accreditation Committee: *A pathway for patients and families facing terminal illness,* Arlington, Va, 1997, National Hospice Organization.

NHO Standards and Accreditation Committee: *Standards of a hospice program of care,* Arlington, Va, 1998, National Hospice Organization. For more information, write to NHO at 1901 North Moore Street, Suite 901, Arlington, VA 22209 (703-243-5900).

NHO Standards and Accreditation Committee, Medical Guidelines Task Force: *Medical guidelines for determining prognosis in selected non-cancer diseases,* Arlington, Va, 1996, National Hospice Organization.

PAIN

Agency for Health Care Policy and Research (AHCPR) (800-358-9295 or 301-495-3453):
Clinical Practice Guideline Number 9: *Management of Cancer Pain;*
Quick Reference Guide for Clinicians; Management of Cancer Pain: Adults;
Patient Guide Managing Cancer Pain.

Cancer Information Service of National Cancer Institute (800-4-CANCER [422-6237]):
Get Relief from Cancer Pain (free pamphlet)
Questions and Answers about Pain Control (free 76-page booklet)
AHCPR Cancer Pain Guidelines (free)

Competency Guidelines for Cancer Pain Management in Nursing Education and Practice Developed by the Wisconsin Center Cancer Pain Initiative (WCPI). Single laser-printed copy available free of charge by writing the WCPI at 1300 University Avenue, Room 4720, Madison WI 53706 or calling 608-262-0978.

Ferrell BR: *Suffering,* Boston, 1996, Jones and Bartlett.

Johanson G: *Physician handbook of symptom relief in terminal care,* ed 4, Santa Rosa, Calif, 1994, Sonoma County Academic Foundation for Excellence in Medicine. (707-527-6223)

Kaye P: *Notes on symptom control in hospice & palliative care,* Essex, Conn, 1990, Hospice Education Institute.

Management of cancer pain. Clinical practice guideline No. 9, Rockville, Md, 1994, Agency for Health Care Policy Research, Public Health Service, U.S. Department of Health and Human Services. AHCPR Publication No. 94-0592.

Principles of analgesic use in the treatment of acute pain and cancer pain, ed 3, Skokie, Ill, 1992, American Pain Society. For more information, write to the American Pain Society at 5700 Old Orchard Road, First Floor, Skokie, IL 60077-1057 (708-966-5595)

For the "Patient Comfort Assessment," write to The Purdue Frederick Company, 100 Connecticut Avenue, Norwalk, CT 06850-3590. Ask for a listing of free resources related to pain and its management available to home care and hospice nurses.

Reese K: Home care 101 part one: understanding and assessing pain at home, *Home Care Nurse News* 2(1):1, 1995.

Reese K: *Home care 101 part two: understanding and assessing pain at home, Home Care Nurse News,* 2(2):1, 1995.

The Roxane Pain Institute for Cancer and AIDS has a 24-hour toll-free number for services to both professionals and patients. For information and reference materials, such as AHCPR materials, call 800-335-9100.

Twycross RG, Lack SA: *Oral morphine: information for patients, families and friends,* Beaconsfield, Bucks, England, 1991, Beaconsfield Publishers. Available from Roxane Laboratories, Columbus, OH 43216 (800-335-9100).

PATIENT RESOURCES

Airline Travel with Oxygen, a booklet by Gail Livingstone, is available from the American Lung Association, 1740 Broadway, New York, NY 10019-4374 (212-315-8700 or fax 212-265-5642).

American Brain Tumor Association, 2720 River Road, Des Plaines, IL 60018 (847-827-9910 or 800-886-2282 [patient line]; fax 847-827-9918). Patient education booklets, listings of support groups, referrals to support organizations, and information about treatment facilities.

Chemotherapy and You: A Guide to Self-Help During Treatment (NIH Publication No. 96-1136; free booklet). Published by the National Cancer Institute of the National Institutes of Health (800-4-CANCER).

Eating Hints for Cancer Patients (NIH Publication No. 95-2079; free booklet). Published by the National Cancer Institute of the National Institutes of Health (800-4-CANCER).

Gone from My Sight: The Dying Experience. This pamphlet may be obtained by writing to Barbara Karnes, RN, P.O. Box 335, Stilwell, KS 66085.

Leukemia Society of America, 600 Third Avenue, New York, NY 10016 (212-573-8484 or 800-955-4LSA [4572]). Web site at www.leukemia.org.

My Friend, I Care: The Grief Experience. This pamphlet may be obtained by writing to Barbara Karnes, RN, P.O. Box 335, Stilwell, KS 66085.

Radiation Therapy and You: A Guide to Self-Help During Treatment (NIH Publication No. 95-2227; free booklet). Published by the National Cancer Institute of the National Institutes of Health (800-4-CANCER).

A Time to Live: Living with a Life-Threatening Illness. This pamphlet may be obtained by writing to Barbara Karnes, RN, P.O. Box 335, Stilwell, KS 66085.

"tlc" Catalog of hats, scarves, hairpieces, and mastectomy bras and clothing from the American Cancer Society. *"tlc,"* Hanover, PA 17333-0080 (800-850-9445).

Traveling with Oxygen is a booklet that lists equipment specifications, requirements, and restrictions concerning availability and use of supplementary oxygen by travelers. Available from American Association for Respiratory Care (AARC) at 11030 Ables Lane, Dallas, TX 75229 (214-243-2272; fax 214-484-2720).

PEDIATRIC

Acute Pain Management in Infants, Children, and Adolescents: Operative and Medical Procedures (AHCPR 92-0020). U.S. Department of Health and Human Services, Agency for Health Care Policy and Research (800-358-9295 or 301-495-3453).

Alex's Journey: The Story of a Child with a Brain Tumor is a booklet from the American Brain Tumor Association, 2720 River Road, Des Plaines, IL 60018 (847-827-9910 or 800-886-2282).

Armstrong-Daily A, Goltzer SZ, editors: *Hospice care for children,* New York, 1993, Oxford University Press. Available from Children's Hospice International: 800-2-4-CHILD or 703-684-0330.

Brenner P, Zarbock S: *Implementation manual: establishing hospice programs to serve children and their families.* Available from Children's Hospice International: 800-2-4-CHILD or 703-684-0330.

Candlelighters Childhood Cancer Foundation (7910 Woodmont Avenue, Suite 460, Bethesda, MD 20814) publishes *The Candlelighter's Quarterly* newsletter, *The CCCF Youth Newsletter,* and other publications. They can also provide contacts for support groups and other resources for children with cancer and their families. For more information, call 800-366-2223 or 301-657-8401.

Children's Hospice/Home Care: An Implementation Manual For Nurses, by I.M. Martinson et al, is available from Children's Hospice International (800-2-4-CHILD or 703-684-0330).

Children's Hospice International (2202 Mt. Vernon Avenue, Suite 3C, Alexandria, VA 22301) offers information, a referral network, and a quarterly newsletter. For more information, call 800-2-4-CHILD or 703-684-0330. Website at www.chionline.org.

Coping with Infant Loss: Grief and Bereavement is a pamphlet available from the American Sudden Infant Death Syndrome Institute, 6065 Roswell Road, Suite 876, Atlanta, GA 30328. For more information, call 404-843-1030 or toll-free 800-232-SIDS (in Georgia 800-847-SIDS).

Funletter is a national activities letter for kids and families living with cancer published by Friends Network, P.O. Box 4545, Santa Barbara, CA 93140. For more information, call 805-565-7031.

Home Care For Seriously Ill Children: A Manual For Parents, by I.M. Martinson and D.G. Moldow, is available from Children's Hospice International (800-2-4-CHILD or 703-684-0330).

The Karing Book: Patient's Pal, by C. Hawkins, is a large three-ring notebook for tracking important medical information. The book attempts to empower parents of very ill children by encouraging their active participation in their child's care. For more information, call 800-9KARING.

Leukemia Society of America, 600 Third Avenue, New York, NY 10016 (212-573-8484 or 800-955-4LSA [4572]). Web site at www.leukemia.org.

Mango Days: A Teenager Facing Eternity Reflects on the Beauty of Life, by P. Smith, is available from Children's Hospice International (800-2-4-CHILD or 703-684-0330).

My Round Rainbow: Helping Children Manage Illness Through Story and Image, by M. Walker, is published by The Children's Hospital, 701 Grove Road, Greenville, SC 296-5601 (864-455-3195).

National Funeral Directors Association offers free brochures, including the following titles: *Will I Ever Stop Hurting? A Parent's Grief* and *When a Baby Has Died* (800-228-6332).

Palliative Pain and Symptom Management for Children and Adolescents is available from Children's Hospice International (800-2-4-CHILD or 703-684-0330).

Radiotherapy Days is a softcover workbook for children undergoing a course of radiation therapy. It presents essential information in a nonthreatening context and was produced by pediatric oncology staff members at the Mount Sinai Medical Center. Copies may be obtained by sending a check (payable to MSMC/Radiotherapy Days) for $5 per copy to the following address:

The Mount Sinai Medical Center
Radiotherapy Days
Department of Pediatric Hematology/Oncology
Box 1208
Attn: Brenda Magalaner
One Gustave L. Levy Place
New York, NY 10029

When Your Child Is Ready To Return to School is a pamphlet from the American Brain Tumor Association, 2720 River Road, Des Plaines, IL 60018 (847-827-9910 or 800-886-2282).

PHYSICIAN RESOURCES

Hospice Care: A Physician's Guide (item #714384) is published by the National Hospice Organization (NHO) (800-646-6460).

NHO's Medical Guidelines for Determining Prognosis in Selected Non-Cancer Diseases is a set of 45 slides that cover general guidelines for determining prognoses and disease-specific guidelines for heart disease, pulmonary disease, dementia, HIV disease, liver disease, renal disease, stroke, and amyotrophic lateral sclerosis. To purchase, call the NHO Store at 800-646-6460, and specify store item number 71476.

SPIRITUAL

Carson VB, editor: *Spiritual dimensions of nursing practice,* Philadelphia, 1989, WB Saunders.

Spiritual Assessment in Pastoral Care: A Guide to Selected Resources by G. Fitchett, is published by The Journal of Pastoral Care Publications (404-320-0195).

Fitchett G: *Assessing spiritual needs: a guide for caregivers,* Minneapolis, 1993, Augsburg Fortress Publishers. For more information, write to the publisher at 426 South Fifth Street, Box 1209, Minneapolis, MN 55440-1209 (612-330-3327).

Fitchett G: The 7 × 7 model for spiritual assessment: an introduction, *Vision,* March 1966, p 10.

Johnson C, McGee M: *How different religions view death and afterlife,* Philadelphia, 1991, The Charles Press.

Journal of Health Care Chaplaincy is a biannual publication available from The Haworth Press, Inc., 10 Alice Street, Binghamton, NY 13904-1580 (800-3-HAWORTH [342-9678]; fax 607-722-6362).

Kalina K: *Midwife for souls: spiritual care for the dying,* Boston, 1993, Pauline Books and Media. A guide for hospice care workers and all who live with the terminally ill. For more information, write the publisher at 50 St. Paul's Avenue, Boston, MA 02130.

Millison M, Dudley J: Providing spiritual support: a job for the hospice professionals, *The Hospice Journal* 84(4):49, 1992.

Reanney D: *After death, a new future for human consciousness,* New York, 1995, William Morrow.

Stepnick A, Perry T: Preventing spiritual distress in the dying client, *J Psychosocial Nurs* 30(1):17, 1992.

VOLUNTEERS

Compton A: The volunteer in bereavement work: tracking the grief process, *The Hospice Journal* 5(1):119, 1989.

Hoad P: Volunteers in the independent hospice movement, *Sociology of Health and Illness* 13:231, 1991.

Stephany T: Identifying roles of hospice workers, *Home Healthcare Nurse* 7:3, 1989.

PART TEN

NANDA-APPROVED NURSING DIAGNOSES

NANDA-APPROVED NURSING DIAGNOSES

Activity intolerance
Activity intolerance, risk for
Adaptive capacity, decreased: intracranial
Adjustment, impaired
Airway clearance, ineffective
Anxiety
Aspiration, risk for
Body image disturbance
Body temperature, altered, risk for
Bowel incontinence
Breast-feeding, effective
Breast-feeding, ineffective
Breast-feeding, interrupted
Breathing pattern, ineffective
Cardiac output, decreased
Caregiver role strain
Caregiver role strain, risk for
Communication, impaired verbal
Community coping, ineffective
Community coping, potential for enhanced
Confusion, acute
Confusion, chronic
Constipation
Constipation, colonic
Constipation, perceived
Coping, defensive
Coping, family: potential for growth
Coping, ineffective family: compromised
Coping, ineffective family: disabling
Coping, ineffective individual
Decisional conflict (specify)
Denial, ineffective
Diarrhea
Disuse syndrome, risk for
Diversional activity deficit
Dysreflexia
Energy field disturbance
Environmental interpretation syndrome, impaired
Family processes, altered
Family processes, altered: alcoholism
Fatigue
Fear
Fluid volume deficit
Fluid volume deficit, risk for
Fluid volume excess
Gas exchange, impaired
Grieving, anticipatory

Grieving, dysfunctional
Growth and development, altered
Health maintenance, altered
Health-seeking behaviors (specify)
Home maintenance management, impaired
Hopelessness
Hyperthermia
Hypothermia
Incontinence, functional
Incontinence, reflex
Incontinence, stress
Incontinence, total
Incontinence, urge
Infant behavior, disorganized
Infant behavior, disorganized: risk for
Infant behavior, organized: potential for enhanced
Infant feeding pattern, ineffective
Infection, risk for
Injury, perioperative positioning: risk for
Injury, risk for
Knowledge deficit (specify)
Loneliness, risk for
Management of therapeutic regimen, community: ineffective
Management of therapeutic regimen, families: ineffective
Management of therapeutic regimen, individual: effective
Management of therapeutic regimen, individual: ineffective
Memory, impaired
Mobility, impaired physical
Noncompliance (specify)
Nutrition, altered: less than body requirements
Nutrition, altered: more than body requirements
Nutrition, altered: risk for more than body requirements
Oral mucous membrane, altered
Pain
Pain, chronic
Parent/infant/child attachment, altered: risk for
Parental role conflict
Parenting, altered
Parenting, altered, risk for
Peripheral neurovascular dysfunction, risk for
Personal identity disturbance
Poisoning, risk for
Post-trauma response
Powerlessness
Protection, altered
Rape-trauma syndrome
Rape-trauma syndrome: compound reaction
Rape-trauma syndrome: silent reaction
Relocation stress syndrome
Role performance, altered

Self-care deficit, bathing/hygiene
Self-care deficit, dressing/grooming
Self-care deficit, feeding
Self-care deficit, toileting
Self-esteem, chronic low
Self-esteem disturbance
Self-esteem, situational low
Self-mutilation, risk for
Sensory/perceptual alterations (specify) (visual, auditory, kinesthetic, gustatory, tactile, olfactory)
Sexual dysfunction
Sexuality patterns, altered
Skin integrity, impaired
Skin integrity, impaired, risk for
Sleep pattern disturbance
Social interaction, impaired
Social isolation
Spiritual distress (distress of the human spirit)
Spiritual well-being, potential for enhanced
Suffocation, risk for
Swallowing, impaired
Thermoregulation, ineffective
Thought processes, altered
Tissue integrity, impaired
Tissue perfusion, altered (specify type) (renal, cerebral, cardiopulmonary, gastrointestinal, peripheral)
Trauma, risk for
Unilateral neglect
Urinary elimination, altered
Urinary retention
Ventilation, inability to sustain spontaneous
Ventilatory weaning response, dysfunction (DVWR)
Violence, risk for: directed at others
Violence, risk for: self-directed

Compiled from *North American Nursing Diagnoses Association: Nursing diagnoses: definitions and classification, 1997-1998,* Philadelphia, 1996, The Association.

APPENDIX A

DRUG FORMULARIES

DRUG CLASSIFICATION FORMULARY

	Generic	Trade	Recommended Dose	Cost
Analgesic	Acetaminophen	Tylenol	325–1000 mg (PO/PR) q 4–6 h prn (max 4 g/24 h)	$
	Acetaminophen/codeine	Tylenol #3	30 mg	$
	Acetaminophen/codeine	Tylenol #4	60 mg	$
	Choline magnesium trisalicylate	Trilisate	750–1500 mg (PO) q 8–12 h	$$
	Hydromorphone	Dilaudid	2–4 mg	$$
	Ibuprofen	Advil/Motrin	200–400 mg (PO) q 4–6 h prn	$
	Indomethacin	Indocin	25–50 mg (PO/PR) q 6–8 h	$$/$$$$
	Morphine concentrate solution	Roxanol	20 mg/ml	$$$$
	Morphine sulfate immediate release		10 mg (SL) tab	$
	Morphine sustained release	MS Contin	15, 30, 60, 100, 200 mg tabs	$$$
	Naproxen	Naprosyn	250–500 mg (PO) q 8–12 h	$$$
	Oxycodone/APAP	Percocet/Roxicet	5/325 mg	$
	Oxycodone/ASA	Percodan	5/325 g	$
	Oxycodone oral solution	Roxicodone	5 mg/5 cc, 20 mg/1 cc	$$$$
	Propoxyphene-n/APAP	Darvocet N-100	100–650 mg	$$
Antacid Combination	Aluminum/magnesium hydroxide simethicone	Maalox Plus or Mylanta	30 cc (PO) q 4 h or prn	$
Antianxiety Agents	Hydroxyzine	Atarax	10 mg (PO) q 4–6 h prn	$$
	Lorazepam	Ativan	0.5–1.0 mg (PO/SL) q 4–6 h prn	$$

Modified from and courtesy of Hospice of the Western Reserve, Inc, Cleveland, Ohio.

Continued

DRUG CLASSIFICATION FORMULARY—cont'd

	Generic	Trade	Recommended Dose	Cost
Antibiotics (Dysuria)	Ciprofloxacin	Cipro	250-500 mg (PO) bid × 7-14 days	$$$$
	Nitrofurantoin	Macrodantin	50-100 mg (PO) qid × 7 days	$$
	Trimethoprim/sulfamethoxazole	Bactrim/Bactrim D	160-800 mg (PO) bid × 10-14 days	$
Anticholinergic Agents	Atropine sulfate		0.4-0.5 mg (SQ) q 4-6 h prm	$
	Hyoscyamine sulfate	Levsin	0.125-0.25 mg (PO/SL) q 4-6 prn	$
Antidepressants	Amitriptyline hydrochloride	Elavil	25 mg (PO) hs/may increase every 3 nights by 25 mg (max 100 mg)	$$
	Desipramine	Norpramin	Begin: 25 mg (PO) hs (frail: 10 mg [PO] hs)	$
			Titrate: Increase 1-2 tabs 2-3 days	
			Target: 100-150 mg (PO) hs	
	Nortriptyline	Pamelor	Begin: 25 mg (PO) hs (frail: 10 mg [PO] hs)	$$$
			Titrate: Increase 1-2 tabs 2-3 days	
			Target: 100-150 mg (PO) hs	
Antiepileptic Agents	Carbamazepine	Tegretol	200 mg (PO) bid to qid	$
	Clonazepam	Klonopin	0.25-0.5 mg (PO) tid	$$
	Phenytoin	Dilantin	100-200 mg (PO) tid	$
	Valproic acid	Depakene	250-500 mg (PO) bid to tid	$$$
Antifungal Agents	Nystatin oral suspension	Mycostatin	5 cc (S&S) qid × 10 days	$$$$

Antinauseant Agents	Chlorpromazine	Thorazine	10 mg (PO) q 8 h prm 12.5-50 mg (PR) q 8 h prm	$/$$$$
	Haloperidol	Haldol	0.5-1.0 mg (PO) q 6 h prm	$
	Lorazepam	Ativan	0.5-1.0 mg (PO/SL) q 4-6 h prm	$$
	Prochlorperazine	Compazine	5-10 mg (PO) q 4 h prm 25 mg (PR) q 6 h prm	$$$/$$$$
Antipsychotic Agents	Chlorpromazine	Thorazine	12.5-50 mg (PO/PR) q 6 h.	$/$$$
	Haloperidol	Haldol	0.5-2.0 mg (PO) q 6 h prm	$$
	Prochlorperazine	Compazine	5-10 mg (PO) q 4 h prm 25 mg (PR) q 6 h prm	$$$/$$$$
Antispasmodic Agents	Oxybutynin hydrochloride	Ditropan	5 mg (PO) bid-tid	$
Antitussive Agents	Benzonatate	Tessalon Perles	1-2 perles (PO) q 4-6 prm	$$$
	Guaifenesin	Robitussin	1-2 tsp (PO) q 4 h prm	$
	Guaifenesin w/codeine phosphate	Robitussin AC	1-2 tsp (PO) q 4 h prm	$
	Guaifenesin w/dextromethorphan	Robitussin DM	1-2 tsp (PO) q 4 h prm	$
Central Nervous System Stimulants	Methylphenidate	Ritalin	5 mg (PO) AM/noon	$
Corticosteroids	Dexamethasone	Decadron	2-4 mg (PO) bid-tid	$$
Gastrointestinal Stimulants	Metoclopramide	Reglan	10-20 mg (PO) q 6 h prm	$$

Modified from and courtesy of Hospice of the Western Reserve, Inc, Cleveland, Ohio.

Continued

DRUG CLASSIFICATION FORMULARY—cont'd

	Generic	Trade	Recommended Dose	Cost
Laxatives/Stool Softeners				
	Bisacodyl suppository	Dulcolax	10 mg (PR) prn	$$
	Docusate sodium w/casanthranol	Peri-Colace	1-2 caps (PO) bid prn (max 6 caps/24 h)	$
	Glycerin suppository		Prn	$
	Lidocaine hydrochloride 2% jelly		Prn for fecal disimpaction	$$
	Loperamide	Imodium Tabs Liquid	2-4 mg (PO) after each loose stool (max 16 mg)	$$$
	Milk of magnesia		30 cc (PO) prn	$
	Mineral oil enema	Fleet's or SS Enema	Prn	$
	Senna concentrate w/docusate	Senokot-S	1-2 tabs (PO) bid prn (max 6 tabs/24 h)	$$$
Sedative/Hypnotic Agents				
	Diphenhydramine hydrochloride	Benadryl	25-50 mg (PO) hs prn	$
	Lorazepam	Ativan	0.5-1.0 mg (PO/SL) hs prn	$$$
	Temazepam	Restoril	15-30 mg (PO) hs prn	$$$
Skeletal Muscle Relaxants				
	Cyclobenzaprine	Flexeril	10 mg (PO) tid	$$$
	Diazepam	Valium	2.5-10 mg (PO) q 4-6 h prn	$
	Methocarbamol	Robaxin	500-750 mg (PO) tid/qid	$$
Miscellaneous Agents				
	Artificial saliva	Xerolube	Prn	$
	Benadryl/Maalox/Xylocaine	BMX	Apply paste to lesions prn	$$

Modified from and courtesy of Hospice of the Western Reserve, Inc, Cleveland, Ohio.

SYMPTOM MANAGEMENT FORMULARY

	Generic	Trade	Recommended Dose	Cost
Agitation/Anxiety	Haloperidol	Haldol	0.5-2.0 mg (PO) q 6 h prn	$
	Lorazepam	Ativan	0.5-1.0 mg (PO/SL) q 4-6 h prn	$$
	Chlorpromazine	Thorazine	12.5-50 mg (PO/PR) q 6 h	$/$$$
Bladder Spasm	Oxybutynin hydrochloride	Ditropan	5 mg (PO) bid-tid	$
	Belladonna/opium suppositories	B&O Supprettes	1 supp (PR) q 6 h prn	$$$$
Copious Secretions	Atropine sulfate		0.4-0.5 mg (SQ) q 4-6 h prn	$
	Hyoscyamine sulfate	Levsin	0.125-0.25 mg (PO/SL) q 4-6 h prn	$
Cough	Guaifenesin	Robitussin	1-2 tsp (PO) q 4 h prn	$$
	Guaifenesin w/codeine phosphate	Robitussin AC	1-2 tsp (PO) q 4 h prn	$
	Guaifenesin w/dextromethorphan	Robitussin DM	1-2 tsp (PO) q 4 h prn	$
	Benzonatate	Tessalon Perles	1-2 perles (PO) q 4-6 prn	$$$
Depression	Desipramine	Norpramin	Begin: 25 mg (PO) hs (frail: 10 mg [PO] hs) Titrate: Increase 1-2 tabs 2-3 days Target: 100-150 mg (PO) hs	$

Continued

Modified from and courtesy of Hospice of the Western Reserve, Inc, Cleveland, Ohio.

SYMPTOM MANAGEMENT FORMULARY—cont'd

	Generic	Trade	Recommended Dose	Cost
Depression—cont'd	Methylphenidate	Ritalin	5 mg (PO) AM/noon	$
	Amitriptyline hydrochloride	Elavil	25 mg (PO) hs/may increase every 3 nights by 25 mg (max 100 mg)	$$
	Nortriptyline	Pamelor	Begin: 25 mg (PO) hs (frail: 10 mg [PO] hs)	$$$
			Titrate: Increase 1-2 tabs 2-3 days [PO] hs	
			Target: 100-150 mg (PO) hs	
Dyspnea	Lorazepam	Ativan	0.5 mg-1.0 mg (PO/SL) q 4-6 h prn	$
	Morphine sulfate		5-10 mg (SL) q 2-3 h prn	$$
Dysuria	Trimethoprim/sulfamethoxazole	Bactrim/Bactrim DS	160-800 mg (PO) bid × 10-14 days	$
	Nitrofurantoin	Macrodantin	50-100 mg (PO) qid × 7 days	$$
	Ciprofloxacin	Cipro	250-500 mg (PO) bid × 7-14 days	$$$$
Elimination (Bowel)	Docusate sodium w/casanthranol	Peri-Colace	1-2 caps (PO) bid prn (max 6 caps 24 h)	$
	Glycerin suppository		prn	$
	Milk of magnesia		30 cc (PO) prn	$
	Oil enema	Fleet's or SS Enema	prn	$
	Bisacodyl suppository	Dulcolax	10 mg (PR) prn	$$
	Lidocaine hydrochloride 2% jelly		prn for fecal disimpaction	$$
	Loperamide	Imodium Tabs/Liquid	2-4 mg (PO) after each loose stool (max 16 mg)	$$$

Fever	Senna concentrate w/docusate	Senokot-S	1-2 tabs (PO) bid prn (max 6 tabs/24 h)	$$$
	Acetaminophen	Tylenol	325-1000 mg (PO/PR) q 4-6 h prn (max 4 g/24 h)	$
	Ibuprofen	Advil/Motrin	200-400 mg (PO) q 4-6 h prn	$
Hiccoughs	Haloperidol	Halodol	0.5-1.0 mg (PO) q 4 h prn	$
	Metoclopramide	Reglan	10-20 mg (PO) q 6 h prn	$$
	Chlorpromazine	Thorazine	12.5-50 mg (PO/PR) q 4-6 h prn	$/$$$$
Indigestion	Aluminum/magnesium hydroxide simethicone	Maalox Plus or Mylanta	30 cc (PO) q 4 h or prn	$
Insomnia	Diphenhydramine hydrochloride	Benadryl	25-50 mg (PO) hs prn	$
	Lorazepam	Ativan	0.5-1.0 mg (PO/SL) hs prn	$$$
	Temazepam	Restoril	15-30 mg (PO) hs prn	$$$
Muscle Spasm	Diazepam	Valium	2.5-10 mg (PO) q 4-6 h prn	$
	Methocarbamol	Robaxin	500-750 mg (PO) tid/qid	$$
	Cyclobenzaprine	Flexeril	10 mg (PO) tid	$$$
Nausea/Vomiting	Haloperidol	Haldol	0.5-1.0 mg (PO) q 6 h prn	$
	Lorazepam	Ativan	0.5-1.0 mg (PO/SL) q 4-6 h prn	$$
	Chlorpromazine	Thorazine	10 mg (PO) q 8 h prn 12.5-50 mg (PO) q 8 h prn	$/$$$$
	Prochlorperazine	Compazine	5-10 mg (PO) q 4 h prn 25 mg (PR) q 6 h prn	$$$/$$$$

Continued

Modified from and courtesy of Hospice of the Western Reserve, Inc, Cleveland, Ohio.

SYMPTOM MANAGEMENT FORMULARY—cont'd

	Generic	Trade	Recommended Dose	Cost
Oral Care	Artificial saliva	Xerolube	Prn	$
	Benadryl/Maalox/Xylocaine	BMX	Apply paste to lesions prn	$$
	Nystatin oral suspension	Mycostatin	5 cc (S&S) qid × 10 days	$$$$
Pain				
First Analgesic Level	Ibuprofen	Advil/Motrin	400-800 mg (PO) q 6-8 h	$
	Choline magnesium trisalicylate	Trilisate	750-1500 mg (PO) q 8-12 h	$$
	Naproxen	Naprosyn	250-500 mg (PO) q 8-12 h	$$$
	Indomethacin	Indocin	25-50 mg (PO/PR) q 6-8 h	$$/$$$$
Second Analgesic Level	Acetaminophen/codeine	Tylenol #3	30 mg	$
	Acetaminophen/codeine	Tylenol #4	60 mg	$
	Oxycodone/APAP	Percocet/Roxicet	5-325 mg	$
	Oxycodone/ASA	Percodan	5-325 mg	$
	Propoxyphene-N/APAP	Darvocet N-100	100-650 mg	$$
	Oxycodone oral solution	Roxicodone	5 mg/5 cc, 20 mg/1 cc	$$$$
Third Analgesic Level	Morphine sulfate immediate release		10 mg (SL) tab	$
	Hydromorphone	Dilaudid	2-4 mg	$$
	Morphine sustained release	MS Contin	15, 30, 60, 100, 200 mg tabs	$$$
	Morphine concentrate solution	Roxanol	20 mg/ml	$$$$
Adjuvant Analgesic	Dexamethasone	Decadron	2-4 mg (PO) bid-tid	$$
Neuropathic Pain	Amitriptyline hydrochloride	Elavil	25 mg (PO) hs/may increase every night by 25 mg (max 100 mg)	$

	Carbamazepine	Tegretol	200 mg (PO) bid-tid	$
Pruritus	Nortriptyline hydrochloride	Pamelor	10-25 mg (PO) tid-qid	$$
	Diphenhydramine	Benadryl	25-50 mg (PO) q 6 h prn or Benadryl ointment q 6 h prn	$
	Hydroxyzine	Atarax	10 mg (PO) q 4-6 h prn	$$
Seizure	Carbamazepine	Tegretol	200 mg (PO) bid to qid	$
	Phenytoin	Dilantin	100-200 mg (PO) tid	$
	Clonazepam	Klonopin	0.25-0.5 mg (PO) tid	$$
	Valproic acid	Depakene	250-500 mg (PO) bid to tid	$$$

Modified from and courtesy of Hospice of the Western Reserve, Inc, Cleveland, Ohio.

APPENDIX B

OASIS

Medicare Home Health Care Quality Assurance and Improvement Demonstration Outcome and Assessment Information Set (OASIS-B)

> This data set should not be reviewed or used without first reading the accompanying narrative prologue that explains the purpose of the OASIS and its past and planned evolution.

Items to be Used at Specific Time Points

Start of Care (or Resumption of Care Following Inpatient Facility Stay):   1-79

Follow-Up: 1-11, 14, 19-21, 23, 26-36, 39-81

Discharge (not to inpatient facility):   1-11, 14, 19-21, 23, 26-36, 39-84, 88-89

Transfer to Inpatient Facility (with or without agency discharge):   1-11, 80-82, 85-89

Death at Home: 1-11, 89

Note: For items 61-77, please note special instructions at the beginning of the section.

DEMOGRAPHICS AND PATIENT HISTORY

1. (M0010) Agency ID: __ __ __ __ __ __ __ __

2. (M0020) Patient ID Number: _____

3. (M0030) Start of Care Date: __ __ / __ __ / __ __ __ __
   month   day   year

4. (M0040) Patient's Last Name: __ __ __ __ __ __ __ __ __ __ __

5. (M0050) Patient State of Residence: __ __

6. (M0060) Patient Zip Code: __ __ __ __ __

7. (M0063) Medicare Number: __ __ __ __ __ __ __ __ __ __ __
   (including suffix if any)
   ☐ NA   -No Medicare

8. (M0066) Birth Date: __ __ / __ __ / __ __ __ __
   month   day   year

9. (M0080) Discipline of Person Completing Assessment:
   ☐ 1-RN   ☐ 2-LPN   ☐ 3-PT   ☐ 4-SLP/ST   ☐ 5-OT   ☐ 6-MSW

10. (M0090) Date Assessment Information Recorded: __ __ / __ __ / __ __ __ __
    month   day   year

11. (M0100) This Assessment is Currently Being Completed for the Following Reason:

    ☐ 1   -   Start of care
    ☐ 2   -   Resumption of care (after inpatient stay)
    ☐ 3   -   Discharge from agency - not to an inpatient facility [Go to M0150]
    ☐ 4   -   Transferred to an inpatient facility - discharged from agency [Go to M0830]
    ☐ 5   -   Transferred to an inpatient facility - not discharged from agency [Go to M0830]
    ☐ 6   -   Died at home [Go to M0906]
    ☐ 7   -   Recertification reassessment (follow-up) [Go to M0150]
    ☐ 8   -   Other follow-up [Go to M0150]

12. (M0130) Gender:

    ☐ 1   -   Male
    ☐ 2   -   Female

13. (M0140) Race/Ethnicity (as identified by patient):

    ☐ 1   -   White, non-Hispanic
    ☐ 2   -   Black, African-American

☐ 3   - Hispanic
☐ 4   - Asian, Pacific Islander
☐ 5   - American Indian, Eskimo, Aleut
☐ 6   - Other
☐ UK - Unknown

14. (M0150) Current Payment Sources for Home Care: (Mark all that apply.)

☐ 0   - None; no charge for current services
☐ 1   - Medicare (traditional fee-for-service)
☐ 2   - Medicare (HMO/managed care)
☐ 3   - Medicaid (traditional fee-for-service)
☐ 4   - Medicaid (HMO/managed care)
☐ 5   - Workers' compensation
☐ 6   - Title programs (e.g., Title III, V, or XX)
☐ 7   - Other government (e.g., CHAMPUS, VA, etc.)
☐ 8   - Private insurance
☐ 9   - Private HMO/managed care
☐ 10 - Self-pay
☐ 11 - Other (specify) _____
☐ UK - Unknown

15. (M0160) Financial Factors limiting the ability of the patient/family to meet basic health needs: (Mark all that apply.)

☐ 0   - None
☐ 1   - Unable to afford medicine or medical supplies
☐ 2   - Unable to afford medical expenses that are not covered by insurance/Medicare (e.g., copayments)
☐ 3   - Unable to afford rent/utility bills
☐ 4   - Unable to afford food
☐ 5   - Other (specify) _____

16. (M0170) From which of the following Inpatient Facilities was the patient discharged <u>during the past 14 days</u>? (Mark all that apply.)

☐ 1   - Hospital
☐ 2   - Rehabilitation facility
☐ 3   - Nursing home
☐ 4   - Other (specify) _____
☐ NA - Patient was not discharged from an inpatient facility [If NA, go to M0200]

17. (M0180) Inpatient Discharge Date (most recent):

__ __ / __ __ / __ __ __ __
month   day   year

☐ UK - Unknown

18. (M0190) Inpatient Diagnoses and three-digit ICD code categories <u>for only those conditions treated during an inpatient facility stay within the last 14 days</u> (no surgical or V-codes):

Inpatient Facility Diagnosis	ICD
a. _____	(__ __ __)
b. _____	(__ __ __)

19. (M0200) Medical or Treatment Regimen Change Within Past 14 Days: Has this patient experienced a change in medical or treatment regimen (e.g., medication, treatment, or service change due to new or additional diagnosis, etc.) within the last 14 days?

☐ 9   - No   [If No, go to M0220]
☐ 1   - Yes

20. (M0210) List the patient's Medical Diagnoses and three-digit ICD code categories <u>for those conditions requiring changed medical or treatment regimen</u> (no surgical or V-codes):

Changed Medical Regimen Diagnosis	ICD
a. _____	(__ __ __)
b. _____	(__ __ __)
c. _____	(__ __ __)

d. _____   (__ __ __)

21. **(M0220) Conditions Prior to Medical or Treatment Regimen Change or Inpatient Stay Within Past 14 Days:** If this patient experienced an inpatient facility discharge or change in medical or treatment regimen within the past 14 days, indicate any conditions with existed <u>prior to</u> the inpatient stay or change in medical or treatment regimen. **(Mark all that apply.)**

☐ 1 - Urinary incontinence
☐ 2 - Indwelling/suprapubic catheter
☐ 3 - Intractable pain
☐ 4 - Impaired decision-making
☐ 5 - Disruptive or socially inappropriate behavior
☐ 6 - Memory loss to the extent that supervision required
☐ 7 - None of the above
☐ NA - No inpatient facility discharge <u>and</u> no change in medical or treatment regimen in past 14 days
☐ UK - Unknown

22. **(M0230/M0240) Diagnoses and Severity Index:** List each medical diagnosis or problem for which the patient is receiving home care and ICD code category (no surgical or V-codes) and rate them using the following severity index. (Choose one value that represents the most severe rating appropriate for each diagnosis.)

0 - Asymptomatic, no treatment needed at this time
1 - Symptoms well controlled with current therapy
2 - Symptoms controlled with difficulty, affecting daily functioning; patient needs ongoing monitoring
3 - Symptoms poorly controlled, patient needs frequent adjustment in treatment and dose monitoring
4 - Symptoms poorly controlled, history of rehospitalizations

(M0230) Primary Diagnosis	ICD	Severity Rating				
a. _____	(__ __ __)	☐ 0	☐ 1	☐ 2	☐ 3	☐ 4

(M0240) Other Diagnoses	ICD	Severity Rating				
b. _____	(__ __ __)	☐ 0	☐ 1	☐ 2	☐ 3	☐ 4
c. _____	(__ __ __)	☐ 0	☐ 1	☐ 2	☐ 3	☐ 4
d. _____	(__ __ __)	☐ 0	☐ 1	☐ 2	☐ 3	☐ 4
e. _____	(__ __ __)	☐ 0	☐ 1	☐ 2	☐ 3	☐ 4
f. _____	(__ __ __)	☐ 0	☐ 1	☐ 2	☐ 3	☐ 4

23. **(M0250) Therapies the patient receives <u>at home</u>: (Mark all that apply.)**

☐ 1 - Intravenous or infusion therapy (excludes TPN)
☐ 2 - Parenteral nutrition (TPN or lipids)
☐ 3 - Enteral nutrition (nasogastric, gastrostomy, jejunostomy, or any other artificial entry into the alimentary canal)
☐ 4 - None of the above

24. **(M0260) Overall Prognosis:** BEST description of patient's overall prognosis for <u>recovery from this episode of illness</u>.

☐ 0 - Poor: little or no recovery is expected and/or further decline is imminent
☐ 1 - Good/Fair: partial to full recovery is expected
☐ UK - Unknown

25. **(M0270) Rehabilitative Prognosis:** BEST description of patient's prognosis for <u>functional status</u>.

☐ 0 - Guarded: minimal improvement in functional status is expected; decline is possible
☐ 1 - Good: marked improvement in functional status is expected
☐ UK - Unknown

26. **(M0280) Life Expectancy:** (Physician documentation is not required.)

☐ 0 - Life expectancy is greater than 6 months
☐ 1 - Life expectancy is 6 months or fewer

27. **(M0290) High Risk Factors characterizing this patient: (Mark all that apply.)**

☐ 1 - Heavy smoking
☐ 2 - Obesity
☐ 3 - Alcohol dependency
☐ 4 - Drug dependency
☐ 5 - None of the above
☐ UK - Unknown

LIVING ARRANGEMENTS

28. (M0300) Current Residence:

    ☐ 1 - Patient's owned or rented residence (house, apartment, or mobile home owned or rented by patient/couple/significant other)
    ☐ 2 - Family member's residence
    ☐ 3 - Boarding home or rented room
    ☐ 4 - Board and care or assisted living facility
    ☐ 5 - Other (specify) _____

29. (M0310) Structural barriers in the patient's environment limiting independent mobility: (Mark all that apply)

    ☐ 0 - None
    ☐ 1 - Stairs inside home which <u>must</u> be used by the patient (e.g., to get to toileting, sleeping, eating areas)
    ☐ 2 - Stairs inside home which are used optionally (e.g., to get to laundry facilities)
    ☐ 3 - Stairs leading from inside house to outside
    ☐ 4 - Narrow or obstructed doorways

30. (M0320) Safety Hazards found in the patient's current place of residence: (Mark all that apply.)

    ☐ 0 - None
    ☐ 1 - Inadequate floor, roof, or windows
    ☐ 2 - Inadequate lighting
    ☐ 3 - Unsafe gas/electric appliance
    ☐ 4 - Inadequate heating
    ☐ 5 - Inadequate cooling
    ☐ 6 - Lack of fire safety devices
    ☐ 7 - Unsafe floor coverings
    ☐ 8 - Inadequate stair railings
    ☐ 9 - Improperly stored hazardous materials
    ☐ 10 - Lead-based paint
    ☐ 11 - Other (specify) _____

31. (M0330) Sanitation Hazards found in the patient's current place of residence: (Mark all that apply.)

    ☐ 0 - None
    ☐ 1 - No running water
    ☐ 2 - Contaminated water
    ☐ 3 - No toileting facilities
    ☐ 4 - Outdoor toileting facilities only
    ☐ 5 - Inadequate sewage disposal
    ☐ 6 - Inadequate/improper food storage
    ☐ 7 - No food refrigeration
    ☐ 8 - No cooking facilities
    ☐ 9 - Insects/rodents present
    ☐ 10 - No scheduled trash pickup
    ☐ 11 - Cluttered/soiled living area
    ☐ 12 - Other (specify) _____

32. (M0340) Patient Lives With: (Mark all that apply.)

    ☐ 1 - Lives alone
    ☐ 2 - With spouse or significant other
    ☐ 3 - With other family member
    ☐ 4 - With a friend
    ☐ 5 - With paid help (other than home care agency staff)
    ☐ 6 - With other than above

SUPPORTIVE ASSISTANCE

33. (M0350) Assisting Person(s) Other than Home Care Agency Staff: (Mark all that apply.)

    ☐ 1 - Relatives, friends, or neighbors living outside the home
    ☐ 2 - Person residing in the home (EXCLUDING paid help)
    ☐ 3 - Paid help
    ☐ 4 - None of the above *[If None of the above, go to M0390]*
    ☐ UK - Unknown *[If Unknown, go to M0390]*

34. (M0360) Primary Caregiver taking <u>lead</u> responsibility for providing or managing the patient's care, providing the most frequent assistance, etc. (other than home care agency staff):

   ☐ 0   -   No one person [If No one person, go to *M0390*]
   ☐ 1   -   Spouse or significant other
   ☐ 2   -   Daughter or son
   ☐ 3   -   Other family member
   ☐ 4   -   Friend or neighbor or community or church member
   ☐ 5   -   Paid help
   ☐ UK -   Unknown [If Unknown, go to *M0390*]

35. (M0370) How often does the patient receive assistance from the primary caregiver?

   ☐ 1   -   Several times during day and night
   ☐ 2   -   Several times during day
   ☐ 3   -   Once daily
   ☐ 4   -   Three or more times per week
   ☐ 5   -   One to two times per week
   ☐ 6   -   Less often than weekly
   ☐ UK -   Unknown

36. (M0380) Type of Primary Caregiver Assistance: (Mark all that apply.)

   ☐ 1   -   ADL assistance (e.g., bathing, dressing, toileting, bowel/bladder, eating/feeding)
   ☐ 2   -   IADL assistance (e.g., meds, meals, housekeeping, laundry, telephone, shopping, finances)
   ☐ 3   -   Environmental support (housing, home maintenance)
   ☐ 4   -   Psychosocial support (socialization, companionship, recreation)
   ☐ 5   -   Advocates or facilitates patient's participation in appropriate medical care
   ☐ 6   -   Financial agent, power of attorney, or conservator of finance
   ☐ 7   -   Health care agent, conservator of person, or medical power of attorney
   ☐ UK -   Unknown

SENSORY STATUS

37. (M0390) Vision with corrective lenses if the patient usually wears them:

   ☐ 0   -   Normal vision: sees adequately in most situations; can see medication labels, newsprint.
   ☐ 1   -   Partially impaired: cannot see medication labels or newsprint but <u>can</u> see obstacles in path and the surrounding layout; can count fingers at arm's length.
   ☐ 2   -   Severely impaired: cannot locate objects without hearing or touching them, <u>or</u> patient nonresponsive.

38. (M0400) Hearing and Ability to Understand Spoken Language in patient's own language (with hearing aids if the patient usually uses them):

   ☐ 0   -   No observable impairment. Able to hear and understand complex or detailed instructions and extended or abstract conversation.
   ☐ 1   -   With minimal difficulty, able to hear and understand most multi-step instructions and ordinary conversation. May need occasional repetition, extra time, or louder voice.
   ☐ 2   -   Has moderate difficulty hearing and understanding simple, one-step instructions and brief conversation; needs frequent prompting or assistance.
   ☐ 3   -   Has severe difficulty hearing and understanding simple greetings and short comments. Requires multiple repetitions, restatements, demonstrations, additional time.
   ☐ 4   -   <u>Unable</u> to hear and understand familiar words or common expressions consistently, <u>or</u> patient nonresponsive.

39. (M0410) Speech and Oral (Verbal) Expression of Language (in patient's own language):

   ☐ 0   -   Expresses complex ideas, feelings, and needs clearly, completely, and easily in all situations with no observable impairment.
   ☐ 1   -   Minimal difficulty in expressing ideas and needs (may take extra time; makes occasional errors in word choice, grammar or speech intelligibility; needs minimal prompting or assistance).
   ☐ 2   -   Expresses simple ideas or needs with moderate difficulty (needs prompting or assistance, errors in word choice, organization or speech intelligibility). Speaks in phrases or short sentences.
   ☐ 3   -   Has severe difficulty expressing basic ideas or needs and requires maximal assistance or guessing by listener. Speech limited to single words or short phrases.
   ☐ 4   -   <u>Unable</u> to express basic needs even with maximal prompting or assistance but is not comatose or unresponsive (e.g., speech is nonsensical or unintelligible).
   ☐ 5   -   Patient nonresponsive or unable to speak.

40. (M0420) Frequency of Pain interfering with patient's activity or movement:

☐ 0 - Patient has no pain or pain does not interfere with activity or movement
☐ 1 - Less often than daily
☐ 2 - Daily, but not constantly
☐ 3 - All of the time

41. (M0430) Intractable Pain: Is the patient experiencing pain that is <u>not easily relieved</u>, occurs at least daily, and affects the patient's sleep, appetite, physical or emotional energy, concentration, personal relationships emotions, or ability or desire to perform physical activity?

☐ 0 - No
☐ 1 - Yes

INTEGUMENTARY STATUS

42. (M0440) Does this patient have a Skin Lesion or an Open Wound? This excludes "OSTOMIES."

☐ 0 - No [If No, go to *M0490*]
☐ 1 - Yes

43. (M0445) Does this patient have a Pressure Ulcer?

☐ 0 - No [If No, go to *M0468*]
☐ 1 - Yes

43a. (M0450) Current Number of Pressure Ulcers at Each Stage: (Circle one response for each stage.)

Pressure Ulcer Stages		Number of Pressure Ulcers				
a)	Stage 1: Nonblanchable erythema of intact skin; the heralding of skin ulceration. In darker-pigmented skin, warmth, edema, hardness, or discolored skin may be indicators.	0	1	2	3	4 or more
b)	Stage 2: Partial thickness skin loss involving epidermis and/or dermis. The ulcer is superficial and presents clinically as an abrasion, blister, or shallow crater.	0	1	2	3	4 or more
c)	Stage 3: Full-thickness skin loss involving damage or necrosis of subcutaneous tissue which may extend down to, but not through, underlying fascia. The ulcer presents clinically as a deep crater with or without undermining of adjacent tissue.	0	1	2	3	4 or more
d)	Stage 4: Full-thickness skin loss with extensive destruction, tissue necrosis, or damage to muscle, bone, or supporting structures (e.g., tendon, joint capsule, etc.).	0	1	2	3	4 or more
e)	In addition to the above, is there at least one pressure ulcer that cannot be observed due to the presence of eschar or a nonremovable dressing, including casts? ☐ 0 - No ☐ 1 - Yes					

43b. (M0460) Stage of Most Problematic (Observable) Pressure Ulcer:

☐ 1 - Stage 1
☐ 2 - Stage 2
☐ 3 - Stage 3
☐ 4 - Stage 4
☐ NA - No observable pressure ulcer

43c. (M0464) Status of Most Problematic (Observable) Pressure Ulcer:

☐ 1 - Fully granulating
☐ 2 - Early/partial granulation
☐ 3 - Not healing
☐ NA - No observable pressure ulcer

44. (M0468) Does this patient have a Stasis Ulcer?

☐ 0 - No [If No, go to *M0482*]
☐ 1 - Yes

44a. (M0470) Current Number of Observable Stasis Ulcer(s):

- ☐ 0 - Zero
- ☐ 1 - One
- ☐ 2 - Two
- ☐ 3 - Three
- ☐ 4 - Four or more

44b. (M0474) Does this patient have at least one Stasis Ulcer that Cannot be Observed due to the presence of a nonremovable dressing?

- ☐ 0 - No
- ☐ 1 - Yes

44c. (M0476) Status of Most Problematic (Observable) Stasis Ulcer:

- ☐ 1 - Fully granulating
- ☐ 2 - Early/partial granulation
- ☐ 3 - Not healing
- ☐ NA - No observable stasis ulcer

45. (M0482) Does this patient have a Surgical Wound?

- ☐ 0 - No [If No, go to *M0490*]
- ☐ 1 - Yes

45a. (M0484) Current Number of (Observable) Surgical Wounds: (If a wound is partially closed but has <u>more</u> than one opening, consider each opening as a separate wound.)

- ☐ 0 - Zero
- ☐ 1 - One
- ☐ 2 - Two
- ☐ 3 - Three
- ☐ 4 - Four or more

45b. (M0486) Does this patient have at least one Surgical Wound that Cannot be Observed due to the presence of a nonremovable dressing?

- ☐ 0 - No
- ☐ 1 - Yes

45c. (M0488) Status of Most Problematic (Observable) Surgical Wound:

- ☐ 1 - Fully granulating
- ☐ 2 - Early/partial granulation
- ☐ 3 - Not healing
- ☐ NA - No observable surgical wound

RESPIRATORY STATUS

46. (M0490) When is the patient dyspneic or noticeably Short of Breath?

- ☐ 0 - Never, patient is not short of breath
- ☐ 1 - When walking more than 20 feet, climbing stairs
- ☐ 2 - With moderate exertion (e.g., while dressing, using commode or bedpan, walking distances less than 20 feet)
- ☐ 3 - With minimal exertion (e.g., while eating, talking, or performing other ADLs) or with agitation
- ☐ 4 - At rest (during day or night)

47. (M0500) Respiratory Treatments utilized at home: (Mark all that apply.)

- ☐ 1 - Oxygen (intermittent or continuous)
- ☐ 2 - Ventilator (continually or at night)
- ☐ 3 - Continuous positive airway pressure
- ☐ 4 - None of the above

ELIMINATION STATUS

48. (M0510) Has this patient been treated for a Urinary Tract Infection in the past 14 days?

- ☐ 0 - No
- ☐ 1 - Yes

☐ NA - Patient on prophylactic treatment
☐ UK - Unknown

49. (M0520) Urinary Incontinence or Urinary Catheter Presence:

☐ 0 - No incontinence or catheter (includes anuria or ostomy for urinary drainage) [If No, go to *M0540*]
☐ 1 - Patient is incontinent
☐ 2 - Patient requires a urinary catheter (i.e., external, indwelling, intermittent, suprapubic) [Go to *M0540*]

50. (M0530) When does Urinary Incontinence occur?

☐ 0 - Timed-voiding defers incontinence
☐ 1 - During the night only
☐ 2 - During the day and night

51. (M0540) Bowel Incontinence Frequency:

☐ 0 - Very rarely or never has bowel incontinence
☐ 1 - Less than once weekly
☐ 2 - One to three times weekly
☐ 3 - Four to six times weekly
☐ 4 - On a daily basis
☐ 5 - More often than once daily
☐ NA - Patient has ostomy for bowel elimination
☐ UK - Unknown

52. (M0550) Ostomy for Bowel Elimination: Does this patient have an ostomy for bowel elimination that (within the last 14 days): a) was related to an inpatient facility stay, or b) necessitated a change in medical or treatment regimen?

☐ 0 - Patient does not have an ostomy for bowel elimination.
☐ 1 - Patient's ostomy was not related to an inpatient stay and did not necessitate change in medical or treatment regimen.
☐ 2 - The ostomy was related to an inpatient stay or did necessitate change in medical or treatment regimen.

NEURO/EMOTIONAL/BEHAVIORAL STATUS

53. (M0560) Cognitive Functioning: (Patient's current level of alertness, orientation, comprehension, concentration, and immediate memory for simple commands.)

☐ 0 - Alert/oriented, able to focus and shift attention, comprehends and recalls task directions independently.
☐ 1 - Requires prompting (cuing, repetition, reminders) only under stressful or unfamiliar conditions.
☐ 2 - Requires assistance and some direction in specific situations (e.g., on all tasks involving shifting of attention), or consistently requires low stimulus environment due to distractability.
☐ 3 - Requires considerable assistance in routine situations. Is not alert and oriented or is unable to shift attention and recall directions more than half the time.
☐ 4 - Totally dependent due to disturbances such as constant disorientation, coma, persistent vegetative state, or delirium.

54. (M0570) When Confused (Reported or Observed):

☐ 0 - Never
☐ 1 - In new or complex situations only
☐ 2 - On awakening or at night only
☐ 3 - During the day and evening, but not constantly
☐ 4 - Constantly
☐ NA - Patient nonresponsive

55. (M0580) When Anxious (Reported or Observed):

☐ 0 - None of the time
☐ 1 - Less often than daily
☐ 2 - Daily, but not constantly
☐ 3 - All of the time
☐ NA - Patient nonresponsive

56. (M0590) Depressive Feelings Reported or Observed in Patient: (Mark all that apply.)

☐ 1 - Depressed mood (e.g., feeling sad, tearful)
☐ 2 - Sense of failure or self reproach

☐ 3 - Hopelessness
☐ 4 - Recurrent thoughts of death
☐ 5 - Thoughts of suicide
☐ 6 - None of the above feelings observed or reported

57. (M0600) Patient Behaviors (Reported or Observed): (Mark all that apply.)

☐ 1 - Indecisiveness, lack of concentration
☐ 2 - Diminished interest in most activities
☐ 3 - Sleep disturbances
☐ 4 - Recent change in appetite or weight
☐ 5 - Agitation
☐ 6 - A suicide attempt
☐ 7 - None of the above behaviors observed or reported

58. (M0610) Behaviors Demonstrated at Least Once a Week (Reported or Observed): (Mark all that apply.)

☐ 1 - Memory deficit: failure to recognize familiar persons/places, inability to recall events of past 24 hours, significant memory loss so that supervision is required
☐ 2 - Impaired decision-making: failure to perform usual ADLs or IADLs, inability to appropriately stop activities, jeopardizes safety through actions
☐ 3 - Verbal disruption: yelling, threatening, excessive profanity, sexual references, etc.
☐ 4 - Physical aggression: aggressive or combative to self and others (e.g., hits self, throws objects, punches, dangerous maneuvers with wheelchair or other objects)
☐ 5 - Disruptive, infantile, or socially inappropriate behavior (excludes verbal actions)
☐ 6 - Delusional, hallucinatory, or paranoid behavior
☐ 7 - None of the above behaviors demonstrated

59. (M0620) Frequency of Behavior Problems (Reported or Observed) (e.g., wandering episodes, self abuse, verbal disruption, physical aggression, etc.):

☐ 0 - Never
☐ 1 - Less than once a month
☐ 2 - Once a month
☐ 3 - Several times each month
☐ 4 - Several times a week
☐ 5 - At least daily

60. (M0630) Is this patient receiving Psychiatric Nursing Services at home provided by a qualified psychiatric nurse?

☐ 0 - No
☐ 1 - Yes

ADL/IADLs

For M0640-M0800, complete the "current" column for all patients. For these same items, complete the "prior" column only at start of care; mark the level that corresponds to the patient's condition 14 days prior to start of care. In all cases, record what the patient is *able to do*.

61. (M0640) Grooming: Ability to tend to personal hygiene needs (i.e., washing face and hands, hair care, shaving or make up, teeth or denture care, fingernail care).

Prior Current
☐ ☐ 0 - Able to groom self unaided, with or without the use of assistive devices or adapted methods.
☐ ☐ 1 - Grooming utensils must be placed within reach before able to complete grooming activities.
☐ ☐ 2 - Someone must assist the patient to groom self.
☐ ☐ 3 - Patient depends entirely upon someone else for grooming needs.
☐ UK - Unknown

62. (M0650) Ability to Dress <u>Upper</u> Body (with or without dressing aids) including undergarments, pullovers, front-opening shirts and blouses, managing zippers, buttons, and snaps:

Prior Current
☐ ☐ 0 - Able to get clothes out of closets and drawers, put them on and remove them from the upper body without assistance.
☐ ☐ 1 - Able to dress upper body without assistance if clothing is laid out or handed to the patient.
☐ ☐ 2 - Someone must help the patient put on upper body clothing.
☐ ☐ 3 - Patient depends entirely upon another person to dress the upper body.
☐ UK - Unknown

63. (M0660) Ability to Dress <u>Lower</u> Body (with or without dressing aids) including undergarments, slacks, socks or nylons, shoes:

Prior Current
- ☐ ☐ 0 - Able to obtain, put on, and remove clothing and shoes without assistance.
- ☐ ☐ 1 - Able to dress lower body without assistance if clothing and shoes are laid out or handed to the patient.
- ☐ ☐ 2 - Someone must help the patient put on undergarments, slacks, socks or nylons, and shoes.
- ☐ ☐ 3 - Patient depends entirely upon another person to dress lower body.
- ☐ UK - Unknown

64. (M0670) Bathing: Ability to wash entire body. <u>Excludes</u> grooming (washing face and hands only).

Prior Current
- ☐ ☐ 0 - Able to bathe self in <u>shower or tub</u> independently.
- ☐ ☐ 1 - With the use of devices, is able to bathe self in shower or tub independently.
- ☐ ☐ 2 - Able to bathe in shower or tub with the assistance of another person:
    - (a) for intermittent supervision or encouragement or reminders, <u>OR</u>
    - (b) to get in and out of the shower or tub, <u>OR</u>
    - (c) for washing difficult to reach areas.
- ☐ ☐ 3 - Participates in bathing self in shower or tub, <u>but</u> requires presence of another person throughout the bath for assistance or supervision.
- ☐ ☐ 4 - <u>Unable</u> to use the shower or tub and is bathed in <u>bed or bedside chair</u>.
- ☐ ☐ 5 - Unable to effectively participate in bathing and is totally bathed by another person.
- ☐ UK - Unknown

65. (M0680) Toileting: Ability to get to and from the toilet or bedside commode.

Prior Current
- ☐ ☐ 0 - Able to get to and from the toilet independently with or without a device.
- ☐ ☐ 1 - When reminded, assisted, or supervised by another person, able to get to and from the toilet.
- ☐ ☐ 2 - <u>Unable</u> to get to and from the toilet but is able to use a bedside commode (with or without assistance).
- ☐ ☐ 3 - <u>Unable</u> to get to and from the toilet or bedside commode but is able to use a bedpan/urinal independently.
- ☐ ☐ 4 - Is totally dependent in toileting.
- ☐ UK - Unknown

66. (M0690) Transferring: Ability to move from bed to chair, on and off toilet or commode, into and out of tub or shower, and ability to turn and position self in bed if patient is bedfast.

Prior Current
- ☐ ☐ 0 - Able to independently transfer.
- ☐ ☐ 1 - Transfers with minimal human assistance or with use of an assistive device.
- ☐ ☐ 2 - <u>Unable</u> to transfer self but is able to bear weight and pivot during the transfer process.
- ☐ ☐ 3 - Unable to transfer self and is <u>unable</u> to bear weight or pivot when transferred by another person.
- ☐ ☐ 4 - Bedfast, unable to transfer but is able to turn and position self in bed
- ☐ ☐ 5 - Bedfast, unable to transfer and is <u>unable</u> to turn and position self.
- ☐ UK - Unknown

67. (M0700) Ambulation/Locomotion: Ability to <u>SAFELY</u> walk, once in a standing position, or use a wheelchair, once in a seated position, on a variety of surfaces.

Prior Current
- ☐ ☐ 0 - Able to independently walk on even and uneven surfaces and climb stairs with or without railings (i.e., needs no human assistance or assistive device).
- ☐ ☐ 1 - Requires use of a device (e.g., cane, walker) to walk alone <u>or</u> requires human supervision or assistance to negotiate stairs or steps or uneven surfaces.
- ☐ ☐ 2 - Able to walk only with the supervision or assistance of another person at all times.
- ☐ ☐ 3 - Chairfast, <u>unable</u> to ambulate but is able to wheel self independently.
- ☐ ☐ 4 - Chairfast, unable to ambulate and is <u>unable</u> to wheel self.
- ☐ ☐ 5 - Bedfast, unable to ambulate or be up in a chair.
- ☐ UK - Unknown

68. (M0710) Feeding or Eating: Ability to feed self meals and snacks. Note: This refers only to the process of <u>eating</u>, <u>chewing</u>, and <u>swallowing</u>, <u>not preparing</u> the food to be eaten.

Prior Current
- ☐ ☐ 0 - Able to independently feed self.
- ☐ ☐ 1 - Able to feed self independently but requires:
    - (a) meal set-up; <u>OR</u>
    - (b) intermittent assistance or supervision from another person; <u>OR</u>
    - (c) a liquid, pureed or ground meat diet.

☐ ☐ 2 - <u>Unable</u> to feed self and must be assisted or supervised throughout the meal/snack.
☐ ☐ 3 - Able to take in nutrients orally <u>and</u> receives supplemental nutrients through a nasogastric tube or gastrostomy.
☐ ☐ 4 - <u>Unable</u> to take in nutrients orally and is fed nutrients through a nasogastric tube or gastrostomy.
☐ ☐ 5 - Unable to take in nutrients orally or by tube feeding.
☐   UK - Unknown

69. (M0720) Planning and Preparing Light Meals (e.g., cereal, sandwich) or reheat delivered meals:

Prior Current
☐ ☐ 0 - (a) Able to independently plan and prepare all light meals for self or reheat delivered meals; <u>OR</u>
          (b) Is physically, cognitively, and mentally able to prepare light meals on a regular basis but has not routinely performed light meal preparation in the past (i.e., prior to this home care admission).
☐ ☐ 1 - <u>Unable</u> to prepare light meals on a regular basis due to physical, cognitive, or mental limitations.
☐ ☐ 2 - Unable to prepare any light meals or reheat any delivered meals.
☐   UK - Unknown

70. (M0730) Transportation: Physical and mental ability to <u>safely</u> use a car, taxi, or public transportation (bus, train, subway).

Prior Current
☐ ☐ 0 - Able to independently drive a regular or adapted car; <u>OR</u> uses a regular or handicap-accessible public bus.
☐ ☐ 1 - Able to ride in a car only when driven by another person; <u>OR</u> able to use a bus or handicap van only when assisted or accompanied by another person.
☐ ☐ 2 - <u>Unable</u> to ride in a car, taxi, bus, or van, and requires transportation by ambulance.
☐   UK - Unknown

71. (M0740) Laundry: Ability to do own laundry—to carry laundry to and from washing machine, to use washer and dryer, to wash small items by hand.

Prior Current
☐ ☐ 0 - (a) Able to independently take care of all laundry tasks; <u>OR</u>
          (b) Physically, cognitively, and mentally able to do laundry and access facilities, <u>but</u> has not routinely performed laundry tasks in the past (i.e., prior to this home care admission).
☐ ☐ 1 - Able to do only light laundry, such as minor hand wash or light washer loads. Due to physical, cognitive, or mental limitations, needs assistance with heavy laundry such as carrying large loads of laundry.
☐ ☐ 2 - <u>Unable</u> to do any laundry due to physical limitation or needs continual supervision and assistance due to cognitive or mental limitation.
☐   UK - Unknown

72. (M0750) Housekeeping: Ability to safely and effectively perform light housekeeping and heavier cleaning tasks.

Prior Current
☐ ☐ 0 - (a) Able to independently perform all housekeeping tasks; <u>OR</u>
          (b) Physically, cognitively, and mentally able to perform <u>all</u> housekeeping tasks but has not routinely participated in housekeeping tasks in the past (i.e., prior to this home care admission).
☐ ☐ 1 - Able to perform only <u>light</u> housekeeping (e.g., dusting, wiping kitchen counters) tasks independently.
☐ ☐ 2 - Able to perform housekeeping tasks with intermittent assistance or supervision from another person.
☐ ☐ 3 - <u>Unable</u> to consistently perform any housekeeping tasks unless assisted by another person throughout the process.
☐ ☐ 4 - Unable to effectively participate in any housekeeping tasks.
☐   UK - Unknown

73. (M0760) Shopping: Ability to plan for, select, and purchase items in a store and to carry them home or arrange delivery.

Prior Current
☐ ☐ 0 - (a) Able to plan for shopping needs and independently perform shopping tasks, including carrying packages; <u>OR</u>
          (b) Physically, cognitively, and mentally able to take care of shopping, but has not done shopping in the past (i.e., prior to this home care admission).

☐ ☐ 1 - Able to go shopping, but needs some assistance:
(a) By self is able to do only light shopping and carry small packages, but needs someone to do occasional major shopping; OR
(b) <u>Unable</u> to go shopping alone, but can go with someone to assist.

☐ ☐ 2 - <u>Unable</u> to go shopping, but is able to identify items needed, place orders, and arrange home delivery.

☐ ☐ 3 - Needs someone to do all shopping and errands.
☐   UK - Unknown

74. (M0770) Ability to Use Telephone: Ability to answer the phone, dial numbers, and <u>effectively</u> use the telephone to communicate.

<u>Prior</u> <u>Current</u>
☐ ☐ 0 - Able to dial numbers and answer calls appropriately and as desired.
☐ ☐ 1 - Able to use a specially adapted telephone (i.e., large numbers on the dial, teletype phone for the deaf) and call essential numbers.
☐ ☐ 2 - Able to answer the telephone and carry on a normal conversation but has difficulty with placing calls.
☐ ☐ 3 - Able to answer the telephone only some of the time or is able to carry on only a limited conversation.
☐ ☐ 4 - <u>Unable</u> to answer the telephone at all but can listen if assisted with equipment.
☐ ☐ 5 - Totally unable to use the telephone.
☐ ☐ NA- Patient does not have a telephone.
☐   UK - Unknown

MEDICATIONS

75. (M0780) Management of Oral Medications: <u>Patient's ability</u> to prepare and take <u>all</u> prescribed oral medications reliably and safely, including administration of the correct dosage at the appropriate times/intervals. <u>Excludes</u> injectable and IV medications. (NOTE: This refers to ability, not compliance or willingness.)

<u>Prior</u> <u>Current</u>
☐ ☐ 0 - Able to independently take the correct oral medication(s) and proper dosage(s) at the correct times.
☐ ☐ 1 - Able to take medication(s) at the correct times if:
(a) individual dosages are prepared in advance by another person; <u>OR</u>
(b) given daily reminders; <u>OR</u>
(c) someone develops a drug diary or chart.
☐ ☐ 2 - <u>Unable</u> to take medication unless administered by someone else.
☐ ☐ NA- No oral medications prescribed.
☐   UK - Unknown

76. (M0790) Management of Inhalant/Mist Medications: <u>Patient's ability</u> to prepare and take <u>all</u> prescribed inhalant/mist medications (nebulizers, metered dose devices) reliably and safely, including administration of the correct dosage at the appropriate times/intervals. <u>Excludes</u> all other forms of medication (oral tablets, injectable and IV medications).

<u>Prior</u> <u>Current</u>
☐ ☐ 0 - Able to independently take the correct medication and proper dosage at the correct times.
☐ ☐ 1 - Able to take medication at the correct times if:
(a) individual dosages are prepared in advance by another person, <u>OR</u>
(b) given daily reminders.
☐ ☐ 2 - <u>Unable</u> to take medication unless administered by someone else.
☐ ☐ NA- No inhalant/mist medications prescribed.
☐   UK - Unknown

77. (M0800) Management of Injectable Medications: <u>Patient's ability</u> to prepare and take <u>all</u> prescribed injectable medications reliably and safely, including administration of correct dosage at the appropriate times/intervals. <u>Excludes</u> IV medications.

<u>Prior</u> <u>Current</u>
☐ ☐ 0 - Able to independently take the correct medication and proper dosage at the correct times.
☐ ☐ 1 - Able to take injectable medication at correct times if:
(a) individual syringes are prepared in advance by another person, <u>OR</u>
(b) given daily reminders.
☐ ☐ 2 - <u>Unable</u> to take injectable medications unless administered by someone else.
☐ ☐ NA- No injectable medications prescribed.
☐   UK - Unknown

EQUIPMENT MANAGEMENT

78. (M0810) Patient Management of Equipment (includes <u>ONLY</u> oxygen, IV/infusion therapy, enteral/parenteral nutrition equipment or supplies): <u>Patient's ability</u> to set up, monitor and change equipment reliably and safely, add appropriate fluids or medication, clean/store/dispose of equipment or supplies using proper technique. (NOTE: This refers to ability, not compliance or willingness.)

- ☐ 0 - Patient manages all tasks related to equipment completely independently.
- ☐ 1 - If someone else sets up equipment (i.e., fills portable oxygen tank, provides patient with prepared solutions), patient is able to manage all other aspects of equipment.
- ☐ 2 - Patient requires considerable assistance from another person to manage equipment, but independently completes portions of the task.
- ☐ 3 - Patient is only able to monitor equipment (e.g., liter flow, fluid in bag) and must call someone else to manage the equipment.
- ☐ 4 - Patient is completely dependent on someone else to manage all equipment.
- ☐ NA - No equipment of this type used in care [If NA, go to M0830]

79. (M0820) Caregiver Management of Equipment (includes ONLY oxygen, IV/infusion equipment, enteral/parenteral nutrition, ventilator therapy equipment or supplies): <u>Caregiver's ability</u> to set up, monitor, and change equipment reliably and safely, add appropriate fluids or medication, clean/store/dispose of equipment or supplies using proper technique. (NOTE: This refers to ability, not compliance or willingness.)

- ☐ 0 - Caregiver manages all tasks related to equipment completely independently.
- ☐ 1 - If someone else sets up equipment, caregiver is able to manage all other aspects.
- ☐ 2 - Caregiver requires considerable assistance from another person to manage equipment, but independently completes significant portions of task.
- ☐ 3 - Caregiver is only able to complete small portions of task (e.g., administer nebulizer treatment, clean/store/dispose of equipment or supplies).
- ☐ 4 - Caregiver is completely dependent on someone else to manage all equipment.
- ☐ NA - No caregiver
- ☐ UK - Unknown

EMERGENT CARE

80. (M0830) Emergent Care: Since the last time OASIS data were collected, has the patient utilized any of the following services for emergent care (other than home care agency services)? (Mark all that apply.)

- ☐ 0 - No emergent care services [If No emergent care and patient discharged, go to M0855]
- ☐ 1 - Hospital emergency room (includes 23-hour holding)
- ☐ 2 - Doctor's office emergency visit/house call
- ☐ 3 - Outpatient department/clinic emergency (includes urgicenter sites)
- ☐ UK - Unknown

81. (M0840) Emergent Care Reason: For what reason(s) did the patient/family seek emergent care? (Mark all that apply.)

- ☐ 1 - Improper medication administration, medication side effects, toxicity, anaphylaxis
- ☐ 2 - Nausea, dehydration, malnutrition, constipation, impaction
- ☐ 3 - Injury caused by fall or accident at home
- ☐ 4 - Respiratory problems (e.g., shortness of breath, respiratory infection, tracheobronchial obstruction)
- ☐ 5 - Wound infection, deteriorating wound status, new lesion/ulcer
- ☐ 6 - Cardiac problems (e.g., fluid overload, exacerbation of CHF, chest pain)
- ☐ 7 - Hypo/Hyperglycemia, diabetes out of control
- ☐ 8 - GI bleeding, obstruction
- ☐ 9 - Other than above reasons
- ☐ UK - Reason unknown

DATA ITEMS COLLECTED AT INPATIENT FACILITY ADMISSION OR DISCHARGE ONLY

82. (M0855) To which Inpatient Facility has the patient been admitted?

- ☐ 1 - Hospital [Go to M0890]
- ☐ 2 - Rehabilitation facility [Go to M0903]
- ☐ 3 - Nursing home [Go to M0900]
- ☐ 4 - Hospice [Go to M0903]
- ☐ NA - No inpatient facility admission

83. (M0870) Discharge Disposition: Where is the patient after discharge from your agency? (Choose only one answer.)

☐ 1 - Patient remained in the community (not in hospital, nursing home, or rehab facility)
☐ 2 - Patient transferred to a noninstitutional hospice [Go to *M0903*]
☐ 3 - Unknown because patient moved to a geographic location not served by this agency [Go to *M0903*]
☐ UK - Other unknown [Go to *M0903*]

84. (M0880) After discharge, does the patient receive health, personal, or support Services or Assistance? (Mark all that apply.)

☐ 1 - No assistance or services received
☐ 2 - Yes, assistance or services provided by family or friends
☐ 3 - Yes, assistance or services provided by other community resources (e.g., meals-on-wheels, home health services, homemaker assistance, transportation assistance, assisted living, board and care)

Go to *M0903*

85. (M0890) If the patient was admitted to an acute care Hospital, for what Reason was he/she admitted?

☐ 1 - Hospitalization for <u>emergent</u> (unscheduled) care
☐ 2 - Hospitalization for <u>urgent</u> (scheduled within 24 hours of admission) care
☐ 3 - Hospitalization for <u>elective</u> (scheduled more than 24 hours before admission) care
☐ UK - Unknown

86. (M0895) Reason for Hospitalization: (Mark all that apply.)

☐ 1 - Improper medication administration, medication side effects, toxicity, anaphylaxis
☐ 2 - Injury caused by fall or accident at home
☐ 3 - Respiratory problems (SOB, infection, obstruction)
☐ 4 - Wound or tube site infection, deteriorating wound status, new lesion/ulcer
☐ 5 - Hypo/Hyperglycemia, diabetes out of control
☐ 6 - GI bleeding, obstruction
☐ 7 - Exacerbation of CHF, fluid overload, heart failure
☐ 8 - Myocardial infarction, stroke
☐ 9 - Chemotherapy
☐ 10 - Scheduled surgical procedure
☐ 11 - Urinary tract infection
☐ 12 - IV catheter-related infection
☐ 13 - Deep vein thrombosis, pulmonary embolus
☐ 14 - Uncontrolled pain
☐ 15 - Psychotic episode
☐ 16 - Other than above reasons

Go to *M0903*

87. (M0900) For what Reason(s) was the patient Admitted to a Nursing Home? (Mark all that apply.)

☐ 1 - Therapy services
☐ 2 - Respite care
☐ 3 - Hospice care
☐ 4 - Permanent placement
☐ 5 - Unsafe for care at home
☐ 6 - Other
☐ UK - Unknown

Go to *M0903*

88. (M0903) Date of Last (Most Recent) Home Visit:

__ __ / __ __ / __ __ __ __
month   day   year

89. (M0906) Discharge/Transfer/Death Date: Enter the date of the discharge, transfer, or death (at home) of the patient.

__ __ / __ __ / __ __ __ __
month   day   year

☐ UK - Unknown

(From Center for Health Policy Research, 1996, Denver, Colorado.)

INDEX